PSYCHIATRY:

1200 QUESTIONS TO HELP YOU PASS THE BOARDS

PSYCHIATRY:
1200 QUESTIONS TO HELP YOU PASS THE BOARDS

MAJU MATHEWS, MD,
MRCPsych, DipPsych
Drexel University College of Medicine
Philadelphia, Pennsylvania

KUMAR BUDUR, MD,
(DCP, IRELAND) (MRCPsych, UK)
Cleveland Clinic Foundation
Cleveland, Ohio

BIJU BASIL, MD, **DipPsych**
Drexel University College of Medicine
Philadelphia, Pennsylvania

MANU MATHEWS, MD
Cleveland Clinic Foundation
Cleveland, Ohio

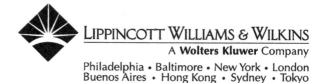

LIPPINCOTT WILLIAMS & WILKINS
A **Wolters Kluwer** Company
Philadelphia • Baltimore • New York • London
Buenos Aires • Hong Kong • Sydney • Tokyo

Acquisitions Editor: Charles W. Mitchell
Managing Editor: Stacey Sebring
Project Manager: Fran Gunning
Manufacturing Manager: Benjamin Rivera
Marketing Manager: Adam Glazer
Production Services: Nesbitt Graphics, Inc.
Printer: Maple Press

© 2005 by LIPPINCOTT WILLIAMS & WILKINS
530 Walnut Street
Philadelphia, PA 19106 USA
LWW.com

Library of Congress Cataloging-in-Publication Data

Psychiatry : 1200 questions to help you pass the boards / Maju Mathews
[et al.].
   p. ; cm.
 Includes index.
 ISBN 0-7817-6106-9 (alk. paper)
 1. Psychiatry—Examinations, questions, etc. I. Mathews, Maju.
 [DNLM: 1. Mental Disorders—Examination Questions. 2.
Psychiatry—Examination Questions. WM 18.2 P9745 2005]
RC457.P7725 2005
616.89'0076—dc22

                                            2004025670

Care has been taken to confirm the accuracy of the information presented and to describe generally accepted practices. However, the authors, editors, and publisher are not responsible for
errors or omissions or for any consequences from application of the information in this book
and make no warranty, expressed or implied, with respect to the currency, completeness, or accuracy of the contents of the publication. Application of the information in particular situation
remains the professional responsibility of the practitioner.

The authors, editors, and publisher have exerted every effort to ensure that drug selection
and dosage set forth in this text are in accordance with current recommendations and practice
at the time of publication. However, in view of ongoing research, changes in government regu-
lations, and the constant flow of information relating to drug therapy and drug reactions, the
reader is urged to check the package insert for each drug for any change in indications and
dosage and for added warnings and precautions. This is particularly important when the recommended agent is a new or infrequently employed drug.

Some drugs and medical devices presented in the publication have Food and Drug
Administration (FDA) clearance for limited use in restricted research settings. It is the responsibility of the health care provider to ascertain the FDA status of each drug or device planned
for use in their clinical practice.

                                            10 9 8 7 6

Contents

Contents v

Preface vi

1. Psychopathology 1

2. Schizophrenia 19

3. Mood Disorders 53

4. Anxiety Disorders 87

5. Geriatric Psychiatry 113

6. Child Psychiatry 123

7. Consultation Liaison Psychiatry 141

8. Forensic Psychiatry 161

9. Substance Use 171

10. Eating Disorders and Sexual Disorders 195

11. Mental Retardation 207

12. Sleep Disorders 217

13. Personality Disorders 223

14. Psychopharmacology 229

15. Psychotherapy 287

16. Psychology 305

17. Emergency Psychiatry 325

18. Neurology 335

19. Miscellaneous Questions 401

Preface

There is a dearth of books aimed at candidates preparing for the Part I Examination of the American Board of Psychiatry and Neurology. A few question and answer textbooks are available, but most of them target a wider audience comprised of medical students, those preparing for USMLE Steps 2 and 3, and residents. The authors hope to fill this void by publishing this book.

This book contains approximately 1200 questions about psychiatry and neurology with detailed answers and explanations, making it one of the very few books in this format exclusively targeted at those preparing for Psychiatry Boards. However, the authors believe that it will also be helpful for psychiatry residents preparing for the PRITE and psychiatrists preparing for recertification exams, and to provide insight for practicing psychiatrists.

This book is divided into 19 chapters, each focusing on a different topic, which makes preparation easier. Special emphasis has been placed on psychopharmacology and neurology, which are a significant part of the Boards.

In addition to being a comprehensive learning tool, this book can be used to identify strengths and weaknesses and the candidate's own command of the subject. This book should ideally be supplemented with readings from more detailed and established psychiatry textbooks.

We wish to thank Charley Mitchell and Stacey Sebring of LWW for their unstinted support and the confidence they placed in us. The authors would also like to thank our spouses Joanne, Kiran, Sajitha, and Shiny for putting up with us during the long hours we spent on this painstaking work.

MAJU MATHEWS
KUMAR BUDUR
BIJU BASIL
MANU MATHEWS

Chapter *1*
PSYCHOPATHOLOGY

QUESTIONS

1. Disorientation to place is seen in
   - **A.** Severe anxiety
   - **B.** Wernicke's encephalopathy
   - **C.** Korsakoff's psychosis
   - **D.** Acute manic episode
   - **E.** Depression

2. Somatic symptoms of severe anxiety include all of the following *except*
   - **A.** Diarrhea
   - **B.** Constipation
   - **C.** Sighing
   - **D.** Hypoventilation
   - **E.** Impotence

3. All of the following are normal experiences *except*
   - **A.** Déjà vu
   - **B.** Jamais vu
   - **C.** Derealization
   - **D.** Hallucinations
   - **E.** Delusional perception

4. Which of the following is true about a primary delusion?
   - **A.** It is always grandiose.
   - **B.** It can occur in normal people.
   - **C.** It is frequently systematized to secondary delusions.
   - **D.** It may be secondary to auditory hallucinations.
   - **E.** It is rarely preceded by delusional mood.

5. Which of the following is true about concrete thinking?
- **A.** It is usually seen in bipolar disorder.
- **B.** It is diagnostic of schizophrenia.
- **C.** It is diagnostic of organic brain disease.
- **D.** It is a defect of conceptual abstract thought.
- **E.** It is always seen in schizophrenia.

6. Psychotic depression is characterized by
- **A.** Circumstantiality
- **B.** Jamais vu
- **C.** Hypnagogic hallucinations
- **D.** Nihilistic delusions
- **E.** Flight of ideas

7. Which of the following is true about pseudohallucinations?
- **A.** They possess the vivid quality of normal perceptions.
- **B.** They are dependent on external stimuli.
- **C.** They cannot be overcome voluntarily.
- **D.** They arise in inner space.
- **E.** They do not appear spontaneously.

8. Obsessions can occur in the form of
- **A.** Cravings
- **B.** Delusions
- **C.** Panic attacks
- **D.** Sexual impulses
- **E.** Hallucinations

9. Pseudodementia is characterized by
- **A.** Abnormal EEG
- **B.** Chronic course
- **C.** Onset with depressive features
- **D.** Localized neurological signs
- **E.** Confabulation

10. Which of the following is true of tangentiality?
- **A.** It is pathognomonic of schizophrenia.
- **B.** It is characteristic of mania.
- **C.** It is a disorder of thought.
- **D.** It is a disorder of perception.
- **E.** It is the same as circumstantiality.

11. Which of the following is true about Capgras syndrome?
   A. It is also called erotomania.
   B. It is also called delusion of doubles.
   C. It is usually associated with brain disease.
   D. It is the same as hysteria.
   E. It is seen in husbands of pregnant women.

12. First-rank symptoms of schizophrenia
   A. Include second-person and third-person hallucinations
   B. Include incongruity of affect
   C. Are diagnostic of schizophrenia
   D. Include passivity phenomena
   E. Are not seen in conditions other than schizophrenia

13. Which of the following is not a Schneider first-rank symptom?
   A. Thought withdrawal
   B. Somatic passivity
   C. Third-person auditory hallucinations
   D. Delusional perception
   E. Thought block

14. Which of the following is true about obsessional thoughts?
   A. They are rarely of a sexual nature.
   B. They are best treated by thought stopping.
   C. Desipramine is the drug of choice.
   D. They always give rise to compulsions.
   E. They are ego-dystonic.

15. Which of the following is true regarding passivity experiences?
   A. They include echo de la pense.
   B. They exclude thought broadcasting.
   C. They are common in bipolar disorder.
   D. They are also called made experiences.
   E. They occur in obsessional states.

16. Frequent wrist cutting is seen in all of the following *except*
  A. Borderline personality disorder
  B. Schizophrenia
  C. Depression
  D. Obsessive-compulsive personality disorder
  E. High states of tension

17. Which of the following is not a disorder of thought process?
  A. Omission
  B. Substitution
  C. Blurring of conceptual boundaries
  D. Knight's move thinking
  E. Paranoid delusions

18. The experience of seeing one's own body projected into external space is called
  A. Reflex hallucination
  B. Autoscopic hallucination
  C. Hypnagogic hallucination
  D. Pseudohallucination

19. Which of the following is true about depersonalization?
  A. It is a psychotic experience.
  B. It is treated with phenobarbitone.
  C. It is usually pleasant.
  D. It is associated with depression.
  E. It is recognized as odd.

20. Which of the following is true about the reliability of psychiatric diagnosis?
  A. It is not increased by training psychiatrists.
  B. It is not important if validity is guaranteed.
  C. It is increased by semistructured interviews.
  D. It is not increased by operational definitions.
  E. It has not been tested internationally.

21. Which of the following is true regarding delusions?
   A. They are usually of a bizarre nature.
   B. They are reality for the patient.
   C. They are held with a conviction that is shakable.
   D. They are usually self-referent.
   E. They may present as obsessive-compulsive disorder.

22. Which of the following is not an experience seen in normal people?
   A. Depersonalization
   B. Déjà vu
   C. Jamais vu
   D. Encapsulated delusions
   E. Ideas of reference

23. Which of the following is not a feature of Gilles de la Tourette syndrome?
   A. Coprolalia
   B. Echopraxia
   C. Echolalia
   D. Coprophagia
   E. Tics

24. Pseudohallucinations occur in all of the following *except*
   A. Long-distance truck drivers
   B. Sensory deprivation
   C. Dreams while asleep
   D. Prisoners in solitary confinement
   E. Dreams while awake

25. Which of the following does not favor a diagnosis of delirium?
   A. Symptoms worsening in the evenings
   B. Visual hallucinations
   C. Misidentification
   D. Delusions of persecution
   E. Improvement at night

26. Verbigeration is seen in
   A. Ganser syndrome
   B. Catatonic schizophrenia
   C. Malingering
   D. Bereavement
   E. Depression

27. The characteristic hallucinations seen in alcoholic hallucinosis are
   A. Tactile
   B. Auditory
   C. Gustatory
   D. Olfactory
   E. Synesthesic

28. Which of the following is false about ideas of reference?
   A. They are always pathological.
   B. They occur in alcoholics.
   C. They are not delusions.
   D. They may improve spontaneously.
   E. They can lead to social isolation.

29. Which of the following is not a type of catatonia?
   A. Echopraxia
   B. Cataplexy
   C. Catalepsy
   D. Psychological pillow
   E. Stupor

30. Schneider first-rank symptoms are
   A. Primary psychological symptoms from which all others are derived
   B. Common in autistic children
   C. Predictive of decline in social functioning
   D. Diagnostic of schizophrenia
   E. Seen in mania

31. In history taking and mental status examination, all of the following are true *except*

    A. Occupational history may give an indication of severity of condition.

    B. Cognitive testing is not indicated if a full history is obtained.

    C. Family history may give a clue about family dynamics.

    D. Mental status examination need not be done in the recommended sequence.

    E. Proverb interpretation demonstrates concrete thinking.

32. Loosening of association is pathognomonic of

    A. Schizophrenia

    B. Mania

    C. Depression

    D. All of the above

    E. None of the above

33. Obsessions in obsessive-compulsive disorder may present as

    A. Hallucinations

    B. Delusions

    C. Mental images

    D. Panic attacks

    E. Thought echo

34. Which of the following conditions does not classically cause emotional lability?

    A. Mania

    B. Severe depression

    C. Pseudobulbar palsy

    D. Hysteria

    E. Delirium

35. Which of the following is not seen in alexithymia?

    A. Lack of empathy

    B. Reduced fantasy thinking

    C. Reduced symbolic thinking

    D. Inability to experience feelings

    E. Difficulty reading

36. Visual hallucinations are most commonly seen in
   A. Late-onset schizophrenia
   B. Temporal lobe dementia
   C. Antihypertensive treatment
   D. Acute organic psychosis
   E. Untreated depression

37. Repetitive, voluntary, purposeful movements are called
   A. Stereotypy
   B. Mannerism
   C. Obsession
   D. Ritual
   E. Automatism

38. The diminution of emotional response is called
   A. Blunting of affect
   B. Flattening of affect
   C. Alexithymia
   D. Depression
   E. Perseveration

39. The most commonly seen symptom in schizophrenia is
   A. Delusion
   B. Visual hallucinations
   C. Auditory hallucinations
   D. Thought withdrawal
   E. Thought echo

40. Perseveration is most commonly seen in
   A. Schizophrenia
   B. Organic brain disorders
   C. Depression
   D. Anxiety
   E. Obsessive-compulsive disorder

41. The experience of seeing one's own body in external space is called
   A. Autoscopic hallucination
   B. Extracampine hallucination
   C. Reflex hallucination
   D. Visual hallucination
   E. Gedankenlautwerden

42. When a person believes that someone known to him has been replaced by a double, the condition is known as
   A. Fregoli syndrome
   B. de Clerambault syndrome
   C. Capgras syndrome
   D. Othello syndrome
   E. Diogenes syndrome

43. Which of the following is a feature of obsessions?
   A. Patient believes they come from an external source.
   B. Patient believes they are logical.
   C. Patient finds them pleasurable.
   D. Patient finds them distressing and unpleasant.
   E. There is no resistance to them.

44. A patient's imitating of the examiner's movements even when asked not to do so is called
   A. Echolalia
   B. Echopraxia
   C. Ambitendence
   D. Waxy flexibility
   E. Mannerism

45. The patient's lack of awareness of his or her illness or condition is called
   A. Anosognosia
   B. Hemisomatognosis
   C. Prosopagnosia
   D. Autotopagnosia
   E. Anton syndrome

46. Presence of insight is suggested by all of the following *except*
   A. Patient recognizes that he is ill.
   B. Patient recognizes that the illness is of a psychological nature.
   C. Patient recognizes that he needs treatment.
   D. Patient is willing to accept help.
   E. Patient agrees with all that the doctor says.

47. Which of the following is a self-rating scale?
   A. Hamilton Depression Rating Scale
   B. Beck Depression Inventory (BDI)
   C. Montgomery-Asberg Depression Rating Scale
   D. Yale-Brown Obsessive-Compulsive Scale
   E. Positive and Negative Syndrome Scale (PANSS)

48. Which of the following is a psychological test to detect organic brain damage?
   A. Cattell P-16
   B. Rorschach test
   C. Stanford-Binet test
   D. New Word Learning Test
   E. Minnesota Multiphasic Personality Inventory (MMPI)

49. Tactile hallucinations are seen in
   A. Dermatitis artefacta
   B. Alcoholic polyneuropathy
   C. Cocaine abuse
   D. Obsessive-compulsive disorder
   E. Panic disorder

50. Nihilistic delusions are most likely to be seen in
   A. Cotard syndrome
   B. Schizophrenia
   C. Capgras syndrome
   D. Fregoli syndrome

ANSWERS

1. **Answer: B.** Disorientation is a sign of confusion and altered levels of consciousness. Among the conditions listed, only Wernicke's encephalopathy is associated with a confusional state. Manic episode, schizophrenia, and anxiety occur on a background of clear consciousness.

2. **Answer: D.** Somatic symptoms of anxiety include gastrointestinal symptoms like dry mouth, swallowing difficulties, diarrhea, and constipation; respiratory symptoms like difficulty inhaling and hyperventilation; cardiovascular symptoms like palpitations and chest discomfort; genitourinary symptoms like frequent micturition, erectile dysfunction, amenorrhea; and neuromuscular system symptoms like tremor, tinnitus, dizziness, and headache.

3. **Answer: E.** In delusional perception, a normal perception acquires a delusional significance. It is a first-rank symptom of schizophrenia. In derealization, objects appear unreal and lifeless. These can be normal phenomena, especially in fatigue. Déjà vu is the recognition of events that are unfamiliar, and jamais vu is failing to recognize events that have been encountered before. Hallucinations of the hypnagogic and hypnopompic variety are not necessarily pathological.

4. **Answer: C.** The concept of primary delusions was introduced by Jaspers. Primary delusions are characterized by their "psychological irreducibility." Secondary delusions emerge from disturbing life experiences or pathological mood states or misperceptions. Primary delusions are usually persecutory. Primary delusions always reflect an illness. "Delusional mood" or "delusional atmosphere" refers to an ensemble of miniscule and almost unnoticed experiences that impart a new and bewildering aspect or meaning to a situation. To the patient, the world seems to be subtly altered; something uncanny seems to be going on in which the patient feels personally involved without knowing how. The delusional atmosphere usually precedes a primary delusion.

5. **Answer: D.** In concrete thinking, the patient cannot keep in mind the abstract use of a notion relevant in a given context and slips into more concrete meanings. In organic mental disorders and subnormality of intelligence, patients may have an inability to think abstractly that may be attributed to a diminished capacity to understand the concept. It is not diagnostic of schizophrenia or organic brain disease, nor is it always seen in schizophrenia.

6. **Answer: D.** In nihilistic delusion, the patient believes that the real world has disappeared completely and that he no longer exists. It is seen in severe depression with psychotic features. In circumstantiality, the patient has to go through many irrelevant details in his conversation before returning to a point. Jamais vu and hypnagogic hallucinations may be normal phenomena. Flight of ideas is classically seen in mania.

7. **Answer: D.** The term "pseudohallucination" is used when a hallucination is recognized as unreal. According to Jaspers, pseudohallucinations are not as tangible and real as hallucinations, though they do appear spontaneously and are discernible from real perception. They can be overcome voluntarily. They arise in inner space and are not dependent on external stimuli.

8. **Answer: D.** Obsessions occur as repeated thoughts, ruminations, memories, images, or impulses that patients know are their own but are unable to prevent. Compulsions are actions, rituals, or behaviors that patient recognize as their own but cannot resist successfully.

9. **Answer: C.** Pseudodementia is a presentation of depression, particularly in the elderly with cognitive impairment. This is not a true dementia, and patients respond to the treatment of depression. Patients typically give "Don't know" answers rather than the confabulation seen in dementia. EEG is normal and there are no localized neurological signs unless another condition is present.

10. **Answer: C.** Tangentiality is a disorder of the thinking process in which ideas deviate toward an obliquely related theme. It may be seen in schizophrenia although it is not pathognomonic of schizophrenia or mania.

11. **Answer: B.** In Capgras syndrome, patients falsely perceive that someone in their environment, usually a close relative or friend, has been replaced by a double. In erotomania, the individual has strong erotic feelings toward another person and has the persistent unfounded belief that the other person is deeply in love with him or her. Erotomania is also called de Clerambault syndrome. The condition seen in husbands of pregnant women is called Couvade syndrome.

12. **Answer: D.** Schneider identified a set of phenomena that he considered strongly indicative of schizophrenia in the absence of brain disease. They are not diagnostic of schizophrenia. They include third-person hallucinations, voices commenting, and audible thoughts. Thought broadcast, withdrawal, and insertion along with made will, made affect, made acts, and somatic passivity are also first-rank symptoms. They may be seen in other organic and affective states.

13. **Answer: D.** Thought block is not a first-rank symptom though thought withdrawal is.

14. **Answer: E.** Obsessional thoughts are recurrent, intrusive, and distressing. Patients realize these are their own thoughts and find them distressing. The obsessional thoughts are commonly of a sexual nature. Thought stopping can be used as an intervention but may not be very effective. Patients respond to medications with an affinity for serotonin receptors, such as clomipramine and SSRIs. The thoughts do not always give rise to compulsions, though they commonly do.

15. **Answer: D.** Passivity experiences are also called made experiences, as the patient perceives them to be under the control of an external force. Echo de la pense (thought echo) is the phenomenon in which the patient hears his thoughts aloud. Thought broadcasting is a passivity phenomenon. Psychotic symptoms are not seen in obsessional states. Passivity phenomena may be seen in bipolar disorder but are not common.

16. **Answer: E.** Frequent wrist cutting is seen in a wide range of psychiatric conditions, including schizophrenia, depression, and bipolar disorder. Patients typically report a relief of tension following the act. It is not associated with obsessive-compulsive disorder.

17. **Answer: E.** Paranoid delusion is a disorder of thought content. The others are examples of disorder of thought process or form.

18. **Answer: B.** This phenomenon is rare and is encountered in a small minority of patients with temporal lobe epilepsy or other organic brain disorders. In reflex hallucination, a stimulus in one sensory modality results in a hallucination in another.

19. **Answer: E.** In depersonalization, one's own feelings are experienced as being detached, distant, not being one's own, lost, or altered. The person recognizes that this is a subjective change and not a change imposed by outside forces. It is experienced as unpleasant and odd. It is associated with depression, anxiety, and use of various substances, especially hallucinogens.

20. **Answer: C.** The reliability of psychiatric diagnosis is increased by the use of semistructured interviews. It is increased by training. Reliability and validity are both important while making a diagnosis. The use of operational criteria like the DSM increases reliability. Most diagnoses have been tested internationally across various cultures.

21. **Answer: B.** There are various definitions of delusions. A delusion is often defined as "a false, unshakable belief that is out of keeping with the patient's social and cultural background." Sometimes, the contents of delusions do not go beyond the impossible and may be true. Thus, delusions may also be defined as "overriding rigid convictions that create a self-evident, private, and isolating reality requiring no proof." Most delusions are not of a bizarre nature, and all delusions are self-referent.

22. **Answer: D.** Encapsulated, overvalued ideas may be seen in normal people. However, delusions are not. Depersonalization, déjà vu, jamais vu, ideas of reference, and hallucinations are all part of normal experience.

23. **Answer: D.** Tourette syndrome begins before age 21 and is characterized by motor tics, vocal tics, coprolalia (utterance of obscenities), copropraxia (obscene gestures), echolalia, echopraxia, and self-injurious behavior. It is not associated with coprophagia. Associated psychiatric conditions include depression, anxiety, personality disorder, ADHD, and obsessive-compulsive disorder.

24. **Answer: C.** The term "pseudohallucination" is used when the hallucinations are recognized as unreal. This term was introduced by Jaspers. Daydreaming can at times have the quality of a pseudohallucination. It is also seen in sensory deprivation states like long-distance truck drivers and prisoners in solitary confinement.

25. **Answer: E.** "Delirium" is a term used to cover all types of acute disturbance of consciousness with general impairment of cognition whether or not the patient was overactive and disturbed. The clinical features are impairment of consciousness with symptoms worse at night; agitation or hypoactivity; labile mood; incoherent speech; abnormalities of perception with visual hallucinations, illusions, and misinterpretation; cognitive dysfunction with impairment of orientation, concentration, and memory with impaired insight. Delusions may be seen, but they are fragmented and unsystematized.

26. **Answer: B.** Verbigeration is a constant repetition of syllables and sound. It is seen in schizophrenia and organic language disorders.

27. **Answer: B.** Auditory hallucinations are the characteristic hallucinations in alcoholic hallucinosis. Auditory hallucinations are present in a clear consciousness without autonomic overactivity. They often begin as simple noises but are gradually replaced by voices that may threaten or abuse the person. Usually the remarks are addressed in the second person. Classified as a substance-induced psychotic disorder, the hallucinations usually respond rapidly to medication and abstinence, and the prognosis is good.

28. Answer: A. Ideas of reference can occur in normal people in the absence of any illness. They are not delusions and may resolve spontaneously. They may result in social isolation due to suspiciousness. They are common in alcoholics.

29. Answer: B. Cataplexy is the loss of muscle tone seen with sleep and narcolepsy. Echopraxia is the imitation of action of others. In catalepsy, uncomfortable and bizarre postures are maintained against gravity or efforts to rectify them. In psychological pillow, the patient holds his head above the level of the bed while lying down. This is a form of catalepsy. In stupor, the patient does not communicate or move though he or she is alert.

30. Answer: E. Schneider first-rank symptoms are phenomena that strongly indicate schizophrenia in the absence of overt brain disease. They have no prognostic value. The presence of more than one first-rank symptom does not increase the probability of schizophrenia. They may be seen in conditions other than schizophrenia; up to one-quarter of patients with mania may have first-rank symptoms.

31. Answer: B. The ability to obtain a good history does not preclude the need for cognitive testing. Occupational history may give an indication of the severity of the condition. Proverb interpretation demonstrates concrete thinking, and mental status exam can be done and recorded in any form.

32. Answer: E. Loosening of association is most commonly seen in schizophrenia; however, it is not pathognomonic of any particular condition.

33. Answer: C. Obsessions, by definition, cannot be psychotic phenomena. They may present as mental imagery.

34. Answer: B. Emotional lability may be seen in mania, pseudobulbar palsy, hysteria, delirium, and mild to moderate depression. However, in severe depression, the patient usually has sustained low moods.

35. Answer: E. Alexithymia is an inability to describe or recognize one's emotions. Patients also have a limited fantasy life, constriction of affective life, reduced symbolic thinking, and an inability to empathize with others. Difficulty reading is not a feature of alexithymia.

36. Answer: D. Visual hallucinations are common in delirium. In fact, they are extremely uncommon in functional psychiatric illnesses. They are not a common feature of late-onset schizophrenia, which is more likely to be characterized by delusions and auditory hallucinations, though visual hallucinations may be present. Frontotemporal dementia presents with disorganized behavior, change in personality, poor insight, emotional blunting, and stereotyped and perseverative behavior. Untreated depression can result in hallucinations, but they are more often auditory.

37. **Answer: B.** This is the definition of mannerism. Stereotypy is the constant repetition of meaningless and purposeless gestures or movements. In automatism, the individual is consciously or unconsciously, but involuntarily, compelled to perform certain motor or verbal acts.

38. **Answer: A.** Diminution of emotional response is called blunting of affect. Flattening of affect is strictly speaking the absence of an emotional response.

39. **Answer: C.** Auditory hallucinations are the most commonly seen symptom in schizophrenia from among the five listed answers.

40. **Answer: B.** Perseveration is the inability to shift from one theme to another. A thought is retained long after it has become inappropriate in the given context. It is seen in organic brain disorders.

41. **Answer: A.** Autoscopy is the experience of seeing one's own body in external space. Extracampine hallucination is the experience of a hallucination outside the field of that particular sense. Reflex hallucination is the presence of hallucinations in one modality when the stimulus is in another modality. Gedankenlautwerden is also called echo de la pense or thought echo.

42. **Answer: C.** In Capgras syndrome, a person believes that someone known to him has been replaced by an exact double. In Fregoli syndrome, the patient believes that one or more individuals have altered their appearance to resemble familiar people, usually to persecute the patient. In de Clerambault syndrome, the patient believes that another person, usually of higher social standing, is in love with him. Othello syndrome is also called pathological or morbid jealousy. Diogenes syndrome is also called senile squalor, characterized by hoarding and self-neglect.

43. **Answer: D.** In obsession, patients realize that the obsessive thoughts are their own and illogical, perceive the thoughts as distressing and unpleasant, and usually try to resist them, though with long-standing illness resistance may be absent.

44. **Answer: B.** Echopraxia is the imitation of movements or actions. Echolalia is the repetition of words. Ambivalence or ambitendence is an inability to make decisions. In waxy flexibility, an awkward posture is held by the patient without distress for longer than would be possible for a normal individual.

45. **Answer: A.** In anosognosia, patients are unaware of their illness or condition. Anton syndrome is a form of cortical blindness in which the patient denies the visual impairment. It is caused by occipital lobe damage that extends from the primary visual cortex into the visual association cortex.

46. Answer: E. Agreement with all that the doctor says does not necessarily demonstrate good insight. The criteria that may be used to judge insight are (a) the patient realizes that he has an illness; (b) the patient recognizes the illness to be of a psychological nature; (c) the patient thinks he needs help with the illness; or (d) the patient is willing to accept help.

47. Answer: B. Beck Depression Inventory (BDI) is a self-rating scale. All the others are clinician-rated or observer-rated scales.

48. Answer: D. The New Word Learning test is a test to detect organic brain damage. Cattell P-16 and MMPI are personality inventories. Rorschach test is a projective test and Stanford-Binet is a test for intelligence.

49. Answer: C. Tactile hallucination is classically seen in cocaine use. Alcoholic polyneuropathy does not cause hallucinations. Obsessive-compulsive disorder or panic disorder is not associated with hallucinations. Dermatitis artefacta is a self-inflicted dermatological injury produced for secondary gain. It is not associated with hallucinations.

50. Answer: A. In Cotard syndrome, the patient has nihilistic delusions, that is, beliefs about the nonexistence of some person or thing. The thoughts are associated with extreme degrees of depressed mood. Comparable ideas concerning failures of bodily function often accompany nihilistic delusions.

Chapter 2
SCHIZOPHRENIA

QUESTIONS

1. A 37-year-old Caucasian male with a history of chronic paranoid schizophrenia is hospitalized for a relapse of symptoms. He is given parenteral haloperidol because he is very agitated and threatening. The patient continues to be belligerent and has to be put in physical restraints. The next day the patient is less agitated and belligerent, but he reports feeling nauseated and tired and toward evening is found to be disoriented to time and place. His laboratory work-up shows an increase in BUN and creatinine. He is diagnosed with acute renal failure and transferred to the medical floor. What could be the cause of his acute presentation?
- **A.** Intramuscular injection
- **B.** Myoglobinuria due to muscle breakdown secondary to struggling when restrained
- **C.** Dystonia secondary to multiple doses of pareneteral antipsychotic
- **D.** All of the above

2. A 32-year-old patient has been under treatment for chronic paranoid schizophrenia. He presents to the ER with a relapse of symptoms and is admitted to the hospital because he is very agitated. He had missed an appointment with his psychiatrist a few days before, although he had his WBC count done the day before that. He is started back on clozapine at the same dosage he was receiving before admission: 450 mg. The next morning he is found unconscious near his bed with a bump on the head. Which of the following could have led to this clinical situation?
- **A.** Starting the patient on clozapine
- **B.** Starting the patient on the same dosage of clozapine as previously
- **C.** Not starting the patient on benztropine
- **D.** None of the above

3. A 58-year-old African American male with a long history of NIDDM develops blindness. Approximately 6 months later, he is brought to the ER by his
girlfriend. According to the girlfriend, the patient has been reporting seeing
burglars breaking into their house. The patient is well oriented to time and
place, and he reports that although he realizes what he is seeing is untrue,
the experience is very unsettling for him. What is this phenomenon called?

    A. Doppelganger

    B. Reflex hallucinations

    C. Charles Bonnet syndrome

    D. Functional hallucinations

4. Which of the following is one of the four *As* identified by Eugene Bleuler as
the primary symptoms of schizophrenia?

    A. Abnormal association

    B. Autistic behavior

    C. Ambivalence

    D. All the above

5. What is the total direct and indirect cost of schizophrenia to the U.S. economy annually?

    A. $100 billion

    B. $50 billion

    C. $65 billion

    D. $40 billion

6. What is the concordance rate for schizophrenia in monozygotic twins?

    A. 90–100%

    B. 10–20%

    C. 30–40%

    D. 40–50%

7. Which of the following cognitive impairments is found in persons with
schizophrenia?

    A. Deficits in information processing

    B. Deficits in executive function

    C. Deficits in language ability

    D. None of the above

    E. All of the above

8. Which season of birth is associated with a higher incidence of schizophrenia?

   A. Spring
   B. Summer
   C. Autumn
   D. Winter

9. Which of the following brain regions has consistently been shown to have abnormal volume measurements?

   A. Occipital and parietal regions
   B. Parietal region
   C. Temporal region
   D. Frontal and temporal regions

10. Which of the following antipsychotics has been used in receptor-binding PET studies of schizophrenia?

   A. Droperidol
   B. Amisulpride
   C. Clozapine
   D. Raclopride

11. Which of the following psychoanalysts introduced the concept of the schizophrenogenic mother?

   A. Bateson
   B. Fromm-Reichmann
   C. Vaughn and Leff
   D. Brown

12. A 28-year-old Southeast Asian man presents to the ER accompanied by his parents. According to family members, the patient has been extremely anxious, not sleeping at night and not going to work regularly. During the interview, the patient reports that he is afraid his penis is becoming small and receding into his body. What is the clinical situation described by this man?

   A. Dhat
   B. Piblokto
   C. Latah
   D. Koro

13. Which French psychiatrist introduced the concept of "folie circulaire" (circular insanity)?

    A. Jean-Pierre Falret

    B. Jules Baillarger

    C. Benjamin Rush

    D. Gabriel Langfeldt

14. A patient with chronic schizophrenia walks the floors of the state hospital where he is an inmate swearing aloud at other inmates. The resident in charge of this patient tells him that he has to earn the right to watch TV from now on. According to the treatment plan submitted to the patient, for every half hour that he is able to prevent himself from using obscenities, he can earn a ticket for a half hour of TV time. What is this treatment plan an example of?

    A. Extinction

    B. Token economy

    C. Counterconditioning

    D. None of the above

15. What is the peak onset of schizophrenia in men?

    A. 22–27 years

    B. 24–31 years

    C. 17–25 years

    D. 26–45 years

16. Which of the following did Bleuler consider a primary symptom of schizophrenia?

    A. Abnormal associations

    B. Autistic behavior

    C. Abnormal affect

    D. Ambivalence

    E. All of the above

17. Which of the following is considered a bad consequence of deinstitutionalization of schizophrenic patients?

    A. Some of the patients were transferred to alternative forms of unregulated custodial care like nursing homes and poorly managed shelter systems.

    B. Some patients were let free into nearby communities, which were unable or unwilling to take care of the released patients.

    C. Responsibility for care was transferred to patients' families, for whom it has become a burden.

    D. Some of the released patients ended up in the prison system.

    E. All of the above

18. For which of the following gene locations is there the strongest research evidence of linkage with schizophrenia in genetic studies of the disorder?

    A. Chromosome 4

    B. Chromosome 8

    C. Chromosome 15

    D. Chromosome 6

19. Which of the following is considered a possible marker distinguishing schizophrenic probands and their biological relatives from controls?

    A. Smooth-pursuit eye movements

    B. Continuous performance tasks

    C. Sensory gating

    D. All of the above

20. Which of the following abnormalities is shown by magnetic resonance imaging (MRI) studies of the brains of schizophrenic patients?

    A. Decreased cortical gray matter in the temporal cortex

    B. Decreased volume of limbic structures

    C. Increased volume of basal ganglia nuclei

    D. All of the above

21. Which of the following areas in the brain shows decreased blood flow during the Wisconsin Card Sorting Test in schizophrenic patients?

    A. Dorsolateral temporal cortex

    B. Parietal cortex

    C. Prefrontal cortex

    D. None of the above

22. A 23-year-old college student is brought to the ER in the early morning by friends who found him behaving strangely. He was very irritable, abusive, and assaultive toward them. He also reported getting special messages from the TV instructing him to perform special missions. What should the psychiatry resident who sees him in the ER do first?

    A. Contact the patient's family to obtain a history regarding mental illness in the family.

    B. Give the patient an injection of long-acting risperidone.

    C. Do a urine drug screen and other laboratory tests.

    D. Place the patient on one-to-one observation.

23. Which of the following neurotransmitters has been implicated in the pathophysiology of schizophrenia?

    A. Glutamate

    B. Serotonin

    C. Dopamine

    D. All of the above

24. The study of which of the following substances of abuse has substantiated the argument that serotonin plays a role in the development of schizophrenia?

    A. PCP

    B. LSD

    C. Marijuana

    D. None of the above

25. Which of the following anesthetic agents has been shown to have a mechanism of action similar to PCP and can lead to the development of schizophrenia-like symptoms?

    A. Midazolam

    B. Fentanyl

    C. Ketamine

    D. None of the above

26. Clonidine has been found by some studies to reduce psychotic symptoms in schizophrenic patients. Which of the neurotransmitters do these studies implicate as playing a role in the development of schizophrenia?

    A. Serotonin

    B. Aspartate

    C. Norepinephrine

    D. Dopamine

27. A 52-year-old woman who is a resident of a state psychiatric hospital is admitted to a private hospital for treatment of her medical problems. When speaking with the resident physician, she claims she is the president of the company that owns the private hospital. However, she willingly takes all the medicines given to her and willingly stays in the room she shares with another patient. What term denotes this phenomenon?

    A. Double depression

    B. Double bookkeeping

    C. Both of the above

    D. None of the above

28. A parent of a schizophrenic patient criticizes the patient, saying that he is not showing any affection toward his parents. The same parent shies away when the patient wants to show affection in public. How did Gregory Bateson describe this kind of family interaction?

    A. Expressed emotions

    B. Double-bind communications

    C. Discursive speech

    D. None of the above

29. Emil Kraepelin described persons with dementia praecox as having a prolonged deteriorating course. What percentage of Kraepelin's sample of patients recovered completely?

    A. None

    B. 10%

    C. 22%

    D. 4%

30. Which of the following described the first-rank symptoms of schizophrenia?

    A. Manfred Bleuler

    B. Kurt Schneider

    C. Ernst Kretschmer

    D. None of the above

31. Which of the following is the most common symptom of acute schizophrenia?

    A. Auditory hallucinations

    B. Delusions of reference

    C. Suspiciousness

    D. Lack of insight

32. Which of the following statements is true regarding periodic catatonia?

    A. It was described by R. Gjessing.

    B. The patients have periodic recurrent incidences of both stuporous and excited catatonic states.

    C. Each episode is associated with a shift in the patient's metabolic nitrogen balance.

    D. All of the above

33. Which of the following forms of schizophrenia has the best prognosis?
  A. Paranoid schizophrenia
  B. Catatonic schizophrenia
  C. Disorganized schizophrenia
  D. Schizophrenia, undifferentiated type

34. A 34-year-old woman is referred to a psychiatrist by her primary care physician. According to her husband, the patient has been behaving differently in the last few months. She is paying less attention to her appearance. She has become less industrious in keeping the house clean and taking care of her children and seems isolated from the family. She doesn't get up until late afternoon. Husband reports that these changes appeared gradually over the last two years and that the patient is showing further deterioration. The patient reports fleeting delusional beliefs and hallucinations. Which of the following is the best diagnosis?
  A. Paranoid schizophrenia
  B. Undifferentiated schizophrenia
  C. Stuporous catatonia
  D. Simple schizophrenia

35. A 42-year-old with schizophrenia keeps repeating certain words in the same fashion. What is this phenomenon called?
  A. Echolalia
  B. Perseveration
  C. Echopraxia
  D. Verbigeration

36. Which of the following stressed the inability of schizophrenics to use their ability of abstraction?
  A. Norman Cameron
  B. Kurt Goldstein
  C. Lidz
  D. None of the above

37. Which of the following is not a feature of Type I schizophrenia, according to Crow's classification?
  A. Acute onset
  B. Predominantly positive symptoms
  C. Insidious onset
  D. Good social functioning

38. Which of the following is a good prognostic indicator for schizophrenia?
- A. Prominent affective symptoms
- B. Insidious onset
- C. Ventriculomegaly
- D. Negative symptoms

39. According to Vaughn and Leff, what is the optimal duration of contact between patients and their family members?
- A. Less than 48 hours per week
- B. Less than 72 hours per week
- C. More than 48 hours per week
- D. Less than 35 hours per week

40. A patient who presents to a clinic describes seeing green ghosts when he hears classical music. What is the phenomenon described by the patient?
- A. Haptic hallucination
- B. Autoscopic hallucination
- C. Hypnagogic hallucination
- D. Reflex hallucination

41. A patient reports to his doctor that enemies from Mars have replaced his wife with an impostor that looks and behaves exactly like his real wife. What is the name of this phenomenon?
- A. Fregoli syndrome
- B. Capgras syndrome
- C. Cotard syndrome
- D. Othello syndrome

42. A patient with a long history of schizophrenia is brought to the hospital by the local fire department's EMTs after his landlord found him standing in bizarre positions for a prolonged period. On examination he is found to be standing in a very uncomfortable position. The ER staff reports that he has maintained this position for the last 40 minutes and has not responded to any attempt to talk to him. What is the most appropriate management?
- A. Haloperidol intramuscularly
- B. ECT
- C. Risperidone orally dissolving tablet
- D. Lorazepam intramuscularly

43. A 35-year-old woman is referred to a psychiatric outpatient clinic by a plastic surgeon. According to the referral letter, this person has consulted three cosmetic surgeons in the last 6 months about what she perceives to be a deformity in her upper lip. All the physicians have told her that there is no deformity and that there is no need for any surgery. But the woman firmly believes that there is a deformity, and this belief has hampered her socially and occupationally. What is the diagnosis?

    A. Hypochondriasis

    B. Somatization

    C. Body dysmorphic disorder

    D. Delusional disorder, somatic type

44. Among the following, which is not a predictor of good response to ECT in patients with schizophrenia?

    A. Recent onset

    B. Shorter duration of illness

    C. Mood incongruent delusions

    D. Presence of affective symptoms

45. Which of the following countries was not part of the International Pilot Study of Schizophrenia conducted by the World Health Organization?

    A. Nigeria

    B. United Kingdom

    C. Taiwan

    D. India

    E. United States

46. Which of the following abnormalities is not seen in schizophrenic patients?

    A. Reduction in the amplitude of P300 wave.

    B. Deficits in smooth-pursuit eye movements (SPEM)

    C. Reduction in blood flow in the prefrontal cortex while taking Wisconsin Card Sorting Test

    D. All of the above

47. Which of the following atypical antipsychotics used in the treatment of schizophrenia is also a norepinephrine reuptake inhibitor?

    A. Aripiprazole

    B. Ziprasidone

    C. Risperidone

    D. None of the above

48. According to Ernst Kretschmer's classification of men into different constitutional groups, which of the following body types has more propensity to develop schizophrenia?
- A. Asthenic
- B. Pyknic
- C. Athletic
- D. None of the above

49. Which of the following did Vaughn and Leff consider to be a component of "expressed emotion"?
- A. Critical comments
- B. Hostility
- C. Overinvolvement
- D. Lack of warmth
- E. All of the above

50. Which of the following is not a poor prognostic indicator for schizophrenia?
- A. Insidious onset
- B. Male sex
- C. Negative symptoms
- D. Short episode
- E. Younger age of onset

51. The term "dementia praecox" was coined by
- A. Emil Kraepelin
- B. Eugene Bleuler
- C. Karl Jaspers
- D. Adolf Meyer
- E. Kurt Schneider

52. For a diagnosis of schizophrenia according to the DSM-IV, how long should the disturbance be present?
- A. 1 month
- B. 3 months
- C. 6 months
- D. 9 months
- E. 1 year

53. For a diagnosis of schizophreniform psychosis according to DSM-IV, how long should the disturbance be present?

    A. 6 months

    B. At least 1 month but less than 6 months

    C. Less than 1 month

    D. 3 months

    E. None of the above

54. The lifetime prevalence of schizophrenia is

    A. 0.2–0.6%

    B. 1%

    C. 0.1–0.5%

    D. 1–2%

    E. 2–3%

55. Which of the following is true regarding schizophrenia?

    A. Prevalence is greater in men than women.

    B. The age of onset is earlier in women.

    C. Women have a poorer prognosis than men.

    D. The age of onset is 5 years earlier in men than in woman.

    E. Men are more likely to have negative symptoms.

56. Which of the following is a positive symptom of schizophrenia?

    A. Avolition

    B. Alogia

    C. Auditory hallucinations

    D. Affective flattening

57. Which of the following suggests schizophrenia?

    A. Perseveration

    B. Autoscopy

    C. Olfactory hallucinations

    D. Asyndetic thinking

    E. Visual hallucinations

58. The most common feature of chronic schizophrenia is
    A. Social withdrawal
    B. Underactivity
    C. Lack of conversation
    D. Few leisure interests
    E. Slowness

59. What percentage of persons with acute schizophrenia experience significant depressive symptoms?
    A. 5%
    B. 10%
    C. 25%
    D. 50%
    E. 75%

60. In persons with schizophrenia, paranoid symptoms are more common in
    A. Children
    B. Young adults
    C. The middle-aged
    D. The elderly
    E. Women

61. The risk of siblings of affected individuals developing schizophrenia is
    A. 5%
    B. 10%
    C. 20%
    D. 40%
    E. 50%

62. The risk of schizophrenia is increased in first-degree relatives of patients with
    A. Depressive disorder
    B. Bipolar disorder
    C. Obsessive-compulsive disorder
    D. Panic disorder
    E. Schizoaffective disorder

63. Fertility rates among schizophrenic patients are

A. Increased

B. Decreased

C. The same as for the general population

D. Subject to improvement with treatment

64. In persons with schizophrenia, brain changes are more evident on

A. The left side of the brain

B. The right side of the brain

C. There is no predisposition to either side of the brain.

D. The cerebellum

65. Psychomotor retardation is associated with increased blood flow in the

A. Left parahippocampal gyrus

B. Caudate nuclei

C. Right anterior cingulate nuclei

D. Right prefrontal cortex

E. Frontal lobes

66. The risk of children developing schizophrenia if both parents have schizophrenia is

A. 5%

B. 17%

C. 46%

D. 72%

E. 100%

67. Enlarged lateral ventricles in schizophrenia are associated with

A. Being female

B. Being male

C. Later age of onset of illness

D. Lack of impairment on neuropsychological testing

E. Good response to treatment

68. The rates of all of these disorders are increased in relatives of persons with schizophrenia *except*

A. Bipolar disorder

B. Schizophrenia

C. Schizoaffective disorder

D. Schizotypal disorder

69. Factors associated with the development of psychosis in persons with complex partial seizures include
   A. Lateral temporal focus
   B. Late onset of seizures
   C. Left-sided seizure focus
   D. Right-sided seizure focus

70. All of the following suggest a viral hypothesis for the etiology of schizophrenia *except*
   A. Increased prevalence in children born during winter
   B. Increased rate of complications during pregnancy
   C. Nonlocalized pathology
   D. Increased prevalence in males

71. All of the following are true regarding chronic institutionalized schizophrenic patients *except*
   A. Patients underestimate their age.
   B. Patients score poorly on IQ tests.
   C. Patients are similar in cognitive deficits to the mentally retarded.
   D. Patients are more likely to be male than female.

72. Which of the following is true regarding depression seen in persons with schizophrenia?
   A. Depression might be an integral part of schizophrenia.
   B. Depressive symptoms may be a response to recovery of insight.
   C. Depression may be a side effect of antipsychotic medications.
   D. Fifty percent of patients with acute schizophrenia have depressive symptoms.
   E. All of the above

73. Which of the following findings is not associated with schizophrenic patients?
   A. High activation levels on the EEG, as judged by reactivity upon opening the eyes
   B. Lower alpha power of the EEG
   C. Increased variability of frequency
   D. Higher wave symmetry than EEGs of control subjects
   E. All of the above

74. Which of the following is true regarding structural changes in the brain in schizophrenic patients?

   A. Reduction in size of hippocampus
   B. Reduction in size of amygdala
   C. Absence of gliosis
   D. Decrease in volume of the hippocampus is restricted to the white matter.
   E. All of the above

75. Which of the following is true regarding the prevalence of schizophrenia in new immigrants to the United States compared to the population in the immigrants' home country?

   A. Prevalence is decreased in migrants from Norway.
   B. Prevalence is increased in migrants from Norway.
   C. Prevalence is increased in migrants from Mexico.
   D. Prevalence is increased in all recent migrant subpopulations.
   E. None of the above

76. Which of the following is *not* true regarding the prevalence of schizophrenia in different social classes?

   A. In most countries there is a higher prevalence in lower socioeconomic classes.
   B. Social causation theory states that lower socioeconomic living condition leads to development of schizophrenia.
   C. Social drift theory proposes that lower socioeconomic status is a consequence of the disease.
   D. There is a higher prevalence in the upper castes of social hierarchy in India.
   E. All of the above

77. Which of the following is associated with increased suicide rates in persons with schizophrenia?

   A. Being young
   B. Being male
   C. Awareness of the deteriorative effects of the illness
   D. Chronic illness with frequent exacerbations
   E. All of the above

78. All of the following statements are true regarding the prevalence of schizo-phrenia in the two sexes *except*

    A. Peak onset in men is at ages 17–25.

    B. Peak onset in women is at ages 24–35.

    C. Male-to-female ratio of incidence is close to 1.

    D. Female schizophrenics are associated with more premorbid asocial characteristics.

    E. Male schizophrenics are associated with more birth complications and cerebral structural changes.

79. Which of the following substances demonstrate effects that support the dopamine hypothesis of schizophrenia?

    A. Cocaine

    B. d-amphetamine

    C. Levodopa

    D. Methylphenidate

    E. All of the above

80. A 19-year-old man was recently discharged from the hospital after treatment for acute schizophrenia. On his follow-up visit 2 weeks later, he reports having stopped taking the prescribed medication. What should be the next step in his treatment?

    A. Start the patient on risperidal consta.

    B. Hospitalize the patient.

    C. Report him to the department of health services.

    D. Inquire about side effects from neuroleptics.

    E. None of the above

81. A 72-year-old patient with over 50 years of being diagnosed with schizo-phrenia is observed to repeat the same words and phrases over and over again for days. What is this phenomenon called?

    A. Echolalia

    B. Echopraxia

    C. Stilted language

    D. Verbigeration

    E. None of the above

82. A 42-year-old female patient with schizophrenia stops in the middle of a sentence while being interviewed. She is not able to explain why she stopped. What is this phenomenon called?

    A. Thought withdrawal

    B. Thought blocking

    C. Thought broadcasting

    D. None of the above

83. Which of the following abnormalities, if present alone without any other symptom, is sufficient for a diagnosis of schizophrenia according to DSM-IV?

    A. Bizarre delusions

    B. Hallucination giving a running commentary about the person's thoughts and actions

    C. Auditory hallucination of two or more voices conversing with each other

    D. All of the above

84. All of the following statements are true regarding tardive dyskinesia *except*

    A. It decreases during sleep.

    B. Oral-facial abnormalities are present in 75% of patients with tardive dyskinesia.

    C. It is reduced by voluntary movement.

    D. 20–30% of patients who have had chronic treatment with antipsychotic medications develop tardive dyskinesia.

    E. It is decreased with emotional arousal.

85. Plasma levels of clozapine should be above what level for an adequate response?

    A. 100 ng/mL

    B. 250 ng/mL

    C. 450 ng/mL

    D. 350 ng/mL

    E. None of the above

86. Which of the following is associated with increased incidence of tardive dyskinesia?

    A. Being elderly

    B. Presence of affective symptoms

    C. Presence of cognitive disorders

    D. Sensitivity to acute extrapyramidal effects

    E. All of the above

87. Which of the following is the least common of the tardive syndromes associated with antipsychotic medications?

    A. Tardive tics

    B. Tardive myoclonus

    C. Tardive akathisia

    D. Tardive dyskinesia

    E. Tardive dystonia

88. Which of the following pharmacological agents is not available as a long-acting intramuscular preparation for treatment of chronic schizophrenia?

    A. Fluphenazine

    B. Haloperidol

    C. Risperidone

    D. Flupenthixol

    E. None of the above

89. Which of the following is not a good prognostic factor for delusional disorder?

    A. Acute onset

    B. Early age of onset

    C. Absence of precipitating factors

    D. Female sex

    E. Being married

90. Which of the following types of delusions has the best prognosis?

    A. Persecutory

    B. Erotomanic

    C. Jealous

    D. Somatic

    E. Grandiose

91. Which of the following has no role in the treatment of delusional disorder?

    A. Risperidone

    B. Pimozide

    C. Fluoxetine

    D. Clozapine

    E. Electroconvulsive therapy (ECT)

92. Which of the following is the most common symptom in persons with delusional disorder?

    A. Delusions of reference

    B. Delusions of persecution

    C. Somatic delusions

    D. Jealous delusions

    E. Delusions of grandeur

93. For a diagnosis of delusional disorder according to DSM-IV, how long must the delusions be present?

    A. 2 weeks

    B. 1 week

    C. 3 months

    D. 1 month

    E. 6 months

94. Who introduced the concept of schizoaffective disorder?

    A. Gabriel Langfeldt

    B. Jacob Kasanin

    C. Kurt Goldstein

    D. None of the above

95. Which subtype of delusional disorder is also known as de Clerambault syndrome?

    A. Persecutory

    B. Erotomanic

    C. Somatic

    D. Grandiose

    E. Jealous

96. Which of the following delusional disorders responds specifically to pimozide?

    A. Persecutory

    B. Erotomanic

    C. Somatic

    D. Grandiose

    E. Jealous

97. Which of the following formal thought disorders is more prevalent in patients with schizophrenia?

    A. Tangentiality

    B. Derailment

    C. Incoherence

    D. Illogicality

    E. Circumstantiality

98. All of the following are true regarding postpartum psychosis *except*

    A. Occurs in approximately in 1 or 2 per 1,000 women after childbirth

    B. The onset can be as early as 48 to 72 hours postpartum

    C. Usually occurs within 2 to 4 weeks of treatment

    D. Has a recurrence rate of less than 50% in future pregnancy

    E. Has increased incidence in patients with history of bipolar disorder

99. What is the rate of infanticide associated with untreated puerperal psychosis?

    A. 10%

    B. 2%

    C. 1%

    D. 4%

    E. None of the above

100. Which of the following can be considered in the differential diagnosis for schizophrenia?

    A. Temporal lobe epilepsy

    B. Acute intermittent porphyria

    C. Neurosyphilis

    D. Systemic lupus erythematosus

    E. All of the above

ANSWERS

1. **Answer: D.** Intramuscular injections can lead to muscle injury and an increase in CPK values. When an agitated patient is put in restraints and struggles against the restraints, the patient may develop physical injuries, which can lead to muscle breakdown. Parenteral injections can lead to acute dystonic reactions, which can also lead to muscle breakdown. Muscle breakdown can lead to myoglobinuria, which in turn can lead to acute renal failure.

2. **Answer: B.** A patient who has been off clozapine for more than 36 hours needs to be put back on the starting dosage and the dose slowly increased. Starting at a higher dosage can lead to orthostatic hypotension and other side effects associated with clozapine.

3. **Answer: C.** Charles Bonnet syndrome is seen in people with recently developed blindness. The person knows that the visual hallucination is not real. A hallucination of one's own body, which leads to the belief that one has a double, is called doppelganger.

4. **Answer: D.** According to Bleuler, the four primary symptoms of schizophrenia are abnormal associations, autistic behavior, abnormal affect, and ambivalence.

5. **Answer: C.** The direct and indirect costs of schizophrenia are estimated to cost the U.S. economy around $65 billion annually. Direct cost to the United States is approximately $20 billion.

6. **Answer: D.** Monozygotic twins have a concordance rate of 40–50% for schizophrenia. The lifetime prevalence of schizophrenia for relatives of schizophrenic patients is 4–5% for parents, around 10% for siblings, 13–15% for children with one parent who has schizophrenia, and around 35% for children of parents who are both schizophrenic.

7. **Answer: E.** Patients with schizophrenia show impaired attention and concentration, information processing, executive functions, and memory and language functions.

8. **Answer: D.** It has been shown that a disproportionate number of children born during winter develop schizophrenia.

9. **Answer: D.** It has consistently been shown persons with schizophrenia have decreased volume of the frontal and temporal regions. Schizophrenia has also been implicated in reduced volume of the superior temporal gyrus, hippocampus, and thalamus.

10. **Answer: D.** Raclopride has been used in quantitative PET studies of occupancy of dopamine receptors in patients with schizophrenia.

11. **Answer: B.** Frieda Fromm-Reichmann propounded the concept of the schizophrenogenic mother, described as being cold, overprotective, moralistic, rejecting, and dominant.

12. **Answer: D.** Koro is a culture-bound syndrome seen in Southeast Asia that involves the fear that the penis is shrinking and receding into the abdomen. Dhat is found among Indian men and involves fears about discharge of semen in urine. Piblokto is seen among Eskimo women and involves the person tearing off her clothing, screaming, and crying and running about wildly in the snow. Latah, which is found in women on the Malay Peninsula, is characterized by echolalia, echopraxia, and other extremely compliant behavior.

13. **Answer: A.** Jules Baillarger described "folie à double forme." Gabriel Langfeldt described schizophreniform psychosis. Benjamin Rush, a signer of the American Declaration of Independence, is considered the father of psychiatry in the United States.

14. **Answer: B.** Token economy involves using contingency management for a group of patients living together in a ward or halfway house. Token economy uses positive reinforcement to encourage desirable behaviors.

15. **Answer: C.** The peak onset of schizophrenia in males is between the ages of 17 and 25 years. Peak onset in females is later, 24 to 35 years.

16. **Answer: E.** Eugene Bleuler divided the symptoms of schizophrenia into primary symptoms and secondary symptoms. His four primary symptoms, also known as the four As of schizophrenia, are abnormal associations, abnormal affect, autistic behavior, and ambivalence. Of these four, Bleuler considered the disconnection between thought process and perception and among thought, emotion, and behavior to be the most important.

17. **Answer: E.** Deinstitutionalization involved transferring the patients from a hospital setting to a community care setting. This movement gained momentum during the 1960s, but it had severe repercussions for the patients and for society. Some of the patients were transferred from hospitals to nursing homes and poorly managed shelter systems. Others were just released into the community. In some situations the responsibility for care was transferred to the patients' families, many of which felt burdened and unable to cope with it. Many patients finally wound up in the prison system.

18. **Answer: D.** Some analyses of genetic linkage strongly indicate that chromosome 6 contributes to the development of schizophrenia.

19. Answer: D. Biological markers of schizophrenia are neurophysiological features that reveal underlying pathophysiology and also serve as diagnostic tests. They help in predicting which persons may develop the disease and also help in predicting prognoses. Among the biological tests for schizophrenia are the following: CAT scan, regional cerebral blood flow, structural MRI, functional MRI, magnetic resonance spectroscopy, evoked potentials, smooth-pursuit eye movement test, tests of continuous performance tasks, and tests of sensory gating.

20. Answer: D. Studies show decreased cortical gray matter in the temporal cortex and limbic structures in persons with schizophrenia. Some studies show that individuals with schizophrenia also have increased numbers of basal ganglia nuclei.

21. Answer: C. Persons with schizophrenia who are doing the Wisconsin Card Sorting Test have been shown to have decreased blood flow in the frontal cortex.

22. Answer: D. The symptoms presented by the patient can be a feature of either acute schizophrenia or substance-induced acute psychosis, so testing the urine for any drugs and getting laboratory tests to rule out other causes of acute psychosis is an absolute necessity. An acutely psychotic patient is very unpredictable and the patient's actions may lead to harm to the patient or others. The first thing to do in this situation is to maintain one-to-one observation of the patient to prevent any harm.

23. Answer: D. According to the dopaminergic theory of schizophrenia, the symptoms of schizophrenia are mainly due to an excess of dopamine. This is also shown by the fact that antipsychotics are mostly dopamine antagonists. Phencyclidine, which exerts its effects through its action on the glutamate receptors, can lead to schizophrenia-like symptoms. The atypical antipsychotics exert their therapeutic effect through serotonin-dopamine antagonism.

24. Answer: B. Lysergic acid diethylamide (LSD) is a hallucinogen that blocks serotonin receptors in the brain. The atypical antipsychotics have been shown to have antagonist properties at both dopamine and serotonin receptors.

25. Answer: C. PCP (phenycyclidine) acts as an antagonist at the NMDA receptor. It is also known by the street names angel dust, dust, wet, killer weed, and purple rain. It was developed in the 1950s as a general anesthetic. PCP use can lead to severe agitation and hallucinations. The anesthetic ketamine acts as an antagonist at the NMDA receptors and can lead to postanesthetic agitation and hallucinatory behavior.

26. Answer: C. Clonidine, a presynaptic alpha-2 agonist, leads to a decrease in the release of norepinephrine. Clonidine's effect of reducing schizophrenic symptoms in some individuals implicates norepinephrine as playing a role in the development of schizophrenia.

27. Answer: B. Some individuals with schizophrenia are totally convinced of the reality of their delusions, but this does not influence their actions and beliefs. This paradox is called double orientation or double bookkeeping.

28. Answer: B. The double-bind communication pattern was described by Bateson and Jackson. In this type of communication pattern, the family members or caretakers of the patient give mutually incompatible messages like the example shown in the question.

29. Answer: D. Kraepelin described dementia praecox as having a chronic deteriorating course, but he also reported that, in his sample of patients, 4% recovered completely and 13% had significant remission.

30. Answer: B. The symptoms Schneider called first-rank symptoms are characteristic of schizophrenia and rarely found in other illnesses. These include hearing thoughts as if spoken aloud, third-person auditory hallucinations, hallucinations in the form of commentary, somatic hallucinations, thought withdrawal or thought insertion, thought broadcasting, delusional perception, and feelings or actions experienced as made or influenced by external agencies.

31. Answer: D. Ninety-seven percent of persons with an acute onset of schizophrenia have lack of insight, 74% have auditory hallucinations, less than 70% have delusions of reference, and around 65% report feeling suspicious.

32. Answer: D. Periodic catatonia, first described by Gjessing, is characterized by periodic recurrent incidences of both stuporous and excited catatonic states. Each episode is associated with a shift in the patient's metabolic nitrogen balance.

33. Answer: A. Persons who develop paranoid schizophrenia have a later onset (usually in their late 20s or in their 30s). By then they have already established an identity. They have completed their education and started working. Their ego resources have been described as better than those of catatonic and disorganized schizophrenics.

34. Answer: D. According to DSM-IV research criteria, persons with simple schizophrenia (simple deteriorative disorder) are characterized by a progressive deterioration over a period of at least 1 year. They show a marked decline in occupational or academic functioning. They show a gradual appearance of and worsening of negative symptoms. They also show a decline in their relationships. Hallucinations and delusions are rare and, even when present, are fleeting.

35. Answer: D. Verbigeration is characterized by use of words in a stereotypical fashion. Echolalia is the repetition of the examiner's words. Perseveration is the repetition of words even after the significance of the same is past. Verbigeration is found exclusively in chronic and regressed patients with schizophrenia.

36. Answer: B. Kurt Goldstein described the thinking of persons with schizophrenia as being very concrete and talked about the decrease in their ability to use abstraction. According to Norman Cameron, overinclusive thinking is a significant feature of persons with schizophrenia. Overinclusion refers to the tendency of these persons to include many irrelevant items in their beliefs and behavior. Lidz did psychoanalytic studies in families of schizophrenic patients and reported two types of abnormal family pattern: marital schism and marital skew.

37. Answer: C. Crow et al. described two types of schizophrenia. Type I is characterized by acute onset, mostly positive symptoms, and good social functioning during periods of remission, and it responds well to treatment with antipsychotics. Type II has an insidious onset, poor prognosis, and mostly negative symptoms.

38. Answer: A. Prominent affective symptoms are a good prognostic indicator. Poor prognostic indicators are insidious onset, male gender, venticulomegaly, social isolation, poor occupational history, earlier onset, negative symptoms, single marital status (widowed, separated, never married, or divorced), and prolonged episode. Good prognostic indicators are acute onset, no prior psychiatric history, paranoid subtype, good social and occupational history, married or in a stable relationship.

39. Answer: D. Vaughn and Leff described the effect of expressed emotion in relatives and patient's response to medications. Spending less than 35 hours per week with relatives was optimal for patients taking antipsychotic medications. According to Vaughn and Leff spending less than 35 hours leads to a relapse rate of 15%. The more time spent with relatives with high expressed emotion, the higher the relapse rate.

40. Answer: D. In reflex hallucination a stimulus in one modality results in hallucinations in another sensory modality. Hypnagogic hallucinations are described in narcolepsy and in normal persons as hallucinations when a person is drifting off to sleep. Autoscopic hallucination is the experience of seeing one's own body projected into external space. If the person is convinced that that he or she has a double, the hallucination is known as "doppelganger." Haptic hallucinations are tactile hallucinations.

41. **Answer: B.** In Capgras syndrome, the patient insists that a friend or family member has been replaced by a double. In Fregoli syndrome, the patient identifies a familiar person in many different strangers. Extremely nihilistic delusion in depressed individuals is known as Cotard syndrome. Delusions of jealousy on the part of husbands about their wives are known as Othello syndrome.

42. **Answer: D.** The patient has catatonic schizophrenia. Intramuscular lorazepam is the treatment of choice for catatonic posturing in schizophrenia.

43. **Answer: D.** This patient firmly believes that there is a deformity in her upper lip even when presented evidence to the contrary. The belief is delusional. In body dysmorphic disorder the belief does not have the delusional intensity.

44. **Answer: C.** Electroconvulsive therapy has been found to be most beneficial in persons with acute onset schizophrenia, persons with shorter episodes, and those with comorbid affective symptoms. Patients should first be treated with antipsychotics. Patients who do not show any response to antipsychotics or who are not able to take antipsychotics would benefit from being treated with ECT.

45. **Answer: E.** The International Pilot Study of Schizophrenia was conducted by the World Health Organization in 1973 to study the diagnosis of schizophrenia in seven countries: Colombia, Czechoslovakia, Denmark, India, Nigeria, Taiwan, and United Kingdom. This study showed that schizophrenic patients in countries like India and Nigeria had better prognoses. This was ascribed to the better family support and less incidence of expressed emotions in these countries.

46. **Answer: D.** P300 is an evoked potential developed after a subject hears a stimulus enmeshed in a series of irrelevant stimuli. This measure is indicative of the auditory information processing. In schizophrenic patients the amplitude of P300 wave is reduced. Smooth-pursuit eye movement (SPEM) abnormalities are found in schizophrenia. These deficits often are explained in the context of the attentional and inhibitory deficits central to schizophrenia psychopathology. Patients with schizophrenia have a decrease in the blood flow in the prefrontal cortex while doing the neuropsychological test called the Wisconsin Card Sorting Test.

47. **Answer: D.** Ziprasidone, besides being a serotonin-dopamine antagonist, also inhibits the reuptake of norepinephrine and serotonin.

48. **Answer: A.** Kretschmer posited three chief constitutional groups: the tall, thin asthenic type; the more muscular, athletic type; and the rotund, pyknic type. He suggested that the lanky asthenics and to a lesser degree the athletic types, were more prone to schizophrenia, while the pyknic types were more likely to develop manic-depressive disorders. His work was criticized because his thinner, schizophrenic patients were younger than his pyknic, manic-depressive subjects, so the differences in body type could be explained by differences in age.

49. **Answer: E.** Expressed emotion is a concept well described by Vaughn and Leff in the 1970s. This concept is characterized by a critical, overinvolved environment experienced by schizophrenic patients either at home or at the caretakers' place, which leads to increased relapse rates. The four components of expressed emotion are the parent's or caretaker's critical comments, hostility, overinvolvement, and lack of warmth.

50. **Answer: D.** Longer episode is considered a poor prognostic indicator. Shorter episodes are associated with a better outcome. The following are considered as poor prognostic indicators for schizophrenia: insidious onset, longer episode, presence of negative symptoms, younger age at onset, enlarged lateral ventricles, single status (widowed, divorced, separated, or never married), poor social skills, poor occupational history, and poor psychosexual development.

51. **Answer: A.** Emil Kraepelin divided mental disorders into dementia praecox and manic-depressive psychosis. He first described dementia praecox in 1893. He elucidated four subtypes: catatonic, hebephrenic, paranoid, and simple.

52. **Answer: C.** For a diagnosis of schizophrenia, the disturbance should be present for at least 6 months. At least two of the following five symptoms must be present for a significant portion of a one-month period: delusions, hallucinations, disorganized speech, disorganized behavior, and negative symptoms (affective flattening, alogia, avolition).

53. **Answer: B.** For a diagnosis of schizophreniform disorder, the episode should last at least 1 month and less than 6 months. If the symptoms last less than 1 month, the episode is classified as "brief psychotic disorder."

54. **Answer: B.** The prevalence of schizophrenia is around 1%.

55. **Answer: D.** Prevalence of schizophrenia is equal in men and women. It has an earlier onset in men. Women have a better prognosis. Men are more likely to have negative symptoms.

56. Answer: C. Alogia, avolition, and affective flattening are considered negative symptoms. Delusions and hallucinations are positive symptoms.

57. Answer: D. Asyndesis describes the lack of connection between two consecutive thoughts and is a characteristic of schizophrenia. Schizophrenic patients have an inability to preserve conceptual boundaries.

58. Answer: A. Social withdrawal is the most common feature of chronic schizophrenia. It is seen in 74% of patients with chronic schizophrenia.

59. Answer: D. Around 50% of patients with acute schizophrenia show significant depressive symptoms. This supports the view that depression is an integral part of schizophrenia. The depressive symptoms remit with the treatment of psychosis.

60. Answer: C. Paranoid symptoms are most common in middle-aged patients with schizophrenia.

61. Answer: B. The prevalence of schizophrenia among siblings of patients with schizophrenia is around 10%. If one parent is schizophrenic, prevalence in a child is around 17%. If both parents have schizophrenia, prevalence in children rises to 46%.

62. Answer: E. The risk of schizophrenia is increased in the first-degree relatives of patients with schizoaffective disorder.

63. Answer: B. Individuals with schizophrenia, especially men, have a low fertility rate. The low male fertility rate is ascribed to the fact that the disease process has an earlier onset in men.

64. Answer: A. The structural abnormality present in persons with schizophrenia is predominantly seen in the left side of the brain.

65. Answer: B. The presence of psychomotor retardation in schizophrenic patients is associated with increased blood flow in the caudate nuclei.

66. Answer: C. Their children have a 46% chance of developing schizophrenia if both parents have schizophrenia.

67. Answer: B. Enlargement of the lateral ventricles is present in 75% of schizophrenic patients. It is more prevalent in males and is associated with earlier onset of illness and impairment shown by neuropsychological testing.

68. Answer: A. The risk of schizophrenia, schizoaffective disorder, and schizotypal personality disorder is increased in the first-degree relatives of patients with schizophrenia. The risk of schizophrenia and mood disorder is increased in relatives of patients with schizoaffective disorder.

69. Answer: C. Left-sided seizure focus is associated with the development of psychosis in patients with complex partial seizures.

70. Answer: D. According to the viral hypothesis of the origin of schizophrenia, the disease process has its origin in viral infection of the child in utero. The following factors have been postulated to support this hypothesis: increased prevalence in children born during winter, increased rate of birth complications in children who later develop schizophrenia, and the potential of the viral hypothesis to explain the symptoms of schizophrenia without overt encephalitis.

71. Answer: C. Institutionalized patients with chronic schizophrenia are characterized by thought disorder and negative symptoms. They show decreased activity, apathy, anhedonia, poor self-hygiene, and social withdrawal. Because onset is earlier in males, and men have a poorer prognosis, the number of chronic institutionalized male schizophrenic patients is higher than the number of females.

72. Answer: E. Depressive symptoms are common in both acute and chronic stages of schizophrenia. Depression may be an integral part of schizophrenia and is present in 50% of patients with acute schizophrenia. Depressive symptoms might also develop as a side effect of the antipsychotic medications. Recovery of insight can also lead to development of depression.

73. Answer: E. The EEGs of schizophrenic patients differ from those of normal controls. According to Nuechterlein KH and Dawson ME, in *Pharmacology: The Fourth Generation of Progress*, ACNP, 2000, one difference is "high activation levels, as judged by reactivity of the EEG upon opening the eyes, among schizophrenic patients in an unmedicated state." Also, schizophrenic patients' EEGs have "lower alpha power, increased variability of frequency, and higher wave symmetry" than those of normal controls.

74. Answer: E. Many structural abnormalities are seen in the brains of patients with schizophrenia. Enlargement of lateral ventricles is the most consistent finding. The other findings seen are smaller size of the hippocampus, thalamus, and amygdala. Neuronal cell architecture abnormalities have been seen in the entorhinal cortex, hippocampus, prefrontal cortex, orbitofrontal cortex, and cingulate cortex.

75. Answer: B. A study by Odegaard showed that there is a greater prevalence of schizophrenia among Norwegian immigrants to the United States than among Norwegians in Norway. An Epidemiological Catchment Area (ECA) study showed that Mexican immigrants in Los Angeles had a lower prevalence than Mexicans in Mexico.

76. Answer: E. Schizophrenia has a higher prevalence in the lower socioeconomic classes of most countries. One exception is India, where there is a higher prevalence in the upper castes of the social hierarchy. Social causation theory states that the lower socioeconomic living condition leads to development of schizophrenia. Social drift theory proposes that lower socioeconomic status is a consequence of the disease.

77. Answer: E. Risk factors for suicide in schizophrenic patients include male sex, age under 30 years, being unemployed, history of depression, history of substance abuse, recent discharge from a hospital, awareness of the deteriorative effects of illness, and frequent exacerbations.

78. Answer: D. Peak onset in men is at ages 17–25; peak onset in women is at age 24–35. The male-to-female ratio of incidence of schizophrenia is close to 1. Male schizophrenics are associated with more premorbid asocial characteristics.

79. Answer: E. Cocaine, d-amphetamine, levodopa, and methylphenidate are all drugs that increase dopaminergic activity in the brain. All four of these drugs can lead to paranoid symptoms similar to those seen in schizophrenia.

80. Answer: D. One of the main reasons for noncompliance with antipsychotic medications is the side effects. Therefore, patients who have stopped taking their prescribed medications should be asked whether they experienced side effects with the medications.

81. Answer: D. Verbigeration involves the senseless repetition of the same words or phrases again and again for long periods of time, sometimes even days. Echolalia involves the repetition of the examiner's words and sentences by the patient.

82. Answer: B. Thought blocking involves a sudden arrest in the train of thought. This leaves a blank and the person is not able to explain how it happened. In thought withdrawal, the person believes that someone or something took away the thought from his mind.

83. Answer: D. A diagnosis of schizophrenia can be made even if only one of the following symptoms is present: bizarre delusions, auditory hallucinations giving a running commentary of the person's thoughts and actions, and two or more voices conversing with each other.

84. Answer: E. Tardive dyskinesia (TD) involves abnormal involuntary movements of mouth, tongue, trunk, and extremities. TD develops in 20% to 30% of patients treated chronically with antipsychotic medications. TD is reduced during voluntary movement and sleep. Emotional arousal increases the movements of TD.

85. Answer: D. Patients show better response to clozapine if the plasma concentration is above 350 ng/mL.

86. Answer: E. Presence of affective symptoms and cognitive disorders increase the risk of developing TD. Being elderly and being sensitive to acute extrapyramidal side effects also are heightened risk factors for the development of TD.

87. Answer: B. Tardive myoclonus is the least common and tardive dyskinesia is the most common.

88. Answer: D. Risperidone, haloperidol, and fluphenazine (Prolixin) are available as long-acting intramuscular preparations. Flupenthixol long-acting preparations are not available in the United States.

89. Answer: C. Presence of precipitating factors is considered a good prognostic factor in addition to acute and earlier onset, being female, and being married.

90. Answer: A. Persecutory delusions have the best prognosis.

91. Answer: E. Antipsychotic medications remain the preferred treatment method for delusional disorder though the response rates are low. ECT gives no benefit unless there is comorbid depression. SSRIs have been shown to reduce delusional beliefs.

92. Answer: B. Delusions of persecution are present in about 83% of patients with delusional order and are the most common.

93. Answer: D. For a diagnosis of delusional disorder, the delusions should be present at least 1 month. The delusions should be nonbizarre.

94. Answer: B. Jacob Kasanin introduced the concept of schizoaffective psychosis. Langfeldt introduced the concept of schizophreniform psychosis.

95. Answer: B. Persons with erotomania have delusions of having secret lovers. The delusion is more prevalent in women and usually involves the belief that a person of higher social standing is in love with the woman. It is also referred to as de Clerambault syndrome.

96. Answer: C. Monosymptomatic hypochondriacal delusion (delusional disorder, somatic type) was reported to respond specifically to a pimozide dose of 4–8 mg/day.

97. Answer: B. Derailment, or loose association, is present in around 45% of patients with schizophrenia and is the most common formal thought disorder in this group of patients.

98. **Answer: D.** Postpartum psychosis has a recurrence rate of around 70% in future pregnancies, and postpartum depression has a recurrence rate of 50%. It occurs in 1 or 2 per 1,000 women after childbirth. Most of the episodes occur within 2 to 4 weeks after childbirth, although the psychosis can occur as early as 48 to 72 hours postpartum.

99. **Answer: D.** Risk of infanticide is estimated to be as high as 4% in untreated puerperal psychosis. The rate of suicide is also very high in this group of patients. Short-term treatment with antipsychotic medication is the most appropriate treatment. ECT is a rapidly effective treatment.

100. **Answer: E.** All of the following illnesses can present with features suggestive of schizophrenia: temporal lobe epilepsy, acute intermittent porphyria, neurosyphilis, and systemic lupus erythematosus.

MOOD DISORDERS

Chapter 3

QUESTIONS

1. All of these people were involved in distinguishing unipolar from bipolar disorders *except*
- A. Kraepelin
- B. Angst
- C. Leonhard
- D. Perris

2. Melancholia is also known as
- A. Reactive depression
- B. Exogenous depression
- C. Endogenous depression
- D. Psychotic depression
- E. Masked depression

3. All of the following are features of endogenous depression *except*
- A. Lack of appetite
- B. Irritability
- C. Weight loss
- D. Psychomotor retardation
- E. Anhedonia

4. One-year prevalence of bipolar affective disorder is
- A. 3%
- B. 2%
- C. 1%
- D. 5%
- E. 10%

5. When compared to patients with unipolar disorder, patients with bipolar disorder have
  - **A.** Less genetic loading
  - **B.** Greater genetic loading
  - **C.** The same genetic loading
  - **D.** No genetic loading

6. According to DSM-IV, rapid-cycling bipolar disorder is characterized by
  - **A.** Four or more mood episodes per year
  - **B.** Four or more mood episodes per month
  - **C.** Four or more episodes of mania or hypomania in a year
  - **D.** Four or more episodes of depression per year

7. All of the following are features of rapid-cycling bipolar disorder *except*
  - **A.** Four or more mood episodes per year
  - **B.** More common in women
  - **C.** Occurs early in the course of illness
  - **D.** Usually resistant to treatment with lithium
  - **E.** Antidepressant-induced hypomania

8. All of the following medications are approved by the FDA for bipolar affective disorder *except*
  - **A.** Lithium
  - **B.** Valproic acid
  - **C.** Olanzapine
  - **D.** Lamotrigine
  - **E.** Carbamazepine

9. The dose of lamotrigine should be lower than the usual dose, if lamotrigine is used in combination with
  - **A.** Valproic acid
  - **B.** Escitalopram
  - **C.** Olanzapine
  - **D.** Lithium
  - **E.** Sertraline

10. Evidence exists for the effectiveness of all of the following antiepileptics as mood stabilizers *except*

- A. Valproic acid
- B. Gabapentin
- C. Lamotrigine
- D. Carbamazepine
- E. Oxcarbamazepine

11. One of the primary reasons for slow titration of lamotrigine when it is used in treatment of bipolar disorder is

- A. Hypotension
- B. Rash leading to Stevens-Johnson syndrome
- C. Extrapyramidal side effects
- D. Sedation
- E. Toxicity

12. Which of the following drugs has been shown to decrease the suicide rate?

- A. Carbamazepine
- B. Olanzapine
- C. Sertraline
- D. Lithium
- E. Valproic acid

13. All of the following are indicators of good response to lithium *except*

- A. Family history of bipolar disorder
- B. Good baseline functioning
- C. Nonrapid cycling
- D. Mixed episode

14. Studies have shown that relapse of bipolar disorder after discontinuation of lithium is

- A. 10% in 1 year
- B. 50% in 1 year
- C. 50% in 6 months
- D. 20% in 6 months
- E. 50% in 2 years

15. According to an ECA study, the lifetime prevalence of depressive illness is
- A. 13%
- B. 70%
- C. 40%
- D. 6%
- E. 3%

16. According to Brown and Harris, all of the following are vulnerability factors for depression in women *except*
- A. Loss of mother before the age of 11
- B. Three or more children under the age of 15
- C. Lack of work outside the house
- D. Lack of anyone in whom to confide
- E. Living in a homeless shelter

17. Who proposed the theory of "learned helplessness" to explain depression?
- A. Wolpe
- B. Seligman
- C. Freud
- D. Beck
- E. Kraepelin

18. The "negative cognitive triad" was proposed by Beck to explain
- A. Anxiety
- B. Depression
- C. Bereavement reaction
- D. Adjustment disorder
- E. Post-traumatic stress disorder

19. A 67-year-old woman with depression and anxiety is prescribed paroxetine and clonazepam by her primary care physician. She also has a history of seizure disorder, which has been stable with phenytoin for many years. A few weeks after she begins taking paroxetine and clonazepam, the patient complains of unsteady gait. Which of the following is the most common cause of ataxia in this patient?
- A. Paroxetine
- B. Clonazepam
- C. Phenytoin
- D. Phenytoin toxicity
- E. All of the above

20. All of the following are true about carbamazepine *except*

   A. Can cause SIADH

   B. Induces its own metabolism

   C. Eliminated by extrahepatic metabolism

   D. Reduces levels of valproic acid

   E. Toxicity is not accurately indicated by plasma level

21. The following are recognized side effects of lithium at therapeutic dose *except*

   A. Thirst

   B. Fine tremors

   C. Polydipsia

   D. Diplopia

   E. Erectile dysfunction

22. A 36-year-old White male patient has been stable on lithium for bipolar illness for the past 4 years. During his routine visit with his primary care provider, he complains of feeling weak and lacking motivation and energy. He also says that he has been feeling particularly cold this winter and wonders if he is getting depressed again. The primary care provider should

   A. Diagnose depression and start the patient on antidepressants

   B. Obtain the patient's lithium levels

   C. Check TSH levels

   D. Discontinue lithium

   E. Refer the patient to a psychiatrist immediately

23. A 23-year-old woman is diagnosed with schizophrenia, paranoid type, following a first episode of psychosis and is started on an atypical antipsychotic. She is worried that the antipsychotics will cause weight gain. Which of the following is the most accurate statement regarding weight gain and antipsychotics?

   A. There is no significant weight gain with antipsychotics.

   B. Weight gain occurs mainly in the first 2 months.

   C. Weight gain is related to the patient's pretreatment BMI.

   D. All antipsychotics cause the same amount of weight gain.

   E. Weight gain is associated with clinical improvement.

24. Which of the following antipsychotics also has an antidepressant effect?

   A. Flupenthixol
   B. Chlorpromazine
   C. Haloperidol
   D. Trifluperazine
   E. Fluphenazine

25. Peripheral neuropathy is a side effect of

   A. SSRI
   B. TCA
   C. SNRI
   D. MAOI
   E. NRI

26. A 48-year-old male patient with difficult-to-treat depression has tried all the antidepressants except MAOIs. He is currently on an SSRI. Which of the following SSRIs needs the longest washout period before switching a patient to an MAOI?

   A. Paroxetine
   B. Fluoxetine
   C. Citalopram
   D. Sertraline
   E. Escitalopram

27. Which of the following tricyclic antidepressants closely resembles an SSRI in its action mechanism?

   A. Amitriptyline
   B. Nortriptyline
   C. Imipramine
   D. Clomipramine
   E. Doxepine

28. Which of the following antidepressant blocks reuptake of dopamine?

   A. Venlafaxine
   B. Bupropion
   C. Buspirone
   D. Mirtazapine
   E. Fluoxetine

29. Which of the following can cause depression?
- A. Methyldopa
- B. Procyclidine
- C. Tryptophan
- D. Flupenthixol
- E. Testosterone

30. Which of the following is used as an augmenting agent in the treatment of depression?
- A. Propranolol
- B. Pindolol
- C. Metaprolol
- D. Sotalol
- E. Labetolol

31. Which of the following are risk factors for tardive dyskinesia?
- A. Old age
- B. Diffuse brain damage
- C. Duration of antipsychotic treatment
- D. Affective psychosis
- E. All of the above

32. All of the following are true about antidepressant discontinuation syndromes *except*
- A. More common with short half-life drugs
- B. Are caused by most antidepressants
- C. May be caused by abrupt discontinuation of antidepressants
- D. Indicate that the patient is dependent on these medicines
- E. Cause irritability, insomnia, and restlessness

33. All of the following are true about zopiclone *except*
- A. Can cause tolerance
- B. Binds preferentially to BDZ receptors
- C. Is a benzodiazepine derivative
- D. Dose should be reduced by half in elderly patients.
- E. Dependence can be an issue if the drug is prescribed for long periods.

34. All of the following are true about dystonia *except*
  A. More common in men than in women
  B. More common in younger than older patients
  C. Is more common than akathisia in patients treated with neuroleptics
  D. Treated with lorazepam or diphenhydramine hydrochloride
  E. Can cause trismus

35. A 37-year-old man is admitted to an acute psychiatric unit for psychosis and agitation, where he is prescribed haloperidol 10 mg IM. Later in the evening, the resident on call is summoned because the patient is noticed to be having rigidity and fever. The resident suspects neuroleptic malignant syndrome (NMS). Which of the following is not a feature of NMS?
  A. Clear consciousness
  B. Rigidity
  C. Elevated temperature
  D. Leukocytosis
  E. Elevated CK

36. All of the following drugs are effective in the treatment of the acute phase of mania *except*
  A. Lithium
  B. Lamotrigine
  C. Olanzapine
  D. Valproic acid
  E. Haloperidol

37. Venlafaxine acts as an antidepressant by
  A. Inhibiting the reuptake of dopamine
  B. Antagonizing H1 receptors
  C. Inhibiting the reuptake of serotonin and noradrenaline
  D. Stimulating the glutamate receptors
  E. Inhibiting the GABA receptors

38. All of the following are true about cyproterone acetate *except*
  A. Used sometimes in the treatment of sexually disinhibited behavior in the context of mental illness
  B. Decreases the erectile response to stimulation
  C. Can be given orally or intramuscularly
  D. More effective in older men
  E. Has been used to control sexual disinhibition in mentally retarded people

39. A 36-year-old woman is diagnosed with bipolar illness and, after a discussion of the risks and benefits, single agrees to take lithium. The psychiatrist advises her to undergo a few tests before starting lithium. All of the following are relevant in this patient *except*

    A. Pregnancy test

    B. TSH

    C. Urea and creatinine

    D. ECG

    E. Liver function tests

40. A 68-year-old man is admitted to an acute psychiatric unit for severe suicidal ideation. He is very much preoccupied with death and refuses to agree to a contract for safety. The diagnostician determines the patient to be severely depressed because of noncompliance with medication and severe social stressors. The patient refuses to take any medication because, he says, "Nothing will change, anyway." He also stops eating and drinking and becomes increasingly dehydrated. A reasonable choice of treatment in this patient would be to

    A. Persuade the patient to take antidepressants

    B. Wait and watch for the patient to change his mind

    C. Restrain the patient and administer intravenous fluids

    D. Prescribe electroconvulsive therapy

    E. Prescribe intensive psychotherapy

41. A 48-year-old man with treatment-resistant schizophrenia has been relatively stable for the past 6 months on clozapine. On a routine follow-up visit, the patient is observed to be depressed and reports lack of appetite and insomnia, among other features of depression. The attending psychiatrist decides to treat the patient with antidepressants. Which of the following antidepressants would mandate particular caution in this patient?

    A. Mirtazapine

    B. Fluoxetine

    C. Sertraline

    D. Citalopram

    E. Trazodone

42. A 28-year-old woman is being assessed for bipolar disorder. She complains of mood swings from time to time ranging from "tearfulness to feeling really good." On further questioning, she reveals that she has not been able to maintain any relationships because of her mood swings and feels empty. She fears abandonment by her friends because of her mood swings but also blames everyone for her "current state." The most important differential diagnosis in this patient is

    A. Major depressive disorder

    B. Borderline personality disorder

    C. Histrionic personality

    D. Depressive personality

    E. Generalized anxiety disorder

43. A 54-year-old with a history of coronary artery disease is diagnosed with psychosis NOS and treatment with an atypical antipsychotic, ziprasidone, is considered. The pharmacist requests an ECG before she can dispense ziprasidone. The most important thing to look at on the ECG is

    A. QTc interval

    B. Heart rate

    C. Signs of ischemia

    D. Signs of old infarction

    E. Signs of hypokalemia

44. Which of the following SSRIs is least likely to cause discontinuation syndrome?

    A. Sertraline

    B. Citalopram

    C. Escitalopram

    D. Paroxetine

    E. Fluoxetine

45. A 32-year-old woman is admitted to an acute psychiatric inpatient unit for severe depression. The patient has been ruminating about suicide and guilt feelings. She believes that she has committed a sin and deserves to be punished. The resident physician thinks that the patient is obsessed with thoughts of guilt and suspects that patient has a primary obsessional disorder. The attending psychiatrist explains that patient is not obsessional but severely depressed because

   A. The patient has suicidal ideation.
   B. The patient has indeed committed a sin.
   C. The patient is not distressed by the guilt feelings and is mood congruent.
   D. The psychiatrist thinks so.
   E. Antidepressants alone were not effective.

46. A 54-year-old woman is diagnosed with seasonal affective disorder and light therapy is prescribed. Ideally the intensity of the light should be

   A. 1,000 lux
   B. 10,000 lux
   C. 100,000 lux
   D. 500 lux
   E. 5,000 lux

47. A 36-year-old man is treated for depression with an SSRI. He has a less than full recovery despite taking the highest recommended dose of the SSRI. The attending psychiatrist is considering using an augmenting agent. All of the following can be used *except*

   A. Thyroxine
   B. Lithium
   C. Tryptophan
   D. Propranolol
   E. Pindolol

48. Which of the following support the serotonin deficiency hypothesis of depression?

   A. Decreased 5HT platelet uptake
   B. Decreased plasma tryptophan levels
   C. Decreased 5HIAA levels in CSF
   D. Blunted 5HT1 mediated prolactin release in response to L-tryptophan
   E. All of the above

49. All of the following support the norepinephrine deficiency hypothesis of depression *except*

   A. Decreased norepinephrine mediated release of growth hormone in response to clonidine
   B. Decreased cAMP turnover in platelets following stimulation with clonidine
   C. Increased platelet alpha 2 adrenergic receptor binding
   D. Increased beta adrenergic receptors in depression and suicides
   E. Decreased levels of cAMP in CSF

50. One of the consistent findings in depression, cortisol secretion abnormality, can be explained by

   A. Primary hypersecretion of cortisol
   B. Primary hypersecretion of ACTH
   C. Primary hypersecretion of CRF by hypothalamus
   D. Positive dexamethasone test
   E. Higher incidence of adrenal tumors in depression

51. All of the following are true regarding sodium and mood disorders *except*

   A. Increased "residual sodium" found in some patients with depression
   B. Decreased "residual sodium" found in some patients with mania
   C. Increased sodium pump activity in the erythrocytes of drug-free manic patients
   D. Increased Na-K pump activity on recovery from depression
   E. Increased Na-K pump activity on recovery from mania

52. According to psychoimmunology, patients with depression are generally more prone to other illnesses because

   A. Patients with depression do not take care of themselves.
   B. Patients with depression do not get adequate care because they have mental illness.
   C. Antibiotics are not as effective in depressed patients compared to other patients.
   D. Hypothalamic-pituitary-adrenal dysfunction causes immune suppression.
   E. Replication of T cells is increased in these patients.

53. All of the following immunologic abnormalities are found in depression *except*

    A. Decreased natural killer cells

    B. Decreased interleukin 2

    C. Decreased absolute neutrophil count

    D. Decreased T-cell replication

    E. Increased monocyte activity

54. A 39-year-old man being treated for major depressive disorder complains of persistent sleep problems since the onset of depression. He is otherwise healthy and does not have any physical health problems. He is referred for a sleep study. The EEG is likely to show all of the following *except*

    A. Decrease in the total duration of deep sleep

    B. Increase in the total duration of REM sleep

    C. Decrease in the latency to the onset of REM sleep

    D. Increased latency to the onset of REM sleep

    E. Impaired sleep continuity

55. All of the following are found in brain imaging studies of persons with depression *except*

    A. Decreased volume of the parietal lobes

    B. Decreased volume of the frontotemporal lobes

    C. Decreased caudate size

    D. Increased ventricular size

    E. Decreased blood flow in the dorsolateral prefrontal cortex

56. The criterion for unintended weight loss used in diagnosis of depression is

    A. Loss of any amount of weight

    B. Loss of 5% or more of the body weight in the past month

    C. Loss of 10% or more of body weight in the past month

    D. Loss of 10% of body weight in the past 2 weeks

    E. Loss of 5% of the body weight in the past 2 weeks

57. "Agitated depression" is a term more commonly used to describe depression in

    A. Young children

    B. Adolescents

    C. Adults

    D. Women

    E. The elderly

58. All of the following are features of "atypical depression" *except*
- A. Intense, unstable emotions
- B. Increased appetite
- C. Increased sleep
- D. Mood reactivity
- E. Rejection sensitivity

59. An obese 24-year-old woman is admitted to the psychiatry inpatient unit following an overdose of Tylenol. She has a history of being impulsive and on occasion has induced vomiting, but these instances were not frequent enough to warrant diagnosis of an eating disorder. Over the course of the next few days of observation, the psychiatrist determines that she is depressed and the treatment team debates over the choice of antidepressants. Which of the following would be the most appropriate in this patient?
- A. Mirtazapine
- B. Bupropion
- C. Venlafaxine
- D. Citalopram
- E. Amitriptyline

60. What does the term "double depression" describe?
- A. Major depressive disorder superimposed on grief reaction
- B. Major depressive disorder superimposed on dysthymia
- C. Major depressive disorder not responding to treatment
- D. Major depressive disorder with psychosis
- E. Major depressive disorder with anxiety

61. How many categories of unipolar depressive disorder are listed by DSM-IV?
- A. 4
- B. 3
- C. 6
- D. 10
- E. 5

62. According to DSM-IV, for a diagnosis of major depressive disorder, the symptoms should be present for a minimum of
- A. 2 months
- B. 6 weeks
- C. 4 weeks
- D. 2 weeks
- E. 6 months

63. All of the following statements are true regarding mood disorders *except*

  A. The interepisode duration in bipolar I disorder increases as the illness progresses.

  B. The interepisode duration in bipolar I disorder decreases as the illness progresses.

  C. The interepisode duration stabilizes at around 6 to 9 months after five or six episodes.

  D. The average duration of an episode is about 6 months in recurrent depression.

  E. Men have more manic episodes on average, and women have more depressed episodes on average.

64. A 34-year-old African American man is admitted to an inpatient psychiatry unit following a suicide attempt. The patient reports many symptoms consistent with major depressive disorder, including lack of interest, feelings of guilt, insomnia, and difficulty concentrating. He states that recently he has been hearing voices telling him that only he can save the world because he has a special gift from God. All of the following support a diagnosis of major depressive disorder, severe, *except*

  A. Voices telling him that he has a special gift

  B. Insomnia

  C. Fatigue

  D. Guilt

  E. The suicide attempt

65. A 56-year-old woman is seen in a psychiatry outpatient clinic because she reports she is "not being able to function." She reports feeling rejected all the time and complains of depressed mood. She also complains of lack of appetite and feeling of heaviness in the arms and legs. She reports sleeping up to 15 hours every day over the past few weeks. Her affect is observed to be reactive when she states that her mother is coming to see her in two weeks. The most appropriate diagnosis is

  A. Major depressive disorder, severe

  B. Borderline personality disorder

  C. Major depressive disorder with atypical features

  D. Generalized anxiety disorder

  E. Malingering

66. A 24-year-old woman is referred to a psychiatrist by her primary care physician for assessment of depression. The mother of a 4-month-old infant, she reports feeling depressed for the past few weeks. The diagnosis of major depressive disorder with postpartum onset is made if the onset of symptoms is within how many weeks of delivery?

    A. 2 weeks

    B. 8 weeks

    C. 10 weeks

    D. 6 weeks

    E. 4 weeks

67. According to DSM-IV, for a mixed manic episode, criteria for both major depressive disorder and mania should be present every day for

    A. 1 day

    B. 1 week

    C. 1 month

    D. 3 days

    E. 2 months

68. All of the following statements are true of the epidemiology of depression *except*

    A. The rates are equal in men and women after the age of 50 years.

    B. Women are twice as affected as men between puberty and 50 years.

    C. Girls are four times more affected than boys before puberty.

    D. Point prevalence of depression is 2–3% for men and 5–9% for women.

    E. Increased rates of depression have been observed over the past 4 to 5 decades.

69. All of the following are true about the course of a major depressive disorder *except*

    A. Five to 10 percent of persons with a single episode will eventually develop bipolar disorder.

    B. Thirty percent of patients recover within 6 months with or without treatment.

    C. The recurrence rate is high, especially after two or more episodes.

    D. Sudden onset of depression is usually associated with a severe psychosocial stressor.

    E. The interepisode interval is less with an increasing number of episodes.

70. All of the following antidepressants increase serotonin neurotransmission by reuptake inhibition *except*

  A. Mirtazapine

  B. Venlafaxine

  C. Fluvoxamine

  D. Citalopram

  E. Sertraline

71. In what proportion of depressed patients does the dexamethasone suppression test reveal decreased cortisol or nonsuppression of cortisol?

  A. 50%

  B. 30%

  C. 80%

  D. 20%

  E. 100%

72. According to lipid homeostasis theory, high levels of cholesterol are found in all of the following conditions *except*

  A. Generalized anxiety disorder

  B. Panic disorder

  C. Obsessive-compulsive disorder

  D. Major depression with increased risk of suicide

  E. Post-traumatic stress disorder

73. A 73-year-old woman with a diagnosis of major depressive disorder fails to respond to treatment with an SSRI. The psychiatrist discusses the option of starting a tricyclic antidepressant. The woman states that "anything" is fine except that she does not like to be sedated by medications. Which of the following tricyclic antidepressants is relatively less sedating?

  A. Doxepine

  B. Amitriptyline

  C. Trimipramine

  D. Nortriptyline

  E. Imipramine

74. Which of the following is a reversible MAOI?

  A. Moclobomide

  B. Tranylcypromine

  C. Phenelzine

  D. L-deprenyl

  E. Maprotiline

75. All of the following are side effects resulting from muscarinic receptor blockade of antidepressants *except*

    A. Orthostatic hypotension

    B. Dry mouth

    C. Constipation

    D. Blurred vision

    E. Urinary retention

76. All of the following cause or contribute to confusion and memory problems following electroconvulsive therapy *except*

    A. Prolonged seizures

    B. Old age

    C. High-intensity stimulus

    D. Inadequate oxygenation

    E. Unilateral electrode placement

77. Which of the following accurately states the role of therapy in depression?

    A. Antidepressants are the treatment of choice in all severities of depression.

    B. Cognitive-behavioral therapy (CBT) is the treatment of choice in all severities of depression.

    C. CBT is as effective as antidepressants in the treatment of mild to moderate depression.

    D. Combined treatment with cognitive-behavioral therapy and antidepressants is no better than either on its own.

    E. Interpersonal therapy offers more rapid response than antidepressants.

78. According to DSM-IV, one of the criteria for dysthymic disorder is that the patient should not be symptom free for more than a certain number of months in a 2-year period (or in a 1 year period in children or adolescents). How many months must the patient be symptom free?

    A. 3 months

    B. 2 months

    C. 1 month

    D. 6 months

    E. 8 months

79. In DSM-IV, the category of depressive disorder not otherwise specified (NOS) is used for all the following disorders *except*

    A. Minor depressive disorder
    B. Adjustment disorder with depressed mood
    C. Recurrent brief depressive disorder
    D. Premenstrual dysphoric disorder
    E. Postpsychotic depressive disorder

80. In what percentage of euthyroid patients with major depression does TRH stimulation reveal blunting of TSH response?

    A. 15%
    B. 5%
    C. 10%
    D. 25%
    E. 1%

81. All of the following are true about the epidemiology of bipolar disorder *except*

    A. High incidence of comorbidity
    B. Lifetime prevalence of about 1% in classic cases
    C. Greater prevalence in women
    D. Average age of onset around 19 to 20 years
    E. Equal incidence in all socioeconomic strata

82. The key difference between mania and hypomania, according to DSM-IV, is

    A. Degree of elevation of mood
    B. Presence of psychosis
    C. Number of episodes
    D. Extent of social and occupational dysfunction
    E. Number of symptoms

83. For a diagnosis of bipolar I disorder according to DSM-IV, which of the following criteria is a must?

    A. At least one hypomanic episode
    B. At least one major depressive disorder episode
    C. Depressed mood for more than 2 years
    D. Numerous periods of hypomania
    E. At least one manic or mixed episode

84. What is the approximate duration of untreated depressive episodes in patients with bipolar disorder?

    A. 3 months

    B. 3 to 6 months

    C. 6 to 12 months

    D. 2 to 4 weeks

    E. 2 months

85. A 29-year-old man is admitted for further evaluation. He was brought to the hospital by his wife, who states that her husband has been demanding more sex, repeating the demand sometimes up to 10 to 15 times per day for the past 8 to 10 days. She also observes that he has been working late into the night, sleeping only 2 to 3 hours, and seems full of energy. He has been talking a lot and has taken on at least four new projects at work during the past 10 days. The woman denies any other physical health problems or drug abuse in her husband. The man himself sees no problem and believes that his wife is "just wasting" his time. As you are assessing the case, his colleague calls you and tells you that the man has been "making a mess" at work for the past few days. What is the most probable diagnosis?

    A. Bipolar II disorder

    B. Bipolar I disorder

    C. Bipolar disorder, mixed type

    D. Cyclothymia

    E. Rapid-cycling bipolar disorder

86. All of the following are known causes of secondary mania *except*

    A. Cocaine

    B. Propranolol

    C. Steroids

    D. Antidepressants

    E. L-dopa

87. In a manic patient, the affect could be

    A. Euphoric

    B. Irritable

    C. Labile

    D. Depressed, in mixed state

    E. All of the above

88. A 29-year-old man comes along with his wife of 4 years to the psychiatric clinic. The patient's wife reports that he has had repeated episodes of "highs and downs" for the last 3 years. The episodes are short, lasting only a few days. These episodes disrupt the patient's work schedule and sometimes the young couple's social life. What is the most appropriate diagnosis?

    A. Bipolar I disorder

    B. Bipolar II disorder

    C. Cyclothymia

    D. Dysthymia

89. Which of the following over-the-counter (OTC) medications is not advisable in a 22-year-old sexually active female college student?

    A. Acetaminophen

    B. Motrin

    C. Loratidine

    D. St. John's wort

90. Following childbirth, a 32-year-old woman has developed severe depression. The woman refuses to eat, is found to be very agitated, and is expressing fears that her baby has an incurable illness. What is the most appropriate treatment at this point?

    A. Tricyclic antidepressants

    B. Wellbutrin

    C. SSRIs and antipsychotics

    D. ECT

91. Which psychologist from the University of Pennsylvania proposed the principle of "low rate of reinforcement" as the cause of depression?

    A. Beck

    B. Seligman

    C. Lewinsohn

    D. Bowlby

92. Some studies of the genetics of bipolar disorder have found that the illness has a higher probability of being transmitted through mothers than through fathers. What is this phenomenon called?

    A. Penetrance

    B. Imprinting

    C. Heterogeneity

    D. None of the above

93. Which of the following sleep abnormalities is found in depressed persons?

   A. Decreased REM sleep latency
   B. Increased REM density
   C. Early morning awakening
   D. All of the above

94. Who coined the term "neurasthenia"?

   A. James Braid
   B. William Cullen
   C. George Beard
   D. Robert Post

95. A 42-year-old presents to the clinic 1 month after his spouse's death. He reports feeling extremely depressed and has a total lack of interest in all activities, decreased ability to go to sleep, and an inability to resume his work. He also reports feeling extremely guilty that he is alive, also reports feelings of worthlessness and hopelessness and says that he gets frequent impulses to commit suicide. Although he has been able to ward off the impulses until now, he reports that he doesn't feel safe. What is the patient suffering from?

   A. Normal sadness
   B. Bereavement
   C. Major depression
   D. Mental fatigue
   E. None of the above

96. What is the lifetime prevalence of dysthymic disorder?

   A. 1%
   B. 10%
   C. 3%
   D. 6%
   E. 15%

97. What percentage of persons with bipolar disorder commit suicide?

   A. Less than 5%
   B. 5–10%
   C. 10–15%
   D. Greater than 20%
   E. None of the above

98. In some depressed persons, the main fold in the upper eyelid is angulated upward and backward at the junction of the inner third with the middle third of the fold. What is this sign called?

    A. Omega sign

    B. Veraguth's fold

    C. Snout spasm

    D. Temple sign

    E. None of the above

99. The loss of a parent before what age is considered as a risk factor for the development of depression in adulthood?

    A. Before 3 years

    B. Before 7 years

    C. Before 11 years

    D. Before 15 years

    E. Before 5 years

100. Which of the following has an equal prevalence in both sexes?

    A. Bipolar I disorder

    B. Dysthymia

    C. Major depressive disorder

    D. All of the above

    E. None of the above

ANSWERS

1. **Answer: A.** Karl Leonhard was one of the first to recognize the differences between unipolar and bipolar disorders. Jules Angst and Carlo Perris also made significant contributions. Emil Kraepelin was involved in distinguishing manic-depressive illness from schizophrenia. In 1899 Kraepelin unified all types of affective disorders under the term "manic-depressive insanity"; despite opposition to it, Kraepelin's unitary concept was adopted worldwide until it was questioned by Angst, Perris, and others.

2. **Answer: C.** Melancholia, also known as endogenous depression, is characterized by anhedonia, loss of appetite, weight loss, early morning awakening, psychomotor retardation, diurnal variation of mood, and lack of reactivity.

3. **Answer: B.** Irritability is a feature of reactive depression. Other features of reactive depression include anxiety, initial insomnia, psychomotor agitation, and persistent reactive mood.

4. **Answer: C.** According to an Epidemiologic Catchment Area (ECA) study, the 1-year prevalence of bipolar disorder is 1%.

5. **Answer: B.** Persons with bipolar disorder have greater genetic loading than those with unipolar disorder. In fact, the risk of bipolar illness in a first-degree relative of a person with bipolar disorder is 7–8%. Concordance rates in monozygotic twins are as high as 80%.

6. **Answer: A.** Rapid-cycling bipolar disorder is characterized by at least four episodes of mood disorder, either depression or hypomania or mania in 1 year. Each episode is characterized either by a switch to opposite polarity or by remission.

7. **Answer: C.** The phenomenon of rapid cycling usually occurs in the later part of bipolar illness and is thought to be due to kindling. More than 50% of rapid cycling is limited to less than 2 years.

8. **Answer: E.** Carbamazepine is not approved by the U.S. Food and Drug Administration for bipolar disorder, although psychiatrists have prescribed it for many years as a mood stabilizer. Lamotrigine is the most recent addition to the list of FDA-approved drugs for bipolar disorder.

9. **Answer: A.** Because valproic acid is a strong inhibitor of hepatic metabolic enzymes, lamotrigine should be started at a low dose and titrated gradually if used in combination with valproic acid. The final dose of lamotrigine is usually half of the usual dose if the drug is prescribed in combination with valproic acid.

10. Answer: B. No studies to date have shown that gabapentin is effective as a mood stabilizer. Although the FDA does not approve carbamazepine and oxcarbamazepine as mood stabilizers, studies have shown them to be beneficial.

11. Answer: B. The incidence of rash leading to Stevens-Johnson syndrome is lowest when the dosage of lamotrigine is increased very slowly.

12. Answer: D. Many naturalistic studies have shown that lithium and clozapine decrease the rate of suicide independent of their mood-stabilizing and antipsychotic properties, respectively.

13. Answer: D. Mixed episode, rapid cycling, substance abuse, and mood disorder secondary to general medical condition respond poorly to lithium.

14. Answer: C. Bipolar disorder has one of the highest rates of relapse, especially after discontinuation of treatment. Therefore, prophylactic treatment is strongly advised if there are more than two episodes.

15. Answer: D. An ECA study showed that the lifetime prevalence of depression was as high as 5.8% and that 70% of women and 40% of men had clinically significant depressive symptoms by the age of 65 years.

16. Answer: E. Brown and Harris studied women in Camberwell, a district of London, in 1978 and enumerated the vulnerability factors for depression in women. However, subsequent studies have only partly replicated their findings.

17. Answer: B. Seligman conducted an experiment with dogs that showed that when an effort is not rewarded repeatedly, the dogs give up. He named the phenomenon "learned helplessness" and proposed that, in human beings, this phenomenon would lead to depression.

18. Answer: B. Beck explained depression in terms of cognitive distortions, maladaptive schemata, and a negative cognitive triad (a negative view of self, world, and future). He is pioneered in the development of cognitive behavioral therapy for depression.

19. Answer: B. Benzodiazepines commonly cause ataxia at therapeutic doses, especially in the elderly. Phenytoin toxicity can cause ataxia and is a possibility in this patient because paroxetine increases the levels of phenytoin. However, this would not be the most common cause of ataxia in this patient.

20. Answer: C. Carbamazepine is a potent inducer of hepatic enzymes and promotes the metabolism of many other drugs, including itself. It is metabolized mainly by CYP3A4 and other oxidative mechanisms in the liver. Plasma levels of carbamazepine are not very useful in determining the degree of carbamazepine toxicity.

21. Answer: D. Thirst, polyuria, and polydipsia are some of the early effects related to Na-K pump changes in the renal tubule. Fine tremors are associated with therapeutic levels, while toxic levels cause coarse tremors. It has been shown that about 7% of male patients report problems with erection when on therapeutic dose of lithium. Lithium causes blurred vision but not diplopia.

22. Answer: C. Patients who are on lithium should have their TSH levels tested before starting lithium and at regular intervals thereafter. Lithium can cause hypothyroidism and therefore TSH should be checked before diagnosing the patient with depression or starting antidepressants.

23. Answer: C. Weight gain with antipsychotics seems to be associated with pretreatment body mass index such that greatest weight gain is seen in patients with the lowest baseline BMI. Although all antipsychotics cause some weight gain, some antipsychotics cause more weight gain than others, though the weight is likely to plateau after 6 months.

24. Answer: A. Flupenthixol, which is a typical antipsychotic, also has an antidepressant effect. Amoxapine is another drug that has both antipsychotic and antidepressant effects.

25. Answer: D. Monoamine oxidase inhibitors (MAOIs) are sometimes associated with peripheral neuropathy, which is thought to be due to pyridoxine deficiency.

26. Answer: B. Norfluoxetine, the active metabolite of fluoxetine, has a half-life of up to 5 to 7 days. Therefore, a washout period of at least 5 weeks is recommended before switching to MAOIs.

27. Answer: D. Clomipramine, although classified as a tricyclic antidepressant, has a strong serotonin reuptake inhibition effect.

28. Answer: B. Bupropion blocks reuptake of both noradrenaline and dopamine. Its unique mechanism of action is said to be particularly useful in persons with psychomotor retardation. Buspirone is a 5HT1A agonist and is effective in anxiety.

29. Answer: A. Methyldopa is an antihypertensive. It is converted to alphamethylnoradrenaline in the central presynaptic neurons, acting as a false neurotransmitter. This reduces overall noradrenergic neurotransmission to the postsynaptic neurons, resulting in depression.

30. Answer: B. Pindolol, which is a 5HT1A antagonist, is used as an augmenting agent in the treatment of depression, particularly with SSRIs.

31. Answer: E. Having an affective psychosis increases the risk of tardive dyskinesia. Increasing age is a much stronger risk factor for men than women. The risk of tardive dyskinesia increases with the duration of antipsychotic treatment.

32. Answer: D. Discontinuation syndrome following cessation of antidepressants does not indicate drug dependence. Patients on antidepressants do not show evidence of tolerance, compulsive desire to take the drug, or difficulty controlling the level of use despite knowledge of harmful effects, etc.

33. Answer: C. Zopiclone is a cylopyrrolone and not a benzodiazepine derivative.

34. Answer: C. Acute dystonia is usually seen in the first few days after starting neuroleptics, although it can occur anytime. Akathisia, which is a subjective sense of psychomotor restlessness, is more common than acute dystonia.

35. Answer: A. Altered sensorium is a common feature with confusion or delirium. NMS is an emergency and needs aggressive treatment. Mortality is high if untreated.

36. Answer: B. Lamotrigine, although one of the drugs approved for the treatment of bipolar disorder, is not effective for the treatment of acute mania. Lamotrigine has to be started in a small dose and has to be titrated gradually over the next few weeks. Data exists about its utility in improving bipolar depression.

37. Answer: C. Venlafaxine inhibits the reuptake of serotonin and noradrenaline in a dose-dependent way in the treatment of depression.

38. Answer: D. Cyproterone acetate is used to reduce sex drive in men who have excessive sex drive and for the treatment of pronounced sexual aggression. It is also prescribed to treat severe hirsutism in women of childbearing age as well as to treat androgenic alopecia in women. Like cimetidine and other similar drugs, cyproterone acetate exerts its effect by blocking binding of dihydrotestosterone (DHT) to its receptors. Cyproterone acetate is found to be most effective in individuals with high testosterone and high sex drive, i.e., young people.

39. Answer: E. Lithium is eliminated almost entirely by the kidneys and does not undergo any hepatic metabolism. Therefore, there is no need for liver function tests. It is always better to get a baseline TSH, an ECG, and urea and creatinine tests. All women of childbearing age should also get a pregnancy test in view of the risk of cardiac defects to the fetus.

40. **Answer: D.** This elderly patient has major depressive disorder, severe, with suicidal ideation. His deteriorating physical health is a real cause of concern and so is his severe suicidal ideation. To obtain response quickly, electroconvulsive treatment is a reasonable option in this patient.

41. **Answer: A.** Mirtazapine can cause neutropenia and agranulocytosis and should be used with caution in patients who are being treated with clozapine.

42. **Answer: B.** In some cases, borderline personality disorder may be very difficult to distinguish from bipolar disorder. Intense mood swings are common in borderline personality, and persons with borderline personality do not have any sustained periods of normal mood in between episodes as seen in bipolar disorder. The patient in question has other traits of borderline personality, including unstable relationships, feelings of emptiness, and fear of abandonment.

43. **Answer: A.** Of all the atypical antipsychotics, ziprasidone is known to cause prolongation of QT interval (prolonged QT interval predisposes to arrhythmias). Although all of the above are important observations to make in an ECG, QTc interval would be the most important.

44. **Answer: E.** All the SSRIs with the exception of fluoxetine can cause discontinuation syndrome because of their short half-life. Norfluoxetine, the active metabolite of fluoxetine, has a half-life of 5 to7 days and "tapers off" on its own.

45. **Answer: C.** This patient is convinced that she has committed a sin and has guilt feelings about it. The feelings are mood congruent and the patient is not distressed by these thoughts and does not resist them. In patients who are depressed and delusional like this, a low-dose antipsychotic is often necessary.

46. **Answer: B.** Ideally, the light should resemble natural light and therefore 10,000 lux is recommended.

47. **Answer: D.** Propranolol is a beta-blocker and in fact can worsen the depression. Pindolol is a 5HT1A antagonist and is used as an augmenting agent in conjunction with an SSRI.

48. **Answer: E.** There is a lot of evidence for the serotonin deficiency hypothesis of depression, including the effectiveness of SSRIs in its treatment.

49. **Answer: E.** Deficiency of norepinephrine has long been thought to be the cause of depression. The efficacy of antidepressants, which specifically inhibit the reuptake of norepinephrine, supports this theory. There is no evidence relating to abnormal cAMP levels in CSF.

50. Answer: C. Primary hypersecretion of cortocotropin-releasing factor (CRF) by the hypothalamus results in increased secretion of ACTH, which in turn leads to elevated cortisol levels. There is no evidence to suggest there is primary hypersecretion of either ACTH or cortisol. Dexamethasone suppression test is positive in 50% of depressed patients and is secondary to increased cortisol levels.

51. Answer: B. Increased "residual sodium" is observed in manic patients, too. The relationship between sodium levels and mood disorders is not well understood, but these are some of the abnormalities found.

52. Answer: D. HPA axis dysfunction leads to increased cortisol level, which is thought to be responsible for various immune system abnormalities found in depression.

53. Answer: C. Absolute neutrophil count is found to be normal in depressed patients. All the other abnormalities mentioned above are thought to be secondary to abnormal HPA axis.

54. Answer: D. In depressive disorder, there is a decrease in the latency to the onset of rapid eye movement (REM) sleep and an increase in the total duration of REM sleep. Slow-wave deep sleep is decreased, and patients do not feel refreshed when they wake up in the morning.

55. Answer: A. Brain imaging studies have shown no consistent abnormalities in the parietal lobes of patients with depression.

56. Answer: B. The weight loss criterion for depression specifies it to be 5% or more of the total body weight in the past month.

57. Answer: E. Depression tends to present differently in different people. Irritability may be the predominant symptom in adolescents, while agitation is a common symptom in the elderly.

58. Answer: A. Intense, unstable emotions are more characteristic of borderline personality disorder than atypical depression.

59. Answer: D. For a patient who is impulsive, amitriptyline, venlafaxine, or bupropion is not a good choice because of the risk of overdose. Mirtazapine can cause significant weight gain and therefore is not indicated when the patient is already obese. Citalopram is one of the SSRIs, which are relatively safe and effective antidepressants.

60. Answer: B. Double depression refers to major depressive disorder superimposed on dysthymia.

61. **Answer: B.** DSM-IV lists three categories of unipolar depressive disorders: major depressive disorder, dysthymia, and depressive disorder not otherwise specified (NOS).

62. **Answer: D.** DSM-IV specifies that five or more of the symptoms should be present for at least 2 weeks and one of the symptoms should be depressed mood or loss of interest or pleasure. Other symptoms are lack of appetite, weight loss or gain, insomnia or hypersomnia, psychomotor agitation or retardation, fatigue or loss of energy, guilt, lack of concentration, suicide ideation, and suicide attempt.

63. **Answer: A.** The interepisode duration in bipolar I disorder *decreases* as the illness progresses.

64. **Answer: A.** DSM-IV specifies that mood-incongruent delusions or hallucinations should not be included to support a diagnosis of major depressive disorder. All the other features listed above support a diagnosis of major depressive disorder.

65. **Answer: C.** Features of atypical depression include reactive mood, increase in appetite or gain in weight, hypersomnia, leaden paralysis, and sensitivity to interpersonal rejection. In the vignette, there is nothing to suggest that this patient has borderline personality disorder or generalized anxiety disorder or is malingering.

66. **Answer: E.** The onset of a depressive episode must occur within 4 weeks of delivery for a diagnosis of major depressive disorder with postpartum onset.

67. **Answer: B.** For a diagnosis of mixed manic episode, a patient should meet the criteria for both mania and major depressive disorder every day for 1 week.

68. **Answer: C.** In the prepubertal age groups, it is the boys who are more prone to depression than girls. However, the lifetime prevalence of depression is almost twice as high in women as in men, and this is thought to be secondary to high estrogen levels in women.

69. **Answer: B.** Up to 50% of patients recover from a depressive episode within 6 months with or without treatment. Recurrence of depression is as high as 80% after three episodes. In up to 80% of sudden-onset depression, a significant psychosocial stressor can be identified in the past 6 months.

70. **Answer: A.** Mirtazapine blocks presynaptic alpha-2 receptors and thereby increases the release of norepinephrine. The released norepinephrine also stimulates central alpha-1 adrenoreceptors located on central serotonergic neurons, leading to release of serotonin. All of the other antidepressants mentioned increase serotonin transmission by reuptake inhibition.

71. Answer: A. The dexamethasone suppression test is positive in about 50% of patients with major depression and 80% of patients with major depression and psychotic features.

72. Answer: D. Several studies have shown low levels of cholesterol in persons with major depressive disorder and an association between low cholesterol and an increased risk of suicide. Some studies have shown a positive correlation between severity of depression and the ratio of omega 6 fatty acids to omega 3 fatty acids in plasma and red blood cell phospholipids.

73. Answer: D. Of all the tricyclic antidepressants, nortriptyline, desipramine, and clomipramine are relatively less sedating. Maprotiline (Ludiomil), a tetracyclic antidepressant, is very sedating.

74. Answer: A. Moclobomide is a reversible and selective inhibitor of MAO-B; phenelzine and tranylcypromine inhibit both MAO-A and MAO-B and are irreversible. Selegiline (L-deprenyl) is an irreversible inhibitor of MAO-B, but at higher doses it inhibits MAO-A too. Maprotiline is a tetracyclic antidepressant.

75. Answer: A. Orthostatic hypotension results from alpha-1 adrenergic blockade and not from muscarinic receptor blockade. All of the other side effects mentioned are from muscarinic receptor blockade.

76. Answer: E. Unilateral electrode placement is associated with less confusion and fewer memory problems. Other factors that can reduce confusion and memory problems include brief pulse stimulation and hyperventilation with 100% oxygenation prior to applying the stimulus.

77. Answer: C. All the evidence to date suggests that any form of therapy is as effective as antidepressants in the treatment of mild to moderate depression. Antidepressants are the treatment of choice in severe depression. Combined treatment with cognitive-behavorial therapy and antidepressants has shown to be better than either individually. It is also used if one modality fails to produce a complete response, if depression is chronic, or if multiple symptoms are present.

78. Answer: B. A person who is symptom-free for more than 2 months does not meet the criteria for dysthymia. Also, there should be no evidence for major depressive disorder for the first 2 years of the disturbance.

79. Answer: B. The category "depressive disorder not otherwise specified (NOS)" is used if the symptoms do not meet criteria for major depressive disorder, dysthymia, adjustment disorder with depressed mood, or adjustment disorder with mixed anxiety and depressed mood.

80. Answer: D. Clinical evaluation of TRH stimulation tests revealed blunting of TSH response in approximately 25% of euthyroid patients with major depression.

81. Answer: C. Bipolar disorder is equally prevalent in both men and women. Up to 60% of individuals with bipolar disorder develop substance abuse at some point, and up to 50% of individuals have anxiety disorder. Although the prevalence of classic bipolar disorder is 1%, the prevalence of all other variants of bipolar disorder is 2% to 5%.

82. Answer: D. In mania, the person affected experiences significant social and occupational dysfunction, which usually results in hospitalization. This is not always the case with hypomania. The number of symptoms, number of episodes, and degree of elevation or psychosis have no bearing on the diagnosis.

83. Answer: E. For the diagnosis of bipolar I disorder, there should be at least one manic or mixed episode; there is no need for depressive or hypomanic episodes. However, for a diagnosis of bipolar II, the patient should never have a manic or mixed episode but should have at least one episode of hypomania and one or more episodes of major depression.

84. Answer: C. In bipolar disorder, depressive episodes tend to last longer than manic episodes. The mean duration of an untreated depressive episode is 6 to 12 months, whereas the mean duration of an untreated manic episode is 3 to 6 months.

85. Answer: B. This patient meets the criteria for mania because he has more than three manic symptoms that have been present for more than 7 days and that are also causing significant problems in his social and occupational functioning.

86. Answer: B. Propranolol, a β-blocker, is a known cause of depression and not mania. Other medications or substances known to cause secondary mania are alcohol, amphetamines, barbiturates, and ACTH.

87. Answer: E. The patient's affect need not be euphoric all the time for a diagnosis of mania. In fact, mixed manic episodes are as common as pure manic episodes.

88. Answer: C. Cyclothymia is characterized by numerous periods with hypomanic symptoms alternating over the course of 2 years with numerous periods of depressive symptoms that do not meet the diagnostic criteria for a major depressive episode. For a diagnosis of cyclothymia, the person must *not* be symptom-free for more than 2 consecutive months and should not have had any major depressive, mixed, or manic episodes during the 2 years.

89. Answer: D. St. John's wort induces enzymes that increase the metabolism of oral contraceptive pills. So it is necessary to discuss the issue of over-the-counter antidepressants like St. John's wort with sexually active women in the reproductive age group.

90. Answer: D. Electroconvulsive therapy is the treatment of choice in patients suffering from postpartum depression. ECT is especially effective in people who are refusing to take any medicines orally. Its fast onset of action can be particularly life saving in women refusing to eat and refusing to take care of their newborn infants and for those harboring murderous impulses toward their newborn children.

91. Answer: C. Lewinsohn propounded the theory of "low rate of reinforcement, or lack of appropriate rewards" as a cause for depression. Martin Seligman propounded the notion of "learned helplessness" as a theory for origin of depression. Beck propounded a cognitive triad of depression consisting of negative views of self, the world, and the future. Bowlby propounded the theory of "object loss" as a cause for depression.

92. Answer: B. Imprinting is the phenomenon by which the probability of the disease depends on whether the gene is inherited from the mother or the father. Other examples of imprinting are Prader-Willi syndrome and Angelman syndrome.

93. Answer: D. Sleep studies of depressed patients show abnormalities such as decreased REM sleep latency, increased REM density, and early morning awakening.

94. Answer: C. "Neurasthenia" is a term coined by George Beard to describe a chronic condition characterized by anxious-depressive symptomatology. In this condition, people are overly anxious with a chronic predisposition to mental fatigue, lethargy, exhaustion, and irritability. This diagnosis is most used in China.

95. Answer: C. According to DSM-IV-TR, the diagnosis of major depressive disorder (MDD) should not be given unless the symptoms are still present 2 months after the loss of a loved one. But if the depression is so severe that the person has thoughts of ending his own life, recurrent feeling of worthlessness, guilt about things other than actions taken or not taken by the survivor at the time of the loved one's death, marked psychomotor impairment, hallucinatory experience other than thinking that he hears or sees the deceased person, then a diagnosis of MDD should be made.

96. Answer: D. Dysthymia has a lifetime prevalence of 6%.

97. Answer: C. It has been shown that 10% to 15% of persons diagnosed with bipolar disorder eventually commit suicide. An estimated 8% to 10% of patients with schizophrenia eventually commit suicide.

98. Answer: B. Veraguth's fold is seen in some depressed patients; in this sign, the main fold in the upper eyelid is angulated upward and backward at the junction of the inner third with the middle third of the fold.

99. Answer: C. The loss of a parent before the age of 11 is considered a risk factor for the development of depression in adulthood.

100. Answer: A. Bipolar I disorder has an equal prevalence in women and men, whereas both dysthymia and major depressive disorder have a higher prevalence among women.

Chapter 4
ANXIETY DISORDERS

QUESTIONS

1. Cessation of diazepam after chronic use may cause all of the following *except*
    - A. Depersonalization and derealization
    - B. Perceptual disturbances
    - C. Anxiety
    - D. Constipation
    - E. Rhinorrhea

2. A 54-year-old man is prescribed buspirone for generalized anxiety disorder. One of the important facts the patient should know about buspirone is that it
    - A. Does not cause dependence
    - B. Acts rapidly to give symptomatic relief
    - C. Causes sedation
    - D. Can cause agitation
    - E. Is effective in low dosages

3. A 26-year-old woman presents who appears to have generalized anxiety disorder with panic attacks. Terrified by the panic attacks, she requests medication, saying: "I need something to control them immediately." She is otherwise fit and healthy and has no history of any substance abuse or dependence. A reasonable approach would be to
    - A. Start the patient on intensive psychotherapy
    - B. Start the patient on a combination of bupropion and clonazepam
    - C. Start the patient on any SSRI
    - D. Start the patient on an SSRI and refer the patient to cognitive-behavorial therapy
    - E. Start the patient on a combination of an SSRI for the long term and low-dose clonazepam for a short duration

4. A 28-year-old female patient is diagnosed with generalized anxiety disorder and substance abuse. A trial of SSRIs fails, and the physician is reluctant to prescribe any benzodiazepines for symptomatic relief in view of the patient's history of substance abuse. He prescribes buspirone. Buspirone acts as a

    A. 5HT2C agonist

    B. 5HT1A agonist

    C. 5HT1A antagonist

    D. GABA agonist

    E. Serotonin reuptake inhibitor

5. Which of the following is true about specific phobias?

    A. More common in men

    B. More common in women

    C. Phobic avoidance uncommon

    D. Onset in adult life

    E. Treatment usually not effective

6. People with anxiety disorders have all of the following cardiac abnormalities *except*

    A. Decreased deceleration after stress

    B. High beat-to-beat fluctuation

    C. Higher baseline heart rate

    D. Higher subjective awareness of heartbeats

    E. Increased deceleration after stress

7. All of the following neurotransmitter abnormalities are detected in anxiety disorders *except*

    A. Increased platelet MAO activity

    B. Increased activity of central noradrenaline

    C. Increased central GABA activity

    D. Increased circulating adrenaline

    E. Increased circulating noradrenaline

8. In patients with anxiety spectrum disorders, all of the following are observed *except*

    A. Decreased skin conductance

    B. Panic in response to sodium lactate infusion

    C. Increased cutaneous blood flow

    D. Decreased splanchnic blood flow

    E. Decreased habituation following electrodermal stimulation

9. All of the following statements are true about mitral valve prolapse (MVP) and panic attacks *except*
   A. The incidence of MVP in the general population is 5–20%.
   B. The incidence of MVP in panic-disorder patients is up to 40–50%.
   C. MVP causes panic attacks.
   D. No evidence suggests MVP causes panic attacks.
   E. MVP and panic may represent part of primary autonomic syndrome.

10. A 34-year-old female patient is referred by her psychiatrist for systematic desensitization therapy because of a specific phobia. However, before she starts therapy, the patient wants to know if there are any factors that would result in a less-than-ideal response in her case. All of the following are predictors of good response *except*
   A. Good relaxation response
   B. Free-floating anxiety
   C. Good motivation
   D. No secondary gain from the phobia
   E. No obsessions

11. A 24-year-old woman is diagnosed with social phobia. All of the following are effective treatments *except*
   A. SSRIs
   B. Flooding
   C. Modeling
   D. Systematic desensitization
   E. ECT

12. Regarding phobias, all of the following are true *except*
   A. The phobia is associated with major depressive disorder.
   B. Patients come from stable families.
   C. Traits are anxiety and dependency.
   D. People with phobias are no different from the general population in terms of education and social class.
   E. Phobias are usually triggered by major life events.

13. All of the following have higher incidence in women than men *except*
   A. Needle phobia
   B. Social phobia
   C. Animal phobia
   D. Hospital phobia
   E. Claustrophobia

14. All of the following theories have been put forward to explain phobias *except*

    A. The concept of "preparedness"

    B. Classic conditioning

    C. Neurodevelopmental theory

    D. Operant conditioning

    E. Observational learning

15. Pathological anxiety is distinguished from a normal emotional response by all of the following characteristics *except*

    A. Autonomy

    B. Physical health status

    C. Intensity

    D. Duration

    E. Behavior

16. Which of the following structures is the main source of the brain's adrenergic innervations?

    A. Nucleus raphe

    B. Locus ceruleus

    C. Nucleus of Meynert

    D. Midbrain

    E. Medial temporal lobe

17. According to Epidemiological Catchment Area studies, which of the following is the most common anxiety disorder in the United States?

    A. Panic disorder

    B. Social phobia

    C. Agoraphobia

    D. Specific phobia

    E. Generalized anxiety disorder

18. A 65-year-old man experiences a panic attack for the first time. He also has angina and COPD. The physician makes a diagnosis of organic anxiety syndrome. All of the following are features of organic anxiety syndrome *except*

    A. Onset of symptoms after 35 years of age

    B. Family history of anxiety disorders

    C. No history of childhood anxiety disorders

    D. Poor response to the usual treatments of panic disorder

    E. No avoidance behavior

19. All of the following are true regarding anxiety seen in primary care settings *except*

A. High rates of anxiety are seen in patients with chest pain, dyspnea, and dizziness.

B. Presenting problem in 11% of patients visiting PCPs

C. Most common psychiatric disorder in PCP's office

D. More than 90% of patients present with somatic symptoms

E. High utilizers of PCPs' time and resources

20. Patients with generalized anxiety disorder have excessive anxiety and worry on more days than not for at least how long?

A. 2 weeks

B. 2 months

C. 6 weeks

D. 6 months

E. 4 weeks

21. All of the following are true about specific phobias *except*

A. If the patient is under 18 years, the phobia should last for longer than 6 months.

B. Natural environment phobias (fear of heights, water) have an onset in childhood.

C. Situational phobias (fear of elevators, airplanes) have an onset in the mid-thirties.

D. Lifetime prevalence is 10%.

E. CBT offers good benefits.

22. A 23-year-old male patient believes he has social phobia and would like to know if the information he has about social phobia is true or not. All of the following facts are true about social phobia *except*

A. Most common anxiety disorder

B. More common in women in clinical samples

C. Onset is usually in adolescence

D. Has two specific subtypes: performance anxiety versus generalized anxiety

E. Most common comorbidities are depression and substance abuse (alcohol or drug abuse)

23. Regarding post-traumatic stress disorder (PTSD), all of the following are true *except*
- A. Symptoms should last for more than 1 month.
- B. There are four subtypes: acute, subacute, chronic, and delayed onset.
- C. Prevalence is about 8% in the general population.
- D. Prevalence is up to 20% in people exposed to combat.
- E. Acute stress disorder is a different diagnosis.

24. The DSM-IV diagnostic criteria for acute stress disorder include most of the criteria for PTSD, but they add and emphasize one of the following groups of symptoms. Which group?
- A. Dissociative symptoms
- B. Psychotic symptoms
- C. Neurotic symptoms
- D. Depressive symptoms
- E. Cognitive symptoms

25. Which of the following people have the highest prevalence of post-traumatic stress disorder?
- A. People involved in traffic accidents
- B. Vietnam veterans
- C. Victims of a violent assault
- D. Torture victims

26. Of all the following factors, which is the most important risk factor for the development of post-traumatic stress disorder?
- A. Individual vulnerability
- B. Nature of the trauma
- C. Sex of the victim
- D. Age of the victim
- E. All of the above are equally important.

27. A 36-year-old woman is diagnosed with post-traumatic stress disorder following a violent assault and rape. Over the next 2 years, although the post-traumatic stress disorder abates, she feels anxious and depressed and starts using alcohol and other illicit drugs. Which of the following is the most common comorbid condition in women with PTSD?

   A. Substance abuse (alcohol or drugs)
   B. Eating disorders
   C. Anxiety disorder
   D. Psychotic disorders
   E. Depression

28. For a diagnosis of chronic PTSD according to DSM-IV, for at least how long must the patient have symptoms of PTSD?

   A. 6 months
   B. 1 year
   C. 2 years
   D. 3 months
   E. 1 month

29. Which of the following SSRIs has been approved by the FDA for the treatment of post-traumatic stress disorder?

   A. Fluvoxamine
   B. Fluoxetine
   C. Sertraline
   D. Citalopram
   E. Escitalopram

30. All of the following therapies have been found to be effective in the treatment of PTSD *except*

   A. Psychosomatic psychotherapy
   B. Psychoanalytic psychotherapy
   C. Cognitive-behavioral psychotherapy
   D. Group therapy
   E. Eye movement desensitization and reprocessing (EMDR)

31. According to DSM-IV, all of the following are the criteria for somatization disorder *except*

    A. Four or more pain symptoms

    B. Two gastrointestinal symptoms that are not pain related

    C. One sexual symptom

    D. One pseudoneurologic symptom

    E. Age of onset after 30 years

32. Which of the following does not suggest a somatization disorder?

    A. Family history of bipolar disorder and histrionic personality

    B. Early onset of symptoms

    C. Chronic course

    D. Involvement of multiple organs

    E. Absence of laboratory, radiologic, and physical abnormalities

33. Which of the following is the most common somatoform disorder?

    A. Conversion disorder

    B. Somatization disorder

    C. Pain disorder

    D. Hypochondriasis

    E. Body dysmorphic disorder

34. All of the following are characteristic features of conversion disorder *except*

    A. Patients are usually suggestible.

    B. Symptoms are initiated or exacerbated following severe stress.

    C. Patients believe that they are severely ill.

    D. Symptoms are not feigned.

    E. Usually occurs between the ages of 10 and 35 years

35. All of the following are true about conversion disorders *except*

    A. About one-third of patients with conversion disorder have concurrent neurological illness.

    B. The symptoms tend to conform to the patient's own idea of illness.

    C. Thirty percent of patients' pseudoseizures are due to a neurological illness.

    D. Remission is usually observed within 2 weeks of hospitalization.

    E. Recurrence rate is as high as 20–25% within the first year.

36. A 36-year-old male patient is admitted to the chronic pain unit for severe, chronic back pain. After extensive evaluations, pain disorder associated with psychological factors and a general medical condition is diagnosed. All of the following are true about pain disorder *except*

   A. A significant psychological stress is often a precipitating factor.
   B. Peak incidence is during third and fourth decade of life.
   C. Men mainly complain of back pain.
   D. Women mainly complain of abdominal pain.
   E. Multidisciplinary treatment approach is best.

37. According to DSM-IV, to diagnose a patient with hypochondriasis, the symptoms should last at least

   A. 2 weeks
   B. 2 months
   C. 6 weeks
   D. 6 months
   E. 1 month

38. All of the following are true about hypochondriasis *except*

   A. It is more common in women.
   B. Onset is in early adulthood.
   C. Course is chronic with waxing and waning of symptoms.
   D. The belief of having a serious disease is not of delusional intensity.
   E. The symptoms can involve more than one system.

39. Factitious disorder with predominant physical signs and symptoms, is also known as

   A. Hypochondriasis
   B. Munchausen syndrome
   C. Munchausen syndrome by proxy
   D. Somatoform disorder
   E. None of the above

40. All of the following are true about factitious disorder *except*

   A. A desire to assume the role of sick patient
   B. No secondary gain
   C. Good prognosis once the condition is diagnosed
   D. Intentional production of signs and symptoms
   E. Exact prevalence is unknown

41. A 28-year-old woman is admitted to a general medical unit for hypo-glycemia. A psychiatry consultation is requested because the patient's story "doesn't fit." The patient tells the psychiatrist how bad the problem is and uses medical jargon. She appears to be an intelligent person with strong dependency needs. The nurse interrupts the psychiatrist and tells him that she found insulin-filled syringes beneath the patient's pillow. This upsets the patient and before anything can be done about it, she elopes from the hospital. The most likely diagnosis in this patient is

    A. Somatization disorder
    B. Hypochondriasis
    C. Factitious disorder
    D. Malingering
    E. Munchausen syndrome by proxy

42. All of the following are true about dissociative amnesia *except*

    A. More common in persons who experienced childhood abuse
    B. Men and women equally affected
    C. Adults less likely to dissociate than children
    D. Dissociative identity disorder more common in men
    E. Dissociation measured clinically by the Dissociative Experience Scale (DES)

43. All of the following are true about dissociative amnesia *except*

    A. Defined in DSM-IV
    B. Equal incidence in men and women
    C. More common in first and second decades of life
    D. Can be global or episodic
    E. Can last up to 5 days

44. A 34-year-old male is seen in the psychiatric emergency room of a city hospital for bizarre presentation. Social worker tells the psychiatrist that after obtaining extensive collateral information, she learned that the patient lives in a nearby town and was "normal" until a severe earthquake hit the town recently. He is not able to recall his personal information, and neither is he able to explain how he traveled the 65 miles from his town or when he arrived in this city. There is no history of any substance abuse and family members are concerned. What is the most likely diagnosis?

    A. Dissociative amnesia
    B. Dissociative fugue
    C. Transient global amnesia
    D. Malingering
    E. Dissociative identity disorder

45. The average number of personality states in dissociative identity disorder is
    A. 3
    B. 13
    C. 30
    D. 33
    E. 10

46. All of the following are true about dissociative identity disorder *except*
    A. More common in men
    B. High comorbid depression
    C. Up to 50% have auditory hallucinations
    D. Very susceptible to hypnosis
    E. Psychotherapy is the treatment of choice

47. All of the following are true about depersonalization disorder *except*
    A. More common in women
    B. Onset usually in late adolescence or early adulthood
    C. May last for weeks in adults
    D. Reality testing impaired
    E. Up to 50% have transient depersonalization symptoms at some point

48. How many anxiety disorders does the DSM-IV-TR list?
    A. 10
    B. 12
    C. 6
    D. 4
    E. 13

49. The only social factor that has been identified as a factor contributing to the development of panic disorder is
    A. Recent history of death in the family
    B. Recent history of separation or divorce
    C. Lack of friends
    D. Unsupportive family
    E. Recent history of witnessing a panic attack

50. Which of the following best describes the relationship between mitral valve prolapse and panic disorder?

    A. No clinical relevance

    B. High clinical relevance

    C. Patients with panic disorder predisposed to develop mitral valve prolapse

    D. High incidence of panic disorder in patients with mitral valve prolapse

    E. Panic disorder well controlled if mitral valve prolapse is corrected

51. A 22-year-old woman is seen in the outpatient clinic for anxiety problems. After the assessment, the psychiatrist tells the patient that she has agoraphobia because she has expressed fear associated with public places. She tells the psychiatrist that her father was killed in a motor vehicle accident when she was 6 years old and wonders if that could be responsible for her problems. All of the following could be the defense mechanisms used in this patient *except*

    A. Symbolization

    B. Avoidance

    C. Undoing

    D. Repression

    E. Displacement

52. The article "Conditioned Emotional Reactions" by John B. Watson explains the behavioral theory of

    A. Panic disorder

    B. Depression

    C. Obsessive-compulsive disorder

    D. Phobia

    E. Post-traumatic stress disorder

53. Which of the following phobias shows a strong familial tendency?

    A. Blood/injection/injury

    B. Animal

    C. Heights/elevators

    D. Spiders/insects

    E. Social

54. The blood/injection/injury phobia is different from other phobias in that
  A. It is twice as common in women.
  B. It has low familial inheritance.
  C. It is characterized by severe tachycardia and hypertensive response.
  D. It is easily treated.
  E. Bradycardia and hypotension often follow the initial tachycardia.

55. Dissociative amnesia, according to DSM-IV, has five subtypes. Which of the following is not one of the subtypes?
  A. Continuous amnesia
  B. Discontinuous amnesia
  C. Localized amnesia
  D. Generalized amnesia
  E. Selective amnesia

56. All of the following statements about dissociative amnesia are true *except*
  A. Amnestic disorders are important differential diagnoses.
  B. SCID-D-R is the only tool available to assess the degree of dissociative amnesia.
  C. Patients often present with anxiety, depression, or history of blank spells.
  D. Implicit-semantic memory is more affected.
  E. Amnesia usually centers around a traumatic event.

57. All of the following culture-bound disorders have fugue as a prominent feature *except*
  A. Dhat
  B. Latah
  C. Amok
  D. Grisi Siknis
  E. Piblokto

58. A 42-year-old male is diagnosed with dissociative fugue after he is found in a nearby town 3 days after his "disappearance." The patient has a hard time understanding the concept of dissociative fugue and would like to "come to terms" with what has happened. The choice of treatment, in this patient would be

A. Antidepressants

B. Benzodiazepines

C. Hypnosis

D. Sodium amobarbital interviews

E. Psychodynamic psychotherapy

59. The term "amaxophobia" implies

A. Fear of dogs

B. Fear of cats

C. Fear of strangers

D. Fear of riding in cars

E. Fear of dirt and germs

60. Severe debilitating OCD in a 42-year-old patient is found to be resistant to pharmacotherapy, psychotherapy, and ECT. The option of psychosurgery is discussed with the patient. The most common psychosurgical procedure for OCD is

A. Cingulotomy

B. Subcaudate tractotomy

C. Caudate nucleus ablation

D. Internal capsule stimulation

E. Frontal tractotomy

61. Following the September 2001 terrorist attacks, the most common psychiatric problem diagnosed in the Manhattan residents was

A. PTSD and depression

B. In PTSD, acrophobia and anxiety

C. Panic disorder and PTSD

D. Depression and anxiety

E. Xenophobia

62. Apart from SSRIs, which have proven efficacy in PTSD, all of the following medications are considered to be useful in the treatment of PTSD *except*
- A. Anticonvulsants
- B. MAOIs
- C. Trazodone
- D. Propranolol
- E. Antipsychotics

63. A 32-year-old man is seen in the psychiatry outpatient clinic after "going crazy." He states that 4 months ago he was involved in an automobile accident and was trapped in his car for several hours. Since then he has not been able to drive and has nightmares about the accident. He also complains of difficulty sleeping and inability to concentrate at work; he says he feels nervous and on edge all the time. The diagnosis is
- A. Acute PTSD
- B. Acute stress disorder
- C. Chronic PTSD
- D. Major depressive disorder
- E. Panic disorder

64. A 38-year-old woman with a diagnosis of acute PTSD completes an MMPI as part of a psychological workup; all of the following scales are likely to be elevated *except*
- A. F: Infrequency scale
- B. SC: Schizophrenia
- C. D: Depression
- D. ES: Ego strength
- E. Ps: Psychaesthenia

65. All of the following are true about post-traumatic stress disorder *except*
- A. Concept was developed after World War I
- B. Also called shell shock
- C. Lifetime prevalence of about 8%
- D. Women more commonly affected than men
- E. Severity of trauma is an important risk factor.

66. All of the following are true about mixed anxiety-depressive disorder *except*
- **A.** Prevalence is unknown.
- **B.** About two-thirds of patients with depressive symptoms have anxiety symptoms.
- **C.** Sertraline is FDA-approved for treatment of this condition.
- **D.** Prognosis is unknown.
- **E.** Criteria include persistent or recurrent dysphoric mood for at least 1 month.

67. All of the following are true about the psychological profile of patients with factitious disorder *except*
- **A.** Poor sense of identity
- **B.** Strong dependence needs
- **C.** Narcissism
- **D.** High frustration tolerance
- **E.** Absence of formal thought disorder

68. All of the following are features of Ganser syndrome *except*
- **A.** Most commonly seen in mentally retarded people
- **B.** Approximate answers
- **C.** Considered by some to be a variant of malingering
- **D.** Classified as a dissociative disorder NOS in DSM-IV
- **E.** Existence of this disorder is controversial

69. The most important feature distinguishing malingering from factitious disorder is
- **A.** Age of onset
- **B.** Secondary gain
- **C.** Intentional production of symptoms
- **D.** Course of illness
- **E.** Response to confrontation

70. The condition "brainwashing" included in DSM-IV under "dissociative disorder, not otherwise specified" is characterized by all of the following *except*

A. It occurs largely in the setting of political reforms.

B. It is seen in people subjected to prolonged and intense coercive persuasion.

C. Patients subjected to brainwashing may undergo considerable harm.

D. Coercive techniques include isolation, degradation, induction of fear, etc.

E. Confrontation of the brainwashed subject is very helpful in treatment.

71. A 24-year-old woman is referred for a psychiatric consultation by a plastic surgeon. She is very angry that the surgeon thinks "It's in my brain" and refused to acknowledge that she has a "crooked nose." The psychiatrist thinks that there is no obvious defect with the patient's nose but reassures her and tries to calm her. After obtaining all the collateral information and extensively interviewing the patient, he diagnoses her with body dysmorphic disorder. All of the following about this disorder are true *except*

A. Suicide is rare.

B. Preoccupation with imagined or slight physical anomaly is markedly excessive.

C. Up to one-third of patients with this disorder may be housebound.

D. Hair, nose, and skin complaints are most common.

E. Comorbid depression and anxiety are common.

72. According to the psychodynamic theory, all of the following defense mechanisms can play a role in the manifestation of body dysmorphic disorder *except*

A. Dissociation

B. Distortion

C. Repression

D. Symbolization

E. Denial

73. All of the following are true about the epidemiology of chronic fatigue syndrome *except*

A. Women are more commonly affected.

B. Incidence is more common in young adults.

C. Incidence is 1 per 100.

D. Prevalence is 0.29% in men.

E. Fatigue is present for more than 6 months.

74. According to psychodynamic theory, all of the following defense mechanisms are possible in factitious disorders *except*

    A. Regression

    B. Identification

    C. Symbolization

    D. Sublimation

    E. Repression

75. The brain-imaging studies in panic disorder implicate pathological involvement of the

    A. Temporal lobe

    B. Frontal lobe

    C. Parietal lobe

    D. Midbrain

    E. Occipitoparietal junction

ANSWERS

1. **Answer: E.** Benzodiazepine withdrawal causes withdrawal symptoms that can last for many days. Apart from anxiety and delirium, it can also cause depression and seizures. Both constipation and diarrhea are recognized features of benzodiazepine withdrawal. Rhinorrhea is a feature of opiate withdrawal.

2. **Answer: A.** Buspirone, an azaspirodecanedione, is a nonbenzodiazepine anxiolytic and doesn't cause any sedation or dependence. However, it takes up to 4 to 6 weeks to work, and the dose has to be titrated up to 30 mg per day.

3. **Answer: E.** Although SSRIs on their own may be effective in anxiety disorders, it takes a while before they can be effective, and therefore clonazepam is often used for symptomatic relief until the SSRIs become effective. Bupropion is activating and can make the anxiety worse.

4. **Answer: B.** Buspirone decreases the symptoms of anxiety by 5HT1A agonistic action. However, it takes a few weeks to act and the dose might have to be titrated up to 30 mg twice a day.

5. **Answer: B.** Specific phobias are the most common phobias and more common in women than men. By definition, avoidance should be present for the condition to be called a phobia. Systematic desensitization, exposure, and response prevention are found to be effective treatments.

6. **Answer: E.** Patients with anxiety disorders have higher baseline heart rates than the norm. The rates continue to be higher after stress; hence, they have decreased deceleration after stress.

7. **Answer: C.** Patients with anxiety disorders have increased levels of activating neurotransmitters like adrenaline and noradrenaline and decreased GABA activity.

8. **Answer: A.** Patients with anxiety spectrum disorders have numerous electrodermal abnormalities, including increased skin conductance, decreased habituation, and higher spontaneous fluctuations.

9. **Answer: C.** Numerous studies have been done to see if there is any causal relationship between MVP and panic but, to date, there is no evidence to prove MVP causes or predisposes patients to have panic attacks.

10. **Answer: B.** Presence of free-floating anxiety is a predictor of a poor response, as it does not allow the patient to relax or divert attention from the phobic stimulus.

11. **Answer: E.** ECT is usually indicated for severe depression not responding to medications. Apart from the above-mentioned treatments, MAOIs have also been found to be effective in the treatment of social phobia.

12. **Answer: A.** Major depressive disorder is no more common in phobia patients than in the general population. There is also an association between phobias and childhood enuresis.

13. **Answer: B.** All anxiety-related problems are more common in women, except social phobia, where the prevalence is equal.

14. **Answer: C.** Neurodevelopmental theory is often used to explain the etiology of schizophrenia.

15. **Answer: B.** Pathological anxiety is autonomous; that is, it may or may not have a trigger. Intensity and duration are out of proportion to real or imagined stressors, and behavior is impaired. Physical health status is not a criterion used to distinguish normal fear from pathological anxiety.

16. **Answer: B.** Locus ceruleus is a small retropontine structure and is the main source of the brain's adrenergic innervations. Stimulation of the center causes panic attacks; blockade of locus ceruleus decreases panic attacks.

17. **Answer: D.** Specific phobia is the most common anxiety disorder; it has a lifetime prevalence of 11%. Social phobia is the next most common.

18. **Answer: B.** Patients with organic anxiety syndrome usually do not have a family history of anxiety disorders. Another feature that helps to distinguish organic anxiety syndrome from primary panic disorder is the absence of triggering factors for the anxiety syndrome.

19. **Answer: C.** Depression is in fact the most common psychiatric disorder seen by primary care physicians. (Source: Sartovius et al. Depression comorbid with anxiety. Results from WHO study on psychological disorders in primary health care. Br J Psychiatry 1996; 168 Suppl 30:538–43.)

20. **Answer: D.** Patients with generalized anxiety disorder have symptoms of excessive worry and anxiety on most days for at least 6 months. They find it hard to control worrying and should have three of the following six symptoms: muscle tension, restlessness, easy fatigability, difficulty concentrating, irritability, and insomnia.

21. **Answer: C.** Situational phobia typically has a bimodal onset, with one peak in childhood and the other in midtwenties.

22. **Answer: B.** Although the prevalence of social phobia is higher in women in both epidemiological and community samples, the prevalence is found to be greater in men in clinical samples. This may be because of increased awareness of the condition because of the pressure to perform.

23. Answer: B. There are three subtypes of PTSD based on duration: Acute symptoms last for less than 3 months. Chronic symptoms last for more than 3 months. Delayed onset symptoms appear more than 6 months after the trauma. In acute stress disorder, symptoms occur within 4 weeks of the traumatic event and last for at least 2 days and a maximum of 4 weeks.

24. Answer: A. The diagnostic criteria for acute stress disorder emphasize dissociative symptoms like depersonalization, derealization, and dissociative amnesia.

25. Answer: D. Torture victims have the highest prevalence of PTSD. The prevalence in Vietnam veterans is about 30%. Prevalence in victims of a violent assault is 20%.

26. Answer: B. The nature of trauma is the most important risk factor for the development of PTSD. Although individual vulnerability is an important risk factor, it seems to play a role in less severe trauma.

27. Answer: E. The most common comorbid condition in women with post-traumatic stress disorder is depression (49%), whereas the most common comorbid condition in men is substance abuse (52%).

28. Answer: D. Presence of symptoms for at least 3 months is required to diagnose chronic PTSD.

29. Answer: C. Although all SSRIs are found to be effective in the treatment of PTSD, only sertraline and paroxetine are FDA-approved.

30. Answer: B. Of all the therapies, cognitive-behavioral therapy has been well studied and is found to be very effective. Psychoanalytic psychotherapy is not indicated in patients with PTSD.

31. Answer: E. For a diagnosis of somatization disorder, the onset of symptoms should be before 30 years of age; the multiple, recurring, physical symptoms usually start in adolescence and the diagnostic criteria are usually met by the age of 25 years.

32. Answer: A. Patients with somatization disorders often have a family history of somatization disorder, antisocial personality, and substance abuse. In fact, 10% to 20% of first-degree female relatives of female patients with somatization disorder develop somatization disorder.

33. Answer: A. Conversion disorder is the most common somatoform disorder; the annual incidence in general population is up to 11 to 300/100,000.

34. Answer: C. Patients with conversion disorder often present with la belle indifference and do not believe they are seriously ill. The reported prevalence rates of conversion disorder vary widely according to different studies. (Source: DSM IV TR, page 496.)

35. Answer: C. More than half of the patients with pseudoseizures have a neurological illness.

36. Answer: D. Women with pain disorder often complain of headaches. Treatment focuses on enabling the patients to live with pain, and patients who continue to work have a better prognosis.

37. Answer: D. For a diagnosis of hypochondriasis, the symptoms should last for at least 6 months and should not be accounted for by another mental disorder.

38. Answer: A. The incidence of hypochondriasis is equal in men and women; the prevalence of hypochondriasis in the general population varies from 3% to 13%.

39. Answer: B. Munchausen syndrome is a psychiatric disorder that causes an individual to self-inflict injury or illness or to fabricate symptoms of physical or mental illness, in order to receive medical care or hospitalization. This is usually a more severe form and accounts for 10% of individuals with factitious disorder.

40. Answer: C. The prognosis in factitious disorder is poor because patients have little insight and go from one hospital to another. Because of this and also because of reluctance of the physicians to diagnose factitious disorder in the absence of thorough knowledge of a patient's history; the prevalence of this disorder is unknown.

41. Answer: C. This patient has most of the features of factitious disorder, such as intentional production of signs and symptoms, enjoying being in a sick role, and no obvious secondary gain. Also patient has other "typical features" like dependency needs and elopement from the hospital as soon as her deception is uncovered.

42. Answer: D. Although men and women are equally affected, dissociative identity disorder is more commonly seen in women, whereas dissociative fugue is more common in men, especially during wartime. It is more common in people with childhood trauma. Dissociation can be measured clinically by the Dissociative Experiences Scale, a 28-item self-report questionnaire.

43. Answer: C. Dissociative amnesia is more common in the third and fourth decades of life. It is defined in DSM-IV as "Inability to recall important personal information, usually of traumatic nature, that is too extensive to be explained by normal forgetfulness." It can last anywhere between 24 hours and 5 days in up to 75% of cases, and it is seen equally in men and women.

44. Answer: B. The most likely diagnosis in this patient would be dissociative fugue. It is commonly seen after natural disasters and in men in their second to fourth decades of life. This is associated with inability to recall one's past. In dissociative amnesia, there is no history of travel away from one's home. In dissociative identity disorder, there are two or more distinct personalities. Malingering is unlikely given the above history.

45. Answer: B. The average number of personality states in dissociative identity disorder is 13; however, they vary from 1 to 50.

46. Answer: A. Although dissociation is equally common in men and women, dissociative identity disorder is more common in women than in men; it is usually diagnosed in the third or fourth decades of life. High rates of depression and auditory hallucination are reported, but they do not have a formal thought disorder; they are also easily hypnotized. Although antidepressants and anti-anxiety agents are used, psychotherapy is the treatment of choice.

47. Answer: D. Reality testing is intact in depersonalization disorders and is an important distinction from other psychotic disorders. Though depersonalization disorder is more common in women, transient depersonalization symptoms are equally common in men and women.

48. Answer: B. DSM-IV-TR lists 12 anxiety disorders: (1) panic disorder with agoraphobia, (2) panic disorder without agoraphobia, (3) agoraphobia without history of panic disorder, (4) specific phobia, (5) social phobia, (6) obsessive-compulsive disorder, (7) post-traumatic stress disorder, (8) acute stress disorder, (9) generalized anxiety disorder, (10) anxiety disorder due to a general medical condition, (11) substance induced anxiety disorder, (12) anxiety disorder NOS.

49. Answer: B. Apart from a recent history of separation or divorce, no other social factor is identified as a contributory factor for the development of panic disorder. It is two or three times more common in women than in men and occurs equally among all races.

50. Answer: A. Historically, there has been a lot of debate and interest concerning a possible association between mitral valve prolapse and panic disorder. However, many studies have found no clinical relevance, and prevalence of panic disorder in patients with mitral valve prolapse is the same as the prevalence of panic disorder in patients without mitral valve prolapse.

51. Answer: C. Repression, displacement, and symbolization could all be the defense mechanisms contributing to agoraphobia in this patient. Undoing is commonly seen in patients with obsessive-compulsive disorder.

52. Answer: D. Watson in his article "Conditioned Emotional Reactions" tried to explain the behavioral factors involved in generating fear or phobia. He described his experiences with Little Albert, an infant with a fear of rats and rabbits.

53. Answer: A. The blood/injection/injury phobia has a particularly high familial tendency. Studies have shown that at least two-thirds to three-fourths of the affected patients have at least one first-degree relative with specific phobia of the same type.

54. Answer: E. Blood/injection/injury phobia is unique in that bradycardia and hypotension follow initial tachycardia. It is almost equally common in men and women and has high familial inheritance. It is also one of the most difficult conditions to treat.

55. Answer: B. DSM-IV defines dissociative amnesia as "inability to recall important personal information, usually of a traumatic or stressful nature, that is too extensive to be explained by normal forgetfulness." It is further classified into five subtypes: (I) continuous amnesia, (II) selective amnesia, (III) localized amnesia, (IV) generalized amnesia, and (V) systematized amnesia.

56. Answer: D. Dissociative amnesia is more likely to involve interruption of episodic-autobiographical memory; that is, historical factual information is commonly affected.

57. Answer: A. Latah and Amok are seen in Western Pacific countries, Grisi Siknis is seen in Nicaragua and Honduras, and Piblokto is seen in Eskimos. All these phobias are characterized by high agitation, fugue, and amnesia for the episode. Dhat, seen in rural Northern India, is guilt, as well as concern about losing energy, associated with masturbation.

58. Answer: E. Psychodynamic psychotherapy is the mainstay of treatment in patients with dissociative fugue; a slow exploratory and expressive therapy combined with a good therapeutic alliance helps. Antidepressants are only useful if there is a comorbid depression. Hypnosis and sodium amobarbital interviews are used if amnesia for identity or autobiographical memory is very dense.

59. Answer: D. The term "amaxophobia" denotes an abnormal and persistent fear of riding in a car. Cynophobia is fear of dogs. Ailurophobia is fear of cats. Xenophobia is fear of strangers. Mysophobia is fear of dirt and germs.

60. **Answer: A.** Cingulotomy is the most common psychosurgical procedure performed for treatment-resistant OCD. It helps in 25–30% of otherwise treatment-resistant OCD. The most common complications of this procedure are seizures.

61. **Answer: A.** A survey conducted 5 to 8 weeks after the 9/11 attacks found a prevalence of 9.8% of either PTSD or clinical depression in Manhattan residents, and another 3.7% of the population met the criteria for both the diagnoses.

62. **Answer: E.** Antipsychotics are not found to be of any value in the treatment of PTSD, and therefore these drugs are used only to control severe aggression or agitation. Apart from MAOIs, anticonvulsants, trazodone, and propranolol, medications like reversible MAOI like moclobomoide and clonidine are also found to be useful.

63. **Answer: C.** The patient has all the signs and symptoms suggestive of PTSD and since the symptoms have lasted for more than 3 months, it is chronic. In acute stress disorder, the symptoms last for less than 4 weeks. The patient does not meet the criteria for diagnosis of major depressive disorder or panic disorder.

64. **Answer: D.** Ego strength is not elevated in acute PTSD. If anything, it is likely to be decreased in comparison with that of the normal population.

65. **Answer: A.** The modern concept of PTSD was developed after the Vietnam war; before this, it was known as shell shock, soldier's heart, irritable heart, and by other names. The lifetime prevalence in general population is about 8%, and an additional 5 to 15% of the population has subclinical forms; the most important risk factors are severity, duration, and proximity of a person's exposure to the trauma.

66. **Answer: C.** Very little is known about the prevalence or the prognosis of mixed anxiety disorder because of confusion about the diagnosis and the common comorbidity of depressive and anxiety symptoms. Venlafaxine has been approved by FDA for the treatment of both depression and generalized anxiety disorder and is considered to be the drug of choice although most of the SSRIs are also effective.

67. **Answer: D.** Patients with factitious disorder have low tolerance for frustration; some of the other features of these patients are normal or above average intelligence quotient, poor sexual adjustment, and elevation of almost all clinical scales on MMPI-2.

68. Answer: A. The existence of the condition called Ganser syndrome is very controversial and many think it to be a variant of malingering. It is typically associated with prison inmates and is characterized by approximate answers. It is thought to be more common in men, and severe personality disorder is a predisposing factor.

69. Answer: B. In malingering, there is an obvious, recognizable goal in producing signs and symptoms. Both conditions are characterized by signs and symptoms that are produced intentionally, but the goal in patients with factitious disorder is to assume a sick role. Confrontation usually is not helpful in factitious disorder, and in malingering the patient just goes to a different hospital.

70. Answer: E. Validation of traumatic experience and cognitive reframing of the traumatic experiences will help in the treatment of this condition. Family therapy and interventions may also be of help. Treating preexisting psychopathology and applying general techniques used in treating post-traumatic stress disorder and dissociative disorders are also helpful.

71. Answer: A. People with body dysmorphic disorder may be so distressed that about one-fifth attempt suicide. Many of these patients go from surgeon to surgeon for corrective surgery and are not satisfied with the surgical outcomes.

72. Answer: E. Denial is not one of the defenses used in body dysmorphic disorder. Psychodynamic theory views this condition as the displacement of a sexual or emotional conflict onto an unrelated body part.

73. Answer: C. Although the exact incidence of chronic fatigue syndrome is unknown, it is estimated at 1 per 1,000. Prevalence in women is twice as common at 0.52%.

74. Answer: D. Sublimation is a mature defense mechanism in which unacceptable aggressive ideas or wishes are rechanneled into another form that are accepted and appreciated by the society.

75. Answer: A. Brain-imaging studies in panic disorder point to pathological involvement of the temporal lobes, particularly the hippocampus. One MRI study reported cortical atrophy in the temporal areas on the right side.

Chapter 5

GERIATRIC PSYCHIATRY

QUESTIONS

1. The percentage of elderly people with depressive symptoms is
- A. 5%
- B. 7%
- C. 15%
- D. 30%
- E. 50%

2. The prevalence of delusions in Alzheimer's and vascular dementia is
- A. 5–10%
- B. 10–15%
- C. 20–50%
- D. 50–60%
- E. 60–95%

3. Which of the following is true about depression in the elderly?
- A. Depressed mood is essential for the diagnosis.
- B. Depression may present with a physical symptom.
- C. The condition is usually reactive to social circumstances.
- D. The condition requires only readjustment of social circumstances.
- E. Depression is rarely comorbid with physical illness.

4. Which of the following is true about depression in the elderly?
- A. Elderly persons may deny their symptoms.
- B. The elderly find it easier to express feelings than the young.
- C. Suicidal plans are rare.
- D. Anxiety features are common.
- E. Wishing to die always indicates depression.

5. Which of the following is true regarding geriatric depression?
   A. Minor depression rarely progresses to major depression.
   B. It always requires antidepressants.
   C. It should not be treated until DSM-IV criteria are met.
   D. It may worsen physical illness.
   E. It is frequently overtreated.

6. Which of the following is *not* true regarding the dexamethasone suppression test?
   A. May be positive in dementia
   B. May be positive in infection
   C. May be positive in diabetes
   D. Is a specific test for depression
   E. May be affected by medication

7. All of the following are risk factors for development of depression in the elderly *except*
   A. Physical illness
   B. Female sex
   C. History of depression
   D. Recent bereavement
   E. Living alone

8. Patients with late-onset depressive disorder have
   A. Decreased likelihood of a history of depression
   B. Decreased risk of developing dementia
   C. Reduced mortality
   D. Decreased structural abnormalities
   E. Good treatment response

9. Which of the following is *not* true about depression in the elderly?
   A. It may present as dementia.
   B. Treatment improves cognition.
   C. Dementia is more common in those living in a community.
   D. Depression in the elderly may be due to cognitive deficits.
   E. Depression is more common in early than late dementia.

10. All of the following suggest a diagnosis of dementia *except*
   A. Impaired memory
   B. Fluctuating level of consciousness
   C. Difficulty dressing
   D. Impaired digit span
   E. Difficulty in finding the way home

11. A 60-year-old male is referred for assessment of his mental state. Which of the following symptoms is most suggestive of pseudodementia?
   A. Aphasia
   B. Agnosia
   C. Rapid onset and progression
   D. Apraxia
   E. Loss of short-term memory

12. Which of the following is true regarding suicide in the elderly?
   A. Suicide is associated with depression in about 40% of patients.
   B. Substance abuse is as common as in the younger age groups.
   C. Attempts are associated with a low degree of intent.
   D. Hypochondriasis and insomnia are rare.
   E. Attempts are a strong predictor of successful suicide.

13. Which of the following is not associated with suicide in the elderly?
   A. Living alone
   B. Bereavement
   C. Frequent suicidal thoughts
   D. Financial worries
   E. Previous suicide attempts

14. All of the following are physical changes in aging women *except*
   A. Shrinkage of the labia
   B. Shorter period of sexual arousal
   C. Thinning of vaginal walls
   D. Vaginal dryness
   E. Dry skin

15. Which of the following is found with use of tricyclics in treatment of depression in the elderly?
- **A.** Decreased plasma half-life
- **B.** Increased steady-state levels
- **C.** Reduced volume of distribution
- **D.** Reduced risk of postural hypotension
- **E.** Reduced sensitivity to antimuscuranic side effects

16. Which of the following is a definite risk factor for Alzheimer's disease?
- **A.** Head injury
- **B.** Age
- **C.** Male sex
- **D.** Aluminum
- **E.** Cigarette smoking

17. All of the following are true regarding dementia *except*
- **A.** Alzheimer's is more common than vascular dementia in Asia.
- **B.** One-fifth of patients with Alzheimer's have cerebral vascular lesions.
- **C.** Following a stroke, about one in four patients develops dementia.
- **D.** Hypertension in early life is a risk factor for dementia.
- **E.** Cigarette smoking in early life is a risk factor for dementia.

18. Which of the following is true regarding late-onset psychosis?
- **A.** First-rank symptoms must be present.
- **B.** There is no enlargement of the ventricles.
- **C.** Delusions are more common than hallucinations.
- **D.** Twenty percent of cases have a family history of schizophrenia.
- **E.** Patients usually have a good premorbid personality.

19. All of the following are true regarding first onset of depression in the elderly *except*
- **A.** Somatic delusions are common.
- **B.** The condition responds to treatment with antidepressants.
- **C.** Life expectancy is reduced.
- **D.** The condition rarely results in suicide.
- **E.** There is less likely to be a genetic predisposition.

20. Which of the following is the characteristic neuroimaging change seen in Alzheimer's?

- A. Deep white matter changes on CT scan
- B. Frontotemporal deficits on SPECT
- C. Reduced ventricular size
- D. Lateral temporal lobe hypertrophy
- E. Periventricular hyperintensities on MRI

21. Which of the following is true regarding psychodynamic therapy in the elderly?

- A. It is not appropriate in patients on antipsychotics.
- B. It is contraindicated in patients with dementia.
- C. Older patients make positive changes more rapidly.
- D. Psychodynamic therapy is less effective in the elderly.
- E. Sexuality should not be addressed in those over 70.

22. In the psychometric testing of older people, all of the following are true *except*

- A. The tests take longer.
- B. Performance may be affected by hearing or visual loss.
- C. A fixed battery of tests is recommended.
- D. More extensive procedures can be used in early dementia.
- E. Tests have shown good reliability.

23. All of the following are true regarding late-onset psychosis in women *except*

- A. Associated with deafness
- B. Characterized by visual hallucinations
- C. More prevalent in lower socioeconomic classes
- D. Family history of schizophrenia may be present
- E. Antipsychotic drugs are ineffective

24. All of the following are features of late-onset psychosis *except*

- A. May precede dementia
- B. Good response to antipsychotics
- C. Positive findings shown on CT scan
- D. Runs a chronic course
- E. More common in men than in women

25. Which of the following is a response to change of sleep patterns in the elderly?

   A. Decreased number of REM episodes
   B. Reduced total REM sleep
   C. Increased amplitude of delta waves
   D. Decreased stages 1 and 2 sleep
   E. Concentration of REM sleep in the latter part of night

ANSWERS

1. **Answer: C.** At any given time, 10–15% of the elderly population suffers from depression as opposed to 5% with dementia.

2. **Answer: C.** The prevalence of delusions, hallucinations, and misidentification syndromes in dementia are 20–50%, 17–36%, and 11–36% respectively.

3. **Answer: B.** Atypical presentations of depressive disorder are relatively common in the elderly. These include pseudodementia, agitation, and paranoid symptoms. Hypochondriacal symptoms and other illness behavior, pseudo personality disorder, and mixed personality disorder are quite common. Readjustment of social circumstances alone is not sufficient, and in patients with established depression, pharmacotherapy and, on occasions, ECT may be required.

4. **Answer: A.** The elderly may deny symptoms of depression and may somatize instead. They find it more difficult to express their feelings than the younger population. Wishing to die is not always a result of depression, as this association has not been found in 20% of suicides and 10% of parasuicides.

5. **Answer: C.** Minor depression, if left untreated, can progress to major depression. Antidepressants may not be required in all cases of depression in the elderly. Treatment should be tailored to meet individual needs. It should be directed at predisposing, precipitating, and perpetuating factors on social, psychological, and biological axes. Where possible, correctable factors should be rectified or adjusted. DSM-IV should be used to make a diagnosis before commencing pharmacologic treatment. Supportive psychotherapy, formal counseling, CBT, and group psychotherapy are effective. Depression in the elderly is frequently undertreated.

6. **Answer: D.** The dexamethasone suppression test is positive in depression; however, it is also positive in a number of other conditions and is not specific to depression.

7. **Answer: E.** Physical illnesses predispose the elderly to develop depression. Up to 50% of medically ill elderly patients suffer from depression. Occult malignancies and drugs like corticosteroids can cause depression. Other factors include anxiety tendencies and avoidant and dependent personality, adverse life events, bereavement, female sex, and feeling lonely (but not necessarily living alone).

8. Answer: A. The prognosis of depression in the elderly is mired in controversy. Post (1962) suggested that with treatment most patients had a good outcome, although only 26% showed full recovery at follow-up and 12% were continually ill. Murphy (1983) found only 35% well at 1-year follow-up; 29% were continually ill and 14% dead at 1-year follow-up. There was a 15% risk of developing dementia.

9. Answer: C. Dementia is more common in those in care. Cognitive impairment resulting from depression is called depressive pseudodementia. Treatment of depression corrects the cognitive impairment. Dementia itself can lead to depression in the earlier stages, when insight is fully or partially preserved. This insight usually is absent in late dementia.

10. Answer: B. A fluctuating level of consciousness suggests delirium rather than dementia. The symptoms of dementia include recent memory impairment, agnosia, dyspraxia, dysphasia, and loss of judgment, self-control, and planning ability. Insight and emotions decline only gradually. Depression is present in 20–40% of early cases. Anxiety, paranoid symptoms, social withdrawal, hoarding of possessions, and change of personality may occur.

11. Answer: C. Pseudodementia is the cognitive changes occurring in depression. It can be differentiated from depression by rapid onset and progression, the manner in which the patient answers questions, a past history of depression, depressed mood, diurnal variation in mood, biological symptoms, islands of normality, and exaggerated presentation of symptoms. The cognitive functions usually return to normal with successful treatment of depression.

12. Answer: E. Depression is associated in up to 80% of suicides. Duration of depression varies from 6 to 12 months. Twenty-five to thirty percent of suicides occur in the first episode of depression. Suicide is more common among men than women. It is associated with bereavement and with living alone whether widowed, single, or divorced. Alcohol or substance abuse is present in up to 44% of cases. The prevalence of schizophrenia and paraphrenia is about 6–17%. Mild dementia is a risk factor. Physical illness is present in up to 65% cases. Hypochondriasis may also be present. The elderly are more likely to succeed in their attempts at suicide, and the intent is usually quite high.

13. Answer: D. Financial worries are not associated with suicide in the elderly.

14. Answer: B. Menopause is associated with hot flashes, depression, vaginal dryness, shrinkage of the labia, dyspareunia, cystocele, urinary frequency/incontinence, and genital tract atrophy.

15. Answer: B. With tricyclics in the elderly, all of the following are increased: plasma half-life, steady-state levels, volume of distribution, incidence of postural hypotension, and susceptibility to antimuscuranic side effects.

16. Answer: B. Age is the only definitive risk factor for dementia. Other risk factors include family history in first-degree relatives, Down syndrome, infections, autoimmune conditions, head injury, aluminum, previous history of depression, advanced age of mother at birth, and thyroid disease.

17. Answer: A. Alzheimer's is more common than vascular dementia in the Western world, where it accounts for more than 50% of cases. In Asia, vascular dementia is more common. Hypertension, cigarette smoking, Oriental diet, male sex, increasing age, heart disease, and hyperlipidemia are the other risk factors for vascular dementia.

18. Answer: C. Typical first-rank symptoms are found in only 30% of cases. A CT scan of the brain may show evidence of organic changes, but the significance is unknown. Delusions are usually persecutory, grandiose, or erotic. Hallucinations are usually auditory. The risk of paraphrenia in first-degree relatives of late paraphrenics is about half that found in first-degree relatives of younger schizophrenics.

19. Answer: D. Hypochondriacal delusions and somatization are common presentations in the elderly. The condition responds well to antidepressants and usually SSRIs, NARI, and reversible MAOIs are better tolerated than tricyclics. Murphy et al. found that mortality is increased in this population. Fifty to eighty percent of patients who complete suicide have a depressive illness.

20. Answer: E. Periventricular hyperintensities are seen on the MRIs of patients with Alzheimer's disease.

21. Answer: C. Psychodynamic therapy may be used on patients who are on antipsychotics as long as the patient is not actively psychotic. It's unlikely to be of benefit in moderate to severe dementia. There is no age limit for addressing issues related to sexuality.

22. Answer: C. Various scales have been developed to provide an accurate assessment of psychological functioning in the elderly. Psychometric tests quantify the level and range of ability. Serial measures can be used to measure the effect of interventions or to measure the progression of the illness over time. These tests have shown good reliability.

23. Answer: A. The common associations of late-onset psychosis are female sex, family history, personality, sensory deprivation (deafness, blindness), social isolation, significant life events, and organic brain changes. Hallucinations are most commonly auditory. In 10–20% of cases, only delusions are present. Symptoms do respond to antipsychotic treatment.

24. Answer: E. The female to male ratio is 9:1. Antipsychotics are effective, and long-term treatment is necessary. A CT scan of the brain shows organic changes.

25. Answer: B. REM sleep duration is reduced in the elderly.

Chapter 6

CHILD PSYCHIATRY

QUESTIONS

1. Which of the following is not a feature of sleep terror disorder?
- A. Occurrence in NREM sleep
- B. Increased muscle tone
- C. Episode duration of 30–40 minutes
- D. Vivid memories of a dream's content

2. Rett syndrome is characterized by all of the following *except*
- A. A genetic basis
- B. Hyperammonemia in some patients
- C. History of PCP abuse in mothers of children who develop the disorder
- D. Stereotypic hand-wringing movements

3. In what percentage of persons with schizophrenia is the onset before the age of 10 years?
- A. Less than 10%
- B. Less than 7%
- C. Less than 3%
- D. Less than 1%

4. An 18-month-old-old girl is separated from her parents for about 1 month following a natural calamity. The child develops severe depression following this episode. What is the name of this phenomenon?
- A. Vulnerable child syndrome
- B. Anaclitic depression
- C. Separation anxiety disorder
- D. None of the above

5. Which of the following is characteristic of encopresis?

    A. The child is at least 4 years old.

    B. The episodes of incontinence occur at least once a month for 3 months.

    C. The child repeatedly passes feces in inappropriate places.

    D. All of the above

6. Which of the following is not correct regarding enuresis in children?

    A. Episodes of urinary incontinence occur at a frequency of twice a week for at least 3 months or they lead to clinically significant distress.

    B. The child is at least 5 years old.

    C. It is more common among boys.

    D. All of the above

7. Which of the following has been found useful in the treatment of enuresis in children?

    A. Desmopressin

    B. Bell and pad method of conditioning

    C. Imipramine

    D. All of the above

8. In children with depression, a decrease in growth hormone secretion has been found after challenge with which of the following substances?

    A. Clonidine

    B. Levodopa

    C. Desmethylimipramine

    D. All of the above

9. Which of the following is a characteristic feature of Kleine-Levin syndrome?

    A. Hyperphagia

    B. Hypersomnia

    C. Loss of sexual inhibitions

    D. Higher incidence in boys

    E. All of the above

10. A 32-year-old mother brings her 7-year-old son to a hospital's emergency department. The child is found to be restless and displaying stereotyped hand movements. The mother reports that he was "normal" until 1 year ago and had achieved childhood developmental milestones at the appropriate times. For the past year, the child has shown progressive deterioration in social interactions and communication abilities and recently has lost control over the bowel training that he had attained earlier. Which of the following is the most appropriate diagnosis?

    A. Rett syndrome

    B. Heller syndrome

    C. Asperger syndrome

    D. Minimal brain damage

11. According to his schoolteacher, an 11-year-old boy doesn't interact with his peers and prefers to be left alone. He is considered to be a whiz kid with numbers. He does not get excited by any of his achievements. His parents also report that he is aloof at home and does not respond to affection from his parents or siblings. He does not have any impairment in language or cognitive functions. What is the most likely diagnosis?

    A. Rett syndrome

    B. Pervasive developmental disorder

    C. Asperger syndrome

    D. Selective mutism

12. Which of the following medications can exacerbate tics in Tourette syndrome?

    A. Pimozide

    B. Pemoline

    C. Clonidine

    D. Naltrexone

13. Which of the following medications should not be used to treat Tourette syndrome?

    A. Clonidine

    B. Zoloft

    C. Wellbutrin

    D. Naltrexone

14. Which of the following tricyclic antidepressants used in treatment of ADHD has led to four reported deaths in children?

    A. Imipramine

    B. Nortriptyline

    C. Desipramine

    D. Maprotiline

15. Which of the following is *not* true for Tourette syndrome?

    A. Has an onset before age 18

    B. Is more prevalent in boys

    C. Has obsessive-compulsive features in 40% of cases

    D. Can be caused by postviral encephalitis

16. Which of the following tests can be used to measure the intellectual ability of children aged 3–7 years?

    A. Wechsler Intelligence Scale for Children, 3rd Edition

    B. Stanford-Binet Test

    C. Wechsler Preschool and Primary Scale of Intelligence–Revised

    D. Bayley Scales of Infant Development

    E. None of the above

17. Guanfacine is used in the treatment of ADHD in children. How does it act?

    A. By stimulating the release of dopamine from presynaptic vesicles

    B. By inhibiting the reuptake of dopamine in the brain

    C. By acting as an agonist at presynaptic alpha-2 receptors

    D. None of the above

18. Which of the following stimulants used in the treatment of ADHD requires monitoring of liver enzymes?

    A. Methylphenidate

    B. Amphetamine

    C. Pemoline

    D. None of the above

19. A 17-year-old girl presents to the ER with her parents. Her parents report that she has been behaving very unusually in the last 6 months. She has started expressing strange beliefs and has become very suspicious of family members and friends, claiming for example that her high school teachers are actually members of a radical group who are enemies of the country. Her physical examination shows a minimal resting tremor and a grayish green ring around the edges of the cornea that is most marked at the superior and inferior pole. The abnormality for this disease condition is located in which chromosome?

A. Chromosome 6

B. Chromosome 13

C. Chromosome 12

D. Chromosome 6

20. Which of the following features can be seen in children exposed to toxic levels of lead?

A. Intellectual impairment

B. Behavior disorder

C. Seizures

D. Decrease in heme production

E. All of the above

21. At what age do children develop the concept of death as permanent?

A. 2–3 years

B. 3–4 years

C. 7–8 years

D. 4–5 years

22. A 4-year-old child whose development was normal until around 3½ years develops difficulty comprehending speech. The child psychiatrist who assessed him believes that he has a severe deficit in comprehension that is new in onset. After 2 months, the patient is found in his bed unresponsive and is found to have passed urine in the bed. He is seen by a neurologist, who orders an EEG; the EEG shows abnormalities in both temporal areas. By now the patient is often found to be irritable, inattentive, and depressed. Which of the following is the most appropriate diagnosis?

A. Gerstmann syndrome

B. Rett syndrome

C. Heller syndrome

D. Landau-Kleffner syndrome

23. The age of incidence of fragile X syndrome decreases in succeeding generations. What is this phenomenon called?
  A. Anticipation
  B. Assimilation
  C. Both of the above
  D. None of the above

24. Which of the following is not considered among the causes of school phobia?
  A. Fear of a strict teacher
  B. Fear of being bullied by another student
  C. Separation anxiety on the parent's part
  D. Separation anxiety on the child's part
  E. None of the above

25. According to Thomas and Chess, which of the following is not a category of temperament?
  A. Adaptability
  B. Intensity
  C. Quality of mood
  D. Rhythmicity
  E. None of the above

26. Which of the following is *not* true regarding gender identity?
  A. Gender identity is the child's perception of self as male or female.
  B. In the majority of children, formation of gender identity starts at age 3–4 years and is complete by age 5–7 years.
  C. Gender identity forms earlier in girls.
  D. Homosexual play in early childhood is indicative of adult sexual orientation.
  E. None of the above

27. Who first described autism?
  A. Kanner
  B. Asperger
  C. Chess
  D. Benham
  E. None of the above

28. Which of the following is *not* true regarding Lesch-Nyhan syndrome?
- A. It is due to a deficiency in HGPRT.
- B. Patients show self-mutilating behavior.
- C. Patients have mild to moderate mental retardation.
- D. There is a decrease in uric acid levels.
- E. There is an accumulation of uric acid.

29. Which of the following is *not* true regarding tuberous sclerosis?
- A. Patients show hyperactivity and impulsivity.
- B. It is an autosomal dominant disorder.
- C. CT scan of the brain shows calcified hamartomas.
- D. Patients develop epilepsy.
- E. It is an autosomal recessive disorder.

30. Which of the following is true about persons with oppositional defiant disorder?
- A. They often lose their tempers.
- B. They deliberately annoy others.
- C. They blame others for their mistakes.
- D. Their symptoms last more than 6 months.
- E. All of the above

31. Who proposed the concept of a "holding environment" in the development of children?
- A. Winnicott
- B. Michael Balint
- C. Margaret Mahler
- D. Melanie Klein
- E. None of the above

32. Which of the following should raise suspicions of child abuse?
- A. Bucket-handle fractures
- B. Inflammatory hair loss
- C. Bilateral black eyes
- D. Retinal hemorrhages
- E. All of the above

33. What percentage of intracranial injuries found in children in the first year of life are due to physical abuse?

    A. <10%

    B. <50%

    C. <60%

    D. >50%

    E. >90%.

34. Which of the following features should raise the suspicion of sexual abuse in children?

    A. Anal dilatation with loss of rectal tone

    B. Incidence of sexually transmitted diseases

    C. Flattened rectal rugae

    D. Inappropriate sexual behavior by children

    E. All of the above

35. Which is the only SSRI authorized by the FDA for the treatment of depression in children?

    A. Fluvoxamine

    B. Fluoxetine

    C. Paroxetine

    D. Sertraline

    E. Escitalopram

36. Which of the following is true regarding obsessive-compulsive disorder in children?

    A. Functional imaging studies show increased glucose metabolism in the orbital frontal and prefrontal cortex, right caudate nucleus, and anterior cingulated gyrus.

    B. There is an increased incidence of neurological signs in children with OCD.

    C. Lifetime prevalence of OCD in children is 2–4%.

    D. Encephalitis, head trauma, and epilepsy can lead to the development of OCD.

    E. All of the above

37. Which of the following presentations is common in patients with pediatric autoimmune neuropsychiatry disorder associated with streptococcal infection?

    A. Depression

    B. Hallucinations

    C. Apathy

    D. Alexithymia

    E. OCD

38. Which of the following is *not* true regarding pervasive developmental disorder (PDD)?

    A. There is a higher incidence in males.

    B. The prevalence of PDD is 4–5 per 10,000.

    C. Persons with PDD fail to develop peer relationships.

    D. Naltrexone helps in improving social interactions.

    E. Persons with PDD exhibit stereotyped and repetitive motor patterns.

39. Which of the following antidepressants has been most implicated with increased rate of suicide in children and adolescents?

    A. Sertraline

    B. Citalopram

    C. Venlafaxine

    D. Fluvoxamine

    E. None of the above

40. Which of the following is true regarding suicide in children?

    A. Suicide is the fourth leading cause of death in children.

    B. Suicide is the third leading cause of death in adolescents.

    C. Less than 25% of the adolescents had expressed suicidal thoughts before committing suicide.

    D. Hanging is the most commonly used method of completed suicides in children.

    E. Adolescent females are more likely to commit suicide by jumping from a high place or taking an overdose of medications.

41. Which of the following is considered a cause in the etiology of reactive attachment disorder in children?
- A. Total disregard for the child's emotional needs
- B. Total disregard for the child's basic physical needs
- C. Inconsistent caregivers
- D. Mental retardation in parents
- E. All of the above

42. Which of the following modalities can be used in the treatment of encopresis?
- A. An educational approach
- B. Investigating for a medical cause of encopresis
- C. Daily timed intervals on the toilet
- D. Psychotherapy in children with concomitant behavioral problems
- E. All of the above

43. Which of the following is true regarding pica?
- A. It entails persistent eating of nonnutritional substances.
- B. The name was introduced by the French physician Ambroise Pare.
- C. The behavior is not culturally appropriate.
- D. Economic deprivation, poor parental support, and disorganized family situations can lead to the development of pica.
- E. All of the above

44. Which of the following is *not* true regarding rumination disorder?
- A. It is characterized by repeated regurgitation and rechewing of food.
- B. Symptoms last at least 3 months.
- C. The disorder is most common in the first year of life.
- D. A disturbed caregiver-infant relationship can lead to the development of rumination disorder.
- E. None of the above

45. What percentage of children diagnosed with conduct disorder go on to develop antisocial personality disorder?
- A. 80%
- B. 50%
- C. 5%
- D. 40%
- E. 25%

46. Which of the following is a feature of residual attention-deficit hyperactivity disorder in adults?

  A. Short temper associated with explosive outbursts
  B. Affective lability
  C. Drug and alcohol use
  D. Marital instability
  E. All of the above

47. What is the mechanism of action of atomoxetine (Strattera)?

  A. Serotonin reuptake inhibition
  B. Norepinephrine reuptake inhibition
  C. Dopamine reuptake inhibition
  D. Increased release of norepinephrine
  E. Increased release of dopamine

48. Which of the following is true regarding ADHD in children?

  A. ADHD is more prevalent in girls.
  B. The symptoms should persist for at least 3 months for a diagnosis of ADHD.
  C. Depression is the most common comorbid condition associated with ADHD.
  D. Oppositional defiant disorder and conduct disorder are the most common comorbid conditions associated with ADHD.
  E. Low-dose atypical antipsychotic medications are the treatment of choice for ADHD.

49. Which of the following is true regarding nightmares?

  A. Patient awakens with detailed recall of frightening dreams.
  B. After awakening, the patient rapidly becomes oriented and alert.
  C. Nightmares occur during REM.
  D. All of the above

50. Which of the following is *not* true regarding Hallervorden-Spatz syndrome?

  A. Onset is usually in childhood or early adolescence.
  B. The disease is transmitted in an autosomal recessive fashion.
  C. CT scan shows increased density in the globus pallidus, indicating iron deposition.
  D. Dystonia is a late feature.
  E. The patient shows choreoathetoid movement.

ANSWERS

1. **Answer: D.** Sleep terror is characterized by repeated episodes of sleep disturbances, manifested mainly as repeated awakening from sleep with a terrified cry. These episodes usually occur in the first third of sleep during NREM sleep and each lasts for approximately 1–10 minutes. Upon awakening, the child is unresponsive and thereafter is confused and disoriented. The child usually is not able to remember the content of the dream in detail.

2. **Answer: C.** The characteristic feature of Rett syndrome is the development of numerous deficits after an initial period of normal functioning following birth. The child has a deceleration of head growth between the ages of 5 and 48 months. The child shows a loss of previously acquired hand skills and subsequently develops stereotyped hand movements like hand wringing. The child also develops deficits in expressive and receptive language.

3. **Answer: D.** The onset of schizophrenia is most common from 17 to 27 years of age in males and in the late 20s to early 30s in females. The incidence of childhood-onset schizophrenia is very low, less than 1%. Four percent of cases occur before 15 years of age.

4. **Answer: B.** Anaclitic depression occurs primarily in infants (6–30 months) who have lost or been separated from their mothers or primary caretakers. The condition was described by Rene Spitz.

5. **Answer: D.** Encopresis is characterized by repeated passage of feces in inappropriate places. This can be both voluntary and involuntary. According to DSM-IV this should occur at least once a month for at least 3 months. The child should be at least 4 years of age. Prevalence is about 1% in 5-year-olds and decreases with increasing age.

6. **Answer: D.** Enuresis is characterized by repeated voiding of urine during the day or at night into bed or clothes. Most of the time it is involuntary, but sometimes it can be intentional. For a diagnosis according to DSM-IV, the voiding of urine should occur at least twice per week for at least 3 months. The chronologic age of the child should be at least 5 years.

7. **Answer: D.** Any medical causes that can lead to enuresis should be eliminated. It should also be determined whether the enuresis is a direct physiologic consequence of any medication such as laxatives. It should be explained to the child and parents that this is a common condition and the child is not to be blamed. In addition to the bell and pad conditioning method, imipramine and desmopressin have been found useful in treatment.

8. Answer: D. Children with depression show a decrease growth hormone secretion when challenged by the following medications: levodopa, clonidine, and desmethylimipramine.

9. Answer: E. Kleine-Levin syndrome is characterized by hypersomnia and hyperphagia, sexual disinhibition, and sometimes psychosis. It has a 3:1 male preponderance. The onset of symptoms usually occurs in adolescence. It is hypothesized that symptoms are related to hypothalamic dysfunction.

10. Answer: B. Childhood disintegrative disorder, known as Heller syndrome, is characterized by a clinically significant loss in previously acquired skills in at least two of the following areas: expressive or receptive language, social skills, bowel or bladder control, play, and motor skills. For a diagnosis according to DSM-IV, the child should have had normal development for at least the first 2 years of life.

11. Answer: C. Asperger syndrome is characterized by significant deficits in social skills, preoccupation with one or more interests, and a lack of significant impairment in language and cognitive function.

12. Answer: B. Pimozide, clonidine, and naltrexone can be used in the treatment of tics. But pemoline is a stimulant that is used in the treatment of ADHD and can exacerbate tics.

13. Answer: C. Wellbutrin, which works by the reuptake inhibition of dopamine, can lead to an exacerbation of tics.

14. Answer: C. Tricyclic antidepressants have been used for the treatment of depression and occasionally ADHD. Among the tricyclic antidepressants, it is desmopressin that has been associated with mortality in children.

15. Answer: D. Tourette syndrome is characterized by multiple motor tics and a few vocal tics. The onset of the disease is usually before 18 years of age, with the average age of onset being around 7 years. This is more common in males. For a diagnosis according to DSM-IV, the tics should have been present for at least 1 year and there should not have been a tic-free period of more than 3 months during that year.

16. Answer: C. Wechsler Preschool and Primary Scale of Intelligence–Revised can be used to measure intelligence in children aged 3–7 years. Bayley Scales of Infant Development can be used in the age group 1–42 months. Stanford-Binet Intelligence Test, 4th edition, can be used in the age range from 2.5 years to adult. Wechsler Intelligence Scale for Children-III can be used in the age range 6–16 years.

17. **Answer: C.** Guanfacine is a presynaptic alpha-2 adrenergic receptor agonist that leads to decreased release of norepinephrine. It has been used in the treatment of ADHD and is less sedating and has a longer half-life than clonidine.

18. **Answer: C.** Pemoline belongs to the class of stimulants and has been used in the treatment of ADHD.

19. **Answer: B.** This patient has Wilson's disease, which is an autosomal recessive disorder of copper metabolism, which can present with movement disorder, personality changes, and psychosis. It usually presents in the first through third decades of life. The genetic defect, which is localized to chromosome 13, leads to a defect in copper-transporting adenosine triphosphatase in the liver, which in turn leads to accumulation of copper in the liver, brain, cornea, and kidney.

20. **Answer: E.** There is no pathognomonic sign of lead toxicity. Children exposed to toxic levels of lead for prolonged periods develop the following features: irritability, sleeplessness, lethargy, poor appetite, headaches, abdominal pain, vomiting, and constipation. In children exposure to toxic levels of lead can also lead to seizure, intellectual impairment, and decreased heme production.

21. **Answer: D.** Children don't develop the concept of permanence of death until around 4 or 5 years of age.

22. **Answer: D.** Landau-Kleffner syndrome (LKS) is a rare form of childhood epilepsy that results in a severe language disorder. The cause of the condition is unknown. All children with LKS have abnormal electrical activity in one and sometimes both temporal lobes, the area of the brain responsible for processing language. This epileptiform activity shows up on an EEG, particularly when the child is asleep. About two-thirds of children with LKS have seizures. Expressive language (the ability to speak) is often seriously affected; some children lose their speech completely. Behavioral problems are common, especially hyperactivity, poor attention, depression, and irritability.

23. **Answer: A.** The phenomenon of the decreasing age of incidence of the disease with each successive generation is known as anticipation. This phenomenon is seen in fragile X syndrome and Huntington's disease.

24. **Answer: E.** School phobia mostly occurs when the child starts going to a school. It can occur as a result of separation anxiety of the child and also as a result of the separation anxiety on the part of the parent. It can be due to a legitimate cause such as a very strict teacher or bullying by other students.

25. Answer: E. Stella Chess and Alexander Thomas in their New York longitudinal study found that temperamental traits could be identified from infancy. The nine traits identified by Chess and Thomas are activity level, distractibility, adaptability, attention span, intensity, threshold of responsiveness, quality of mood, rhythmicity, and approach/withdrawal. They postulated that temperament has a genetic base and these traits could also be altered by environmental factors.

26. Answer: D. Gender identity is the child's perception of self as male or female. For majority of children, formation of gender identity starts at the age of 3–4 and is complete by 5–7. Gender identity occurs earlier in girls. Homosexual play in early adulthood is not indicative of adult sexual orientation.

27. Answer: A. Leo Kanner first described features of autism. Anne Benham developed the scale for Infant and Toddler Mental Status Exam. Chess and Thomas described the nine temperamental traits. It was Hans Asperger who first described the Asperger syndrome.

28. Answer: D. Lesch-Nyhan syndrome is caused by a deficiency of hypoxanthine-guanine phosphoribosyl transferase (HPRT). It is genetic in origin, with the pathology located at Xq26–27. It leads to an accumulation of uric acid. Patients show self-mutilating behavior like biting or chewing on their bodies.

29. Answer: E. Tuberous sclerosis is a neurocutaneous syndrome characterized by hamartomas in the brain, kidney, heart, and skin. The hamartomas in the brain are seen as subepindymal calcified nodule on CT and MRI. Persons with tuberous sclerosis also have mental retardation, show features of aggression and impulsivity, and develop seizures. This is inherited as an autosomal dominant disorder.

30. Answer: E. According to DSM-IV, the pattern of negativistic, hostile, and defiant behavior should last for at least 6 months. Children with ODD often lose their temper, argue with adults, actively defy or refuse to comply with adults' rules, deliberately annoy people, and are often angry and spiteful.

31. Answer: A. Donald Winnicott described the concept of a "holding environment," the psychic space created by the mother between herself and the infant that makes it possible for the child to develop his or her awareness as a separate person. Margaret Mahler described the evolution of object relations and described the concept of separation and individuation. Melanie Klein developed a theory of internal object relations and used "play therapy" to learn about the internal fantasies of children. Klein also described the paranoid-schizoid position and depressive position. Balint described the concept of "basic fault" in the development of child.

32. Answer: E. Physical abuse of a child is something for which psychiatrists should have a low threshold of suspicion. Impressions of the human hand on the skin, old and new bruises, immersion burns, intracranial injuries, bilateral black eye, inflammatory hair loss, subgaleal hematomas, and bucket-handle or corner fractures are some of the features that should raise the suspicion of physical abuse if seen in children.

33. Answer: E. Ninety-five percent or more of the intracranial injuries seen in children younger than 1 year are due to physical abuse. Physical abuse can include violent shaking or slamming. This can lead to subdural bleeding. It can also lead to retinal hemorrhage.

34. Answer: E. The following physical findings should raise suspicions of sexual abuse: labial and perineal tears, anal dilatation with loss of rectal tone, flattened rectal rugae, and occurrence of sexually transmitted diseases. Age-inappropriate sexual behavior is also indicative of sexual abuse.

35. Answer: B. Although all SSRIs are used in the treatment of depression in children, only fluoxetine has FDA authorization. Paroxetine and venlafaxine have been found to cause increased agitation in children and therefore contribute to increased suicidal thoughts and attempts.

36. Answer: E. Childhood OCD has a prevalence of 2–4%. Onset of OCD can follow encephalitis, head trauma, and epilepsy, which supports a neurobiological etiology of OCD. PET studies show increased glucose metabolism in the orbitofrontal region of the brain, prefrontal cortex, caudate nucleus, and anterior cingulated gyrus. Children with OCD have a higher incidence of neurological soft signs.

37. Answer: E. Pediatric autoimmune neuropsychiatric disorder associated with streptococcal infection is characterized by the presence of OCD and tics. It develops as a sequela to group A-beta hemolytic streptococcal infection.

38. Answer: E. Pervasive developmental disorder is characterized by delay and deviation in social and communication skills. PDD has a prevalence of 4–5 per 10,000 births. PDD is more prevalent among boys. Naltrexone helps in reducing the hyperactivity and inattention associated with PDD but does not have any effect on social interactions.

39. Answer: E. Paroxetine has been implicated in an increased incidence of suicide rates in children and adolescents. Some countries have issued warnings regarding the use of paroxetine in that age group. Recently venlafaxine was also barred from use in children. On September 17, 2004, an FDA panel voted to advise the agency to require a "black box" warning to highlight the potential risk to depressed pediatric patients. The safety concerns applied to Prozac, Paxil, Wellbutrin, Zoloft, Celexa, Effescor, Luvox, Remeron, and Serzone.

40. Answer: C. Suicide is the fourth leading cause of death in children and the third leading cause in adolescents. Hanging is the most commonly used method in younger children, while hanging and firearms are used with equal frequency in adolescents. More than 65% of the adolescents who complete suicide had expressed suicidal thoughts beforehand.

41. Answer: E. Reactive attachment disorder (RAD) is described by DSM-IV as "markedly disturbed and developmentally inappropriate social relatedness in most contexts." RAD begins before the age of 5 years and is typified by deviant social characteristics like being excessively inhibited, hypervigilant, or ambivalent. The disorder can be precipitated by abuse as well as neglect. Lack of a consistent caregiver, mental retardation, and poor parenting skills can lead to the development of RAD.

42. Answer: E. The first approach in treating encopresis is education. The parents (or other caregiver) and the child should both be educated about the nature of the condition, and it should be stressed to both the child and parents that the condition is not the child's or parents' fault. The child should be investigated for possible medical causes of the encopresis. Daily timed intervals at the toilet are an effective method of treatment. Pharmacotherapy is not very well studied, nor has it been found effective. Behavioral management is still the mainstay of treatment.

43. Answer: E. Pica is characterized by the persistent eating of nonnutritious substances. Economic deprivation, poor parental support, and disorganized family situations can lead to the development of pica. Among the substances ingested by children with this condition are dirt, paint, hair, sand pebbles, uncooked rice, and paper. Ingesting these substances can lead to infections as well as intestinal obstructions. The treatment is mainly behavioral and includes physical restraints, aversive behavioral therapy, and time-outs.

44. Answer: B. Rumination disorder is characterized by repeated regurgitation and rechewing of the regurgitated food. For a diagnosis according to DSM-IV, the disorder should be present for 1 month.

45. Answer: D. Approximately 40% of children diagnosed with conduct disorder will go on to have a diagnosis of antisocial personality disorder in adulthood. There is not much evidence that conduct disorder is treatable.

46. Answer: E. ADHD can persist into adulthood. There is not much data on the prevalence of ADHD in adults, but it is estimated that ADHD traits persist in 10–50% of adults who had ADHD as children. The characteristics of adult ADHD are motor hyperactivity, attention deficits, affective lability, short temper, explosive outbursts, loss of control, emotional overreactivity, disorganized behavior, inability to complete tasks, impulsivity, marital instability, and alcohol and drug use.

47. **Answer: B.** Atomoxetine works by inhibiting the reuptake of norepinephrine. It is used for treatment of ADHD. It should not be taken along with an MAOI or within 2 weeks of stopping an MAOI. Growth should be monitored during treatment with atomoxetine.

48. **Answer: D.** ADHD is more prevalent among boys. The symptoms must be present for at least 6 months to meet the criteria for a diagnosis of ADHD according to DSM-IV. ODD and conduct disorder are the most common co-morbid conditions associated with ADHD. The treatment of choice for ADHD in children is behavioral management along with a stimulant like methylphenidate, dexamphetamine, or pemoline. More recently approved by the FDA is treatment with the nonstimulant medication atomoxetine, a selective norepinephrine reuptake inhibitor. Alpha-2 agonists like clonidine and guanfacine.

49. **Answer: D.** Nightmares are frightening dreams that occur during REM sleep. The child having a nightmare awakens from the dream frightened. The child remembers the content of the dream unlike in night terror. Ten to fifty percent of children in the age range 3–6 years have occasional nightmares. The child rapidly becomes oriented and alert after waking up from sleep.

50. **Answer: D.** Hallervorden-Spatz disease is a hereditary disease with genetic pathology located at chromosome 20 p. The onset of the disease is usually in childhood or early adolescence. Initial features include dystonia, rigidity, difficulty with gait and speech. Seizures and retinitis pigmentosa are also seen. A CT scan of the brain shows iron deposition in the brain, especially in the globus pallidus.

Chapter 7

CONSULTATION LIAISON PSYCHIATRY

QUESTIONS

1. What is the most common cause of hyperthyroidism?
   A. Hashimoto's thyroiditis
   B. Grave's disease
   C. Administration of exogenous thyroid
   D. TSH-secreting pituitary adenoma
   E. Hydatidiform mole

2. Which of the following is not the role of the psychiatry liaison consultant?
   A. Comprehensive assessment of the patient
   B. Accurate note keeping
   C. Detailed psychodynamic formulation
   D. Documentation of plans for follow-up

3. Which of the following is true regarding mental disorders in patients with epilepsy?
   A. Ictal psychosis is more common than interictal psychosis.
   B. Violence is common during a seizure.
   C. Rates of attempted suicide are increased in people with epilepsy.
   D. Mood symptoms are more common than schizophrenia-like symptoms.

4. In which of the following regions of the brain is a tumor most likely to cause psychiatric symptoms?
   A. Frontal
   B. Parietal
   C. Temporal
   D. Occipital

5. What is the most common reason for psychiatric consultation in rehabilitation medicine?

    A. Anxiety

    B. Pain

    C. Depression

    D. Psychosis

6. What is the most common psychiatric manifestation of Cushing syndrome?

    A. Mania

    B. Psychosis

    C. Depression

    D. Panic attacks

    E. Anxiety

7. With which of the following is exogenous administration of steroids most commonly associated?

    A. Mania

    B. Psychosis

    C. Depression

    D. Panic attacks

    E. Anxiety

8. What is the most common psychiatric condition seen in patients with hyperparathyroidism?

    A. Mania

    B. Depression

    C. Psychosis

    D. Anxiety

    E. Panic attacks

9. Which of the following is *not* true regarding diabetes mellitus?

    A. Dementia is less common.

    B. There is a negative correlation between depression and good diabetic control.

    C. In ketoacidotic coma, the level of consciousness correlates with plasma osmolality.

    D. MAOIs potentiate the effect of oral hypoglycemic drugs.

10. Which of the following is not a psychiatric manifestation of hyperthyroidism?

   A. Depression
   B. Anxiety
   C. Schizophrenia-like symptoms
   D. Opiate dependence
   E. Cognitive impairment

11. All of the following are associated with psychiatric illness with steroid treatment *except*

   A. Male sex
   B. Higher dose
   C. Longer duration of therapy
   D. Previous psychiatric illness
   E. Depressed mood

12. Which of the following is true regarding SSRIs used in treatment of premenstrual dysphoric disorder?

   A. They cannot be combined with hormonal treatments.
   B. They are poorly tolerated.
   C. They inhibit ovulation.
   D. They can be used exclusively in the luteal phase.
   E. They have few side effects.

13. Which of the following is true regarding pituitary disease?

   A. There is an increased rate of mania in hypopituitarism.
   B. Libido is increased in acromegaly.
   C. Psychosis is common in acromegaly.
   D. Increased energy and activity are seen in hypopituitarism.
   E. Symptoms of hypopituitarism fully resolve with treatment.

14. All of the following are associated with vitamin B12 deficiency *except*

   A. Macrocytic anemia
   B. Depression
   C. Polyneuropathy
   D. Dementia
   E. Memory impairment

15. All of the following are symptoms of Wilson's disease *except*
   A. Cognitive impairment
   B. Visual symptoms
   C. Epilepsy
   D. Changes in personality
   E. Rigidity and dystonia

16. All of the following are symptoms of premenstrual dysphoric disorder *except*
   A. Pelvic discomfort
   B. Irritability
   C. Occurrence of the disorder soon after menstruation
   D. Carbohydrate craving
   E. Occurrence of the disorder for 2 consecutive months

17. Which of the following is true about premenstrual dysphoric disorder?
   A. It is seen in 10% to 20% of women.
   B. It indicates abnormal ovarian function.
   C. Symptoms are more severe in a middle-aged woman.
   D. It is linked to abnormal central serotonergic function.
   E. It is not associated with sexual abuse.

18. All of the following are true of porphyria *except*
   A. Peripheral neuropathy may be seen.
   B. Elevated ceruloplasmin is seen.
   C. Benzodiazepines may be used.
   D. Symptoms may resemble schizophrenia.
   E. Acute intermittent porphyria is the most common form.

19. Which of the following inborn errors of metabolism can *not* be treated by diet?
   A. Homocystinuria
   B. Lesch-Nyhan syndrome
   C. Phenylketonuria
   D. Galactosemia

20. Which of the following is true about prion diseases?
   A. It is more common in men.
   B. Patients usually have a normal EEG.
   C. There is a reduced risk with E4 apolipoprotein allele.
   D. It is encoded on chromosome 10.
   E. The familial form is autosomal recessive.

21. Which of the following is *not* true regarding affective disorder in patients on renal dialysis?
   A. Adjustment disorder can lead to behavioral problems.
   B. Major depression is the most common psychiatric diagnosis.
   C. Adjustment disorders can influence physical outcome.
   D. Adjustment disorders may become chronic.
   E. Lack of energy and insomnia are less indicative of depression than in patients who are not on dialysis.

22. Which of the following is not true regarding cognitive therapy in liaison settings?
   A. It teaches techniques to deal with future problems.
   B. It can modify negative automatic thoughts about physical illness.
   C. It helps patients regain control of their illness.
   D. It is supported by evidence in liaison settings.
   E. It is directed by therapists' perception of the patient's problems.

23. Which of the following is true regarding denial in patients on renal dialysis?
   A. It is rarely present.
   B. It may cause problems with compliance.
   C. It is always pathological.
   D. If denial is low, less mood dysfunction occurs.
   E. High denial results in rapid readjustment.

24. Which of the following is not useful in diagnosing depression in the patient on a medical inpatient unit?
   A. Hopelessness
   B. Morning depression
   C. Depressed mood
   D. Sleep disturbance
   E. Suicidal thoughts

25. Which of the following is true about the treatment of depression in diabetes mellitus?

    A. Fluoxetine is the preferred drug.

    B. Tricyclic antidepressants can cause hypoglycemic episodes.

    C. Tricyclic antidepressants should be avoided even in well-controlled diabetes mellitus.

    D. Sodium valproate can give false-positive urine tests for glucose.

    E. Amitriptyline is contraindicated in diabetic neuropathy.

26. Which of the following is true regarding the treatment of depression in hepatic disease?

    A. Tricyclic antidepressants are safe in the presence of liver disease.

    B. Lithium is the mood stabilizer of choice in the presence of liver disease.

    C. SSRIs are contraindicated in liver disease.

    D. MAOIs are safe in hepatitis B.

    E. Half-lives of drugs are reduced in liver disease.

27. Which of the following is true regarding delirium?

    A. It rarely involves mood symptoms.

    B. It includes a narrow range of psychiatric symptoms.

    C. Clouding of consciousness is sufficient for the diagnosis.

    D. Attention disturbance is the core cognitive disturbance.

    E. Sleep–wake cycle is preserved.

28. Which of the following is true of hypoactive delirium?

    A. Psychotic symptoms are rare.

    B. It responds poorly to antipsychotics.

    C. It is frequently missed in practice.

    D. It has a better prognosis than agitated delirium.

    E. Patient is commonly unarousable.

29. Which of the following is true regarding the management of delirium?

    A. Iatrogenic causes are rare.

    B. Involvement of the patient in management should be discouraged.

    C. Antipsychotics are effective due to their sedative actions.

    D. Reduction of risk factors can prevent further episodes.

30. Wernicke's syndrome can cause all of the following *except*

   A. Ataxia

   B. Diplopia

   C. Peripheral neuropathy

   D. Dysphasia

   E. Confusion

31. Which of the following is true of Korsakoff syndrome?

   A. It can be caused by continuous vomiting.

   B. Confabulation is always present.

   C. Disorientation is usually present.

   D. Clouding of consciousness is characteristic.

   E. Immediate memory is affected.

32. HIV can manifest as all of the following *except*

   A. Hypomania

   B. Alzheimer's dementia

   C. Depression

   D. Transient panic attacks

   E. Schizophreniform psychosis

33. Which of the following is true concerning AIDS encephalitis?

   A. The EEG is normal in the early stages.

   B. Frank dysphoria is common.

   C. Insight is preserved until late.

   D. Memory is usually preserved.

   E. Treatment does not alter course of disease.

34. Which of the following is true about suicide in medically ill patients?

   A. Most terminally ill patients develop a psychiatric disorder.

   B. Most terminally ill patients are at risk of suicide.

   C. Anger is an important factor in suicide.

   D. Mental illness is not common in patients who commit suicide.

35. What is the risk of completed suicide in a person who has made a previous suicide attempt?

    A. 2 times

    B. 25 times

    C. 50 times

    D. 100 times

36. All of the following are exceptions to confidentiality between psychiatrist and the patient *except*

    A. Child abuse

    B. Danger to self or others

    C. Intent to commit a crime

    D. Communication with other physicians not involved in the care of the patient

    E. Competency procedures

37. Which of the following is true regarding competency?

    A. Most depressed patients are mentally incompetent.

    B. Cognitively impaired patients do not have the capacity to make decisions.

    C. Competency is a clinical determination.

    D. Capacity and competency are the same.

    E. Capacity to consent is specific to the issue and the situation.

38. Which of the following is true regarding advance directives?

    A. Advance directives are a means for people to indicate their wishes and decisions about future healthcare in the event of their incompetency.

    B. Power of attorney is valid even if the person becomes incompetent.

    C. Durable power of attorney empowers an agent to make only business decisions on behalf of the patient.

    D. The determination of a patient's competence is specified in a durable power of attorney and healthcare proxy statutes.

39. The use of seclusion and restraint is contraindicated for all of the following *except*

    A. To prevent harm to the patient or others

    B. To assist the staff during staff shortages

    C. To assist in treatment

    D. To prevent significant disruption to a treatment program

    E. To decrease sensory stimulation

40. Which of the following is characteristic of depression associated with medical illness?

    A. Earlier age of onset

    B. Increased rate of family history of depression

    C. Decreased rate of alcoholism in family members

    D. Greater likelihood of suicide

    E. Poor response to ECT

41. Which of the following is true regarding psychiatric illness in cancer patients?

    A. Twenty-five percent of patients with cancer develop a psychiatric illness.

    B. Depression is the most common psychiatric diagnosis.

    C. Suicide is rare among patients with cancer.

    D. Patients with pancreatic cancer are at highest risk of suicide.

42. Which of the following is the most common course of mania in patients with cancer?

    A. Bipolar I disorder

    B. Cerebral metastasis

    C. Diencephalic tumors

    D. Corticosteroid use

    E. Bipolar II disorder

43. Depression following stroke is associated with lesion in which of the following regions of the brain?

    A. Left occipital

    B. Left temporal

    C. Left frontal

    D. Right parietal

    E. Right frontal

44. Which type of dementia is typically seen in patients with HIV?

    A. Alzheimer's dementia

    B. Subcortical dementia

    C. Lewy body dementia

    D. Infectious dementia

    E. Vascular dementia

45. What is the most common neuropsychiatric complication in hospitalized patients with AIDS?

    A. Depression

    B. Dementia

    C. Psychosis

    D. Mania

    E. Delirium

46. Which of the following is commonly seen in AIDS dementia complex?

    A. Psychosis

    B. Aphasia

    C. Agnosia

    D. Word-finding difficulties

47. Which of the following is associated with high HIV risk behaviors?

    A. Marijuana

    B. Alcohol

    C. LSD

    D. Crack cocaine

48. What proportion of people with chronic pain also have an axis I psychiatric disorder?

    A. 5%

    B. 10%

    C. 25%

    D. 50%

    E. 75%

49. Which of the following is true about ECT?

    A. It can be administered to patients with epilepsy.

    B. It is contraindicated in patients with Parkinson's disease.

    C. Seizures are the most common cause of death in patients given ECT.

    D. The use of bilateral electrodes reduces the risk of cognitive deficits.

    E. ECT should be used after medication failure in catatonia.

50. What is the most commonly used neuroleptic agent in the intensive care
unit?

    A. Risperidone

    B. Haloperidol

    C. Olanzapine

    D. Chlorpromazine

ANSWERS

1. **Answer: B.** Hyperthyroidism is the condition resulting from the effect of excessive amounts of thyroid hormone on body tissues. Grave's disease is the most common cause of hyperthyroidism. Hashimoto's thyroiditis causes hypothyroidism. Excess ingestion of thyroid hormone is relatively common when patients are given higher doses than that necessary to maintain a euthyroid state. TSH-secreting pituitary adenoma is very rare.

2. **Answer: C.** A detailed psychodynamic formulation is not appropriate in the consultation liaison setting. Suggestions about managing troublesome and disruptive behaviors are helpful.

3. **Answer: C.** Interictal psychotic states are more common than ictal psychosis. An estimated 10–30% of all patients with complex partial epilepsy have psychotic symptoms. Risk factors are female gender, lefthandedness, onset of seizures during puberty, and a left-sided lesion. Mood symptoms like depression and mania are seen less often than schizophrenia-like symptoms. There is an increased incidence of attempted suicide in patients with epilepsy.

4. **Answer: A.** Approximately 50% of patients with brain tumors experience psychiatric symptoms. In approximately 80%, the tumors are located in the frontal or limbic region. Meningiomas are likely to cause focal symptoms by compressing a limited region of the cortex, whereas gliomas are likely to cause diffuse symptoms.

5. **Answer: C.** Depression is the most frequent reason for psychiatric consultation in rehabilitation medicine. It is associated with longer duration of inpatient rehabilitation, deficient self-care, and delay in resumption of premorbid social activities.

6. **Answer: C.** The most common psychiatric manifestation of Cushing syndrome is depression. Cushing syndrome refers to a diverse symptom complex due to excess steroid hormone production by the adrenal cortex or sustained administration of glucocorticoids. The depressive symptoms are moderate to severe in 50% of patients. Many patients also experience psychotic features. In patients who demonstrate depression, it may be necessary to institute therapy for the depression itself while awaiting the eventual resolution of the manifestation of Cushing syndrome.

7. **Answer: A.** Exogenous administration of steroids is most commonly associated with mania. It can also cause psychosis, depression, panic attacks, or anxiety.

8. Answer: B. Depression is common in patients with hypercalcemia. The severity of symptoms intensifies as the level of hypercalcemia increases. Delirium, psychosis, and cognitive impairment are more commonly seen in patients who have calcium levels more than 50 mg per dl. Depressive symptoms, but not cognitive symptoms, tend to resolve with treatment. Cognitive symptoms may improve; however, residual symptoms may remain.

9. Answer: A. Dementia is more common in persons with diabetes mellitus. There is a negative correlation between emotional symptoms and diabetic control. Patients exhibiting persistent psychiatric symptoms who receive psychiatric intervention may have less disease morbidity. Between one-third and two-third of patients with diabetes mellitus have some kind of psychiatric disorder, ranging from anxiety and depression to substance abuse.

10. Answer: D. Hyperthyroidism is associated with a variety of psychiatric manifestations including anxiety, depression, psychosis, and cognitive impairment. More than 90% of patients presenting with depression and anxiety who do not have a preexisting psychiatric condition will experience resolution of the symptoms during the course of treatment for hyperthyroidism. Opiate dependence is not known to be associated with hyperthyroidism.

11. Answer: A. Psychiatric illness with steroid use is associated with female sex, high doses of steroids, longer duration of treatment, previous history of psychiatric illness, and depressed mood.

12. Answer: D. Most serotonin-enhancing antidepressants have been shown to be effective in the treatment of premenstrual dysphoric disorder in comparison with placebo. Some SSRIs given in the latter half of the cycle can be as effective as continuous daily doses. In the case of citalopram, half-cycle dosing was found to be better than daily dosing. It has been postulated that some woman may have reduced serotonergic activity across the menstrual cycle as a trait, and during the luteal phase, further abnormalities of serotonergic function may occur. The beneficial effects of SSRIs on dysphoric symptoms are evident soon after initiation of treatment. They are generally well tolerated and do not interfere with ovulation.

13. Answer: E. Symptoms of hypopituitarism generally fully resolve with treatment. There is an increased rate of lethargy and depression in hypopituitarism. Libido is reduced in acromegaly, and psychosis is not common.

14. Answer: B. Vitamin B12 deficiency can cause macrocytosis, polyneuropathy, dementia, and memory impairment. Its association with depression is not established.

15. Answer: B. Wilson's disease is a rare autosomal recessive disorder that occurs between the first and third decades of life. It is characterized by the excess deposition of copper in the liver and brain. It tends to present as liver disease in adolescence and neuropsychiatric disease in young adults. The neurologic manifestations are related to basal ganglia dysfunction and include resting, postural, or kinetic tremor; rigidity; and dystonia of the bulbar musculature with dysarthria and dysphagia. Psychiatric features include behavioral and personality changes and emotional lability. The pathognomonic sign is the brownish Kayser-Fleischer ring in the cornea.

16. Answer: C. The essential features required for a diagnosis of premenstrual dysphoric disorder (PMDD) are symptoms of marked and persistent anger or irritability, depressed mood, anxiety, and affective lability that have occurred regularly during the last week of luteal phase in most menstrual cycles during the last year. Premenstrual dysphoric disorder diagnosis requires that symptoms be present for a minimum of 2 consecutive months. PMDD must also be differentiated from premenstrual exacerbation or magnification of other conditions.

17. Answer: D. A number of studies have consistently demonstrated an important role for serotonin in the pathophysiology of PMDD. Patients have lower whole-blood serotonin levels and lower platelet serotonin uptake during the premenstrual phase. Estimates of prevalence vary with severe symptoms reported in 4–7% of women. The presence of PMDD does not indicate abnormal ovarian function, and women with PMDD show no consistent differences in basal levels of ovarian hormones. Younger age has been associated with more severe symptoms. It is also associated with low levels of education. Past sexual abuse is reported by a significant proportion of women seeking treatment for PMDD.

18. Answer: B. Acute intermittent porphyria is the most common form of porphyria. It is an autosomal dominant condition. Clinical illness usually develops in women. Many drugs may precipitate attacks including alcohol, barbiturates, carbamazepine, tricyclic antidepressants, phenytoin, and valproic acid. Patients present with abdominal pain, autonomic and peripheral neuropathy, seizures, psychosis, and abnormalities of the basal ganglia. Benzodiazepines are generally considered to be safe for use in porphyria.

19. Answer: B. Lesch-Nyhan syndrome is an X-linked recessive condition that affects boys exclusively. Infants with Lesch-Nyhan syndrome develop attacks of hypertonia within a few weeks of birth. They also develop spasticity with ataxia and choreoathetosis. Most children have severe mental retardation and become wheelchair bound. They also show verbal and physical aggression and self-injurious behavior. The condition is not treated by dietary control. Treatment by dietary modification is a part of the treatment for homocystinuria, phenylketonuria, and galactosemia.

20. Answer: A. Prion diseases are called subacute spongiform encephalopathies. They are associated with the accumulation in the brain of abnormal partially protease-resistant glycoproteins known as prion proteins. The human prion diseases can be divided into inherited, sporadic, and acquired forms. CJD is a rapidly progressive multifocal dementia with myoclonus. Onset occurs between 45 and 75 years of age. The clinical progression is typically over weeks, progressing to akinetic mutism and death within 2 to 3 months. Patients with progressive dementia and two or more of the following signs in the setting of an EEG finding of pseudoperiodic sharp wave activity nearly always have CJD: myoclonus; cortical brightness; pyramidal, cerebellar, or extrapyramidal signs; or akinetic mutism. The familial form of prion disease, called Gerstmann-Sträussler-Scheinker syndrome, has an onset in the third and fourth decades of life and is characterized by cerebellar ataxia with pyramidal features and dementia. It is an autosomal dominant disorder.

21. Answer: B. The most common psychiatric diagnoses in patients on renal dialysis are adjustment disorders (30%), mood disorders (24%), and organic mental disorders. Symptoms useful in identifying major depressive disorders are low mood, reduced interest, feelings of worthlessness, excess guilt, anorexia, weight loss, and slow thoughts. Symptoms not useful in making a diagnosis are lack of energy, insomnia, and reduced libido, because these occur in end-stage renal disease. Behavioral problems such as self-neglect, social withdrawal, and noncompliance with treatment are common and can affect physical outcome.

22. Answer: D. Cognitive therapy can be used in the treatment of psychological problems related to physical illness. Patients' attitude about their illness is of considerable importance to the outcome. The less control patients perceive themselves as having in a situation, the more depressed they are likely to be. Therapy involves the patient and therapist understanding the patient's perception of problems. As well as assessing cognition, it is important to target physical symptoms and problems that can be assessed and baselines accorded to measure future change. Therapy should improve patients' sense of control over their physical state and educate them in techniques they can use to deal with problems in the future.

23. Answer: B. Denial is a defense mechanism often used by patients with end-stage illness. Some patients may use this more than others. Patients with low denial scores have been found to have greater interpersonal sensitivity and greater mood and sleep dysfunction than those with high denial scores. Automatic thoughts in patients with low denial tend to focus on their losses, leading to affective disturbance. Therefore, denial may be adaptive in complementing a patient's ability to break the cycle of automatic thoughts that may lead to affective problems, allowing gradual adjustment to occur.

24. Answer: D. Depression is more difficult to diagnose in patients with physical illness. Depressed mood, hopelessness, and morning depression have been shown to be effective as differentiating symptoms to distinguish depression from the effects of physical illness. Sleep disturbance, anorexia, lethargy, and psychomotor retardation may be due to physical illness.

25. Answer: D. SSRIs can reduce serum glucose by up to 30% and cause appetite suppression resulting in weight loss. Fluoxetine should be avoided owing to its increased potential for hypoglycemia. Tricyclic antidepressants can increase serum glucose levels, increase appetite, and decrease the metabolic rate. These are generally safe unless the diabetes mellitus is poorly controlled or is associated with significant cardiac or renal disease. Amitriptyline and imipramine can be used to treat painful diabetic neuropathy. Sodium valproate may give false-positive results on urine tests for glucose in patients with diabetes mellitus. Lithium can be used safely in patients without renal disease.

26. Answer: B. Antidepressants are predominantly metabolized in the liver and so have increased half-lives with reduced clearance. As the dose of drug toxicity increases with disease severity, lower starting and total doses of medications are recommended. Paroxetine prescribed at the lower end of the dose range is probably the safest option. The sedative and constipating side effect of tricyclic antidepressants may unmask or precipitate hepatic encephalopathy. MAOIs are hepatotoxic and may precipitate coma. As lithium undergoes minimal hepatic metabolism, it is the mood stabilizer of choice in liver disease.

27. Answer: D. Delirium is a constellation of physical, biological, and psychological disturbances. Impaired attention is considered the core cognitive disturbance. In addition, most patients experience disturbances of memory, orientation, language, mood, thinking, perception, motor behavior, and the sleep–wake cycle. Although individual delirium symptoms are nonspecific, their pattern is highly characteristic with acute onset, fluctuant course, and transient nature. Delirium is commonly seen in general hospital settings with a point prevalence of 10–30%. It is more frequent among older patients and those with preexisting cognitive impairment and medical or surgical problems.

28. Answer: C. Delirium is frequently missed in clinical practice. Cases of hypoactive delirium are more likely to be missed. Prognosis is poorer for hypoactive delirium than agitated delirium. Patients are usually arousable although they are lethargic. Psychotic symptoms are common and show good response to antipsychotics and treatment of the underlying condition.

29. Answer: D. Delirium is associated with longer hospital stays, reduced independence after discharge, and increased mortality. Involvement of relatives and patients should be encouraged. Antipsychotics have an effect that goes beyond their sedative actions. Iatrogenic causes are common in the etiology of delirium. Reduction of risk factors can be useful in preventing further episodes.

30. Answer: D. Wernicke's encephalopathy is characterized by confusion, ataxia, nystagmus, and ophthalmoplegia. Ophthalmoplegia responds rapidly to treatment with high-dose vitamins. These features are also associated with a peripheral neuropathy. Dysphasia is not a feature of Wernicke's encephalopathy.

31. Answer: A. Korsakoff syndrome is caused by thiamine deficiency, the most common cause of which is alcohol abuse. Continuous vomiting can also cause it. Confabulation is a feature and may be present. Patient is usually not disoriented and retains a clear consciousness. There is usually an anterograde memory loss.

32. Answer: B. HIV can manifest as dementia. However Alzheimer's is a distinct type of dementia and is not due to HIV.

33. Answer: C. Insight is characteristically preserved in AIDS encephalitis until late in the course of the disease. The EEG is normal from an early stage. Frank dysphoria is uncommon. Cognitive deficits may be apparent fairly early on in the illness. Treatment has a favorable impact on the outcome of the disease.

34. Answer: C. Most terminally ill people do not develop depressive disorder and suicidal thoughts. Anger is an important factor in suicide. Suicides are usually committed by medically ill patients who have morbid, often unrecognized, psychiatric illnesses.

35. Answer: D. History of suicide attempts is an important predictor of future suicide. One of every hundred persons who survive a suicide attempt will die by suicide within one year of their index attempt, a risk that is 100 times that for the general population. Of those who complete suicide, 25% to 50% have tried it before.

36. Answer: D. Once the doctor–patient relationship is created, the clinician assumes a duty to safeguard the patient's disclosures. This duty is not absolute and in some circumstances, breaking confidentiality is both ethical and legal.

37. Answer: E. The presence of mental illness or cognitive impairment does not necessarily render the person incompetent. Competency is a legal decision, whereas capacity is a clinical determination. Competency is not a scientifically determinable state and it is situation specific. The person must be examined to determine whether specific functional incapacities render the person incapable of making a particular kind of decision or performing a particular type of task.

38. Answer: A. Advanced directives provide a method for individuals, while competent, to choose alternative healthcare decision makers in the event of their future incompetency. An ordinary power of attorney becomes null and void if the person becomes incompetent. A durable power of attorney is constrained to empower an agent to make healthcare decisions. The healthcare proxy is a legal instrument akin to the durable power of attorney but specifically created for the delegation of healthcare decisions.

39. Answer: A. Restraints and seclusion are appropriate only when a patient presents a risk of harm to self or others and less restrictive alternatives are not available. Restraints are contraindicated in patients with extremely unstable medical or psychiatric conditions, in patients with severe drug reactions, in those with delirium or dementia who are unable to tolerate reduced stimulation, for punishment of the patient, or for the convenience of the healthcare staff.

40. Answer: C. Depression secondary to medical illness has some distinct clinical features. It is more likely to begin at a later age, respond to ECT, and present with impaired cognition. It is less likely to be associated with a family history of alcoholism or dependence and is less likely to result in suicide.

41. Answer: C. The incidence of psychiatric illness is high in patients with cancer, and about half of them develop a diagnosable psychiatric disorder. The prevalence of adjustment disorder is highest, at more than 25%. The next most common is depression, which occurs in approximately 8–14% of patients. Suicide is rare among patients with cancer. Men with head and neck cancer may be at the highest risk of suicide.

42. Answer: D. Mania is rarely related to cancer itself. Corticosteroids are the most frequent cause of mania in patients with cancer. Diencephalic tumors and cerebral metastasis can rarely cause mania.

43. Answer: C. The association between lesion location and depression following a stroke is controversial. Some studies support the contention that the risk of depression is higher the closer the lesion is to the left frontal pole, with left anterior frontal lesions being the most highly associated with depression. There is also evidence that left frontal cortical and left basal ganglia strokes produce depression to a greater degree than do lesions in the right side of the brain.

44. Answer: B. The dementia associated with HIV is typically a subcortical dementia with difficulties with attention and concentration and speed of processing.

45. Answer: E. Delirium is the neuropsychiatric complication that occurs frequently in hospitalized patients with AIDS. Patients with advanced systemic disease and HIV dementia are at high risk for delirium. In the management of delirium, the primary goal is identification and treatment of underlying factors. Specific medications associated with delirium include narcotics, benzodiazepines, anticholinergics, antihistamines, and steroids. Symptomatic treatment with neuroleptics may be necessary to control agitation and help resolve confusion.

46. Answer: D. AIDS dementia complex (ADC) is characterized by cognitive, affective, behavioral, and motor dysfunction. Patients describe short-term memory loss, word-finding difficulties, and difficulty with sequential tasks. They also report depressed mood, social withdrawal, and reduced energy. Patients also describe slowing of their movements, clumsiness, and gait disturbances. Aphasia and agnosia are rare, as is psychosis except in end-stage AIDS dementia complex.

47. Answer: D. Substance-related disorders occur frequently in patients with HIV disease. The prevalence of substance-related disorders in ambulatory patients with HIV who are referred for psychiatric evaluations may be about 45%. Noninjection psychoactive drugs impair the use of judgment and may lead to recidivism due to behavioral changes toward low HIV risk behaviors. Some studies have shown such an effect with alcohol use. Crack cocaine and inhalant abuse are commonly associated with high HIV risk behaviors.

48. Answer: C. About 25% of people with chronic pain also have an axis I disorder. Despite the psychiatric morbidity associated with chronic pain, emotional symptoms are more often a consequence of pain than an antecedent to pain.

49. Answer: A. Patients with concurrent psychiatric illness and epilepsy may be safely treated with ECT. Patients should continue to receive their anticonvulsant medication during ECT; higher stimulus settings are typically necessary. ECT is effective for the mood and motor symptoms in patients with Parkinson's disease. Cardiac complications are the most common cause of death in patients who receive ECT. The use of unilateral electrodes is associated with reduced cognitive deficits. ECT may be used as a first-line treatment in patients with catatonia and should be considered the treatment of choice once the diagnosis of catatonia is made and the patient does not respond to lorazepam.

50. Answer: B. Haloperidol is the most commonly used neuroleptic in the intensive care unit. It is also safe and effective when administered intravenously. Pharmacologic treatment can usually be safely discontinued once the patient is symptom-free for 24 to 48 hours.

Chapter 8

FORENSIC PSYCHIATRY

QUESTIONS

1. To prove malpractice, the plaintiff must prove all of the following *except*
   A. There was a duty of care.
   B. There was a deviation from the standard of care.
   C. The patient died.
   D. The deviation caused the damage.

2. What is the duty to protect a potential victim of a patient called?
   A. Tarasoff I
   B. Tarasoff II
   C. M'Naughten Rule
   D. Model Penal Code
   E. Durham Rule

3. All of the following are criteria used to determine competency *except*
   A. Understanding the information
   B. Communication of choice
   C. Appreciation of risks and benefits
   D. Rational decision making
   E. Agreement with the doctor

4. Which of the following is the term that denotes decision making by a substitute acting on behalf of an individual unable to act on his or her own behalf?
   A. Power of attorney
   B. Parenting
   C. Guardianship
   D. Befriending
   E. Substituted judgment

5. What is the intent to commit a crime or a guilty mind called?
   A. Actus reus
   B. Mens rea
   C. Haggis
   D. Habeus corpus
   E. Respondeat superior

6. Which of the following renders a person incompetent to stand trial?
   A. Presence of mental illness
   B. Diagnosis of schizophrenia
   C. Mental retardation
   D. Acceptance of guilt
   E. Inability to understand the charges

7. All of the following are elements of the insanity defense *except*
   A. Presence of a mental disorder
   B. Denial of guilt
   C. Presence of defect of reason
   D. Inability to refrain from the act
   E. Not knowing that it was wrong

8. All of the following substances are associated with violence in nonpsychotic patients *except*
   A. Alcohol
   B. Amphetamines
   C. Caffeine
   D. Marijuana
   E. Nicotine

9. All of the following are important in the risk assessment of violent offenders with schizophrenia *except*
   A. Treatment compliance
   B. Index offense
   C. Number of first-rank symptoms
   D. A past history of offense
   E. Insight

10. All of the following are management strategies for stalkers that are associated with a favorable outcome *except*
   A. Management of comorbid substance use
   B. Treatment of underlying mental disorder
   C. Understanding the motivation of the stalker
   D. Mediation sessions between stalker and victim
   E. Increased empathy for the victim

11. All of the following are true about violence associated with schizophrenia *except*
   A. It increases with comorbid substance use.
   B. It occurs in about 20% of patients before their first admission.
   C. It is always psychotically motivated.
   D. It can result in homicide followed by suicide.

12. Which of the following is a short-term predictor of violence?
   A. Dementia
   B. Obsessive-compulsive personality traits
   C. Female gender
   D. Compliance with the treatment
   E. Alcohol intoxication

13. For an adult who lacks the capacity to make healthcare decisions, which of the following is true?
   A. The doctor cannot do anything.
   B. The patient's parents can give consent.
   C. The patient's children can give consent.
   D. The doctor can lawfully proceed with treatment if it is in the best interest of the patient.
   E. An advance directive is useless in such a situation.

14. Which of the following is true regarding most criminal offenders with mental disorders?
   A. They commit offenses directly related to their symptoms.
   B. They should receive treatment rather than punishment.
   C. They have committed serious offenses.
   D. They suffer from a personality disorder.
   E. They require examination by a specialist forensic psychiatrist.

15. All of the following are associated with criminal behavior *except*
- **A.** Personality disorder
- **B.** Social anxiety disorder
- **C.** Alcohol and drug dependence
- **D.** Mental retardation
- **E.** Schizophrenia

16. What is the most common offense committed by women?
- **A.** Homicide
- **B.** Infanticide
- **C.** Assault
- **D.** Shoplifting
- **E.** Hit and run

17. Which of the following is true?
- **A.** Most criminals are of markedly low intelligence.
- **B.** The majority of delinquent youth are mentally retarded.
- **C.** Sexual offenses are overly represented in people with mental retardation.
- **D.** People with mental retardation who commit crimes are less likely to be caught.
- **E.** People with mental retardation rarely indulge in arson.

18. Which psychiatric disorder is most commonly associated with homicide followed by suicide?
- **A.** Schizophrenia
- **B.** Personality disorder
- **C.** Heroin dependence
- **D.** Depression
- **E.** Pathological jealousy

19. Which of the following is *not* true regarding fitness to plead?
- **A.** The defendant should understand the nature of the charge.
- **B.** Defendants should understand that what they did was wrong.
- **C.** The defendants should be able to instruct counsel.
- **D.** The defendant understands the difference between pleading guilty and pleading not guilty.
- **E.** The defendant can follow the evidence presented in court.

20. What is the most useful predictor of future violence?

    A. Lack of regret

    B. Morbid jealousy

    C. Past history of suicide attempts

    D. History of past violence

    E. History of alcohol dependence

21. Which of the following is *false* regarding the mental competency of persons making their wills?

    A. Persons making their wills should know the extent of their property.

    B. They should understand that they are making a will.

    C. They should be able to identify their natural beneficiaries.

    D. They should bequeath their property to their natural beneficiaries.

22. Which of the following is the term denoting a person's performing actions for another's benefit without that person's consent?

    A. Paternalism

    B. Autonomy

    C. Beneficence

    D. Justice

    E. Utilitarianism

23. Which of the following is the most common role of a psychiatrist in court?

    A. Witness of fact

    B. Expert witness

    C. Cross-examiner

    D. Attorney

    E. Court-mandated evaluator

24. Which of the following is known as the "right–wrong test"?

    A. M'Naughten Rule

    B. Model Penal Code

    C. Durham Rule

    D. Irresistible impulse

    E. Guilty but insane

25. Which of the following denotes the advance selection of a substitute decision maker to act on one's behalf in the event that one should become incompetent?

    A. Power of attorney

    B. Guardianship

    C. Durable power of attorney

    D. Advance directive

ANSWERS

1. **Answer: C.** To prove malpractice, the plaintiff must establish by a preponderance of evidence that there existed a duty of care, there was a deviation from the standard of care, the patient was damaged, and the deviation directly caused the damage.

2. **Answer: B.** Tarasoff I is the duty to warn. Tarasoff II is the duty to protect.

3. **Answer: E.** Agreement with the doctor is not used to determine competency.

4. **Answer: C.** Guardianship is a method of substitute decision making for people unable to act on their own behalf.

5. **Answer: B.** *Mens rea* is evil intent. *Actus reus* is voluntary conduct. Both of them must be present to determine if a crime has been committed.

6. **Answer: E.** To be able to stand trial, individuals have to understand and appreciate the charges against them, be able to appraise the legal defense available, understand court procedure, have the capacity to challenge prosecution witnesses realistically, and have the capacity to testify relevantly.

7. **Answer: B.** Denial of guilt is not an element of the insanity defense.

8. **Answer: E.** Nicotine or cigarette smoking is not associated with increased rates of violence.

9. **Answer: C.** The number of first-rank symptoms does not bear a direct relationship to the risk a person poses. Command hallucinations are associated with an increased risk of violence. The severity and nature of the index offense, a history of past offenses, noncompliance with treatment, lack of insight, and psychopathy all correlate with risk.

10. **Answer: D.** Mediation sessions between stalker and victim are not useful in the management of stalking.

11. **Answer: C.** Violence in patients at schizophrenia is not always due to psychosis. There's an increased incidence of violence with comorbid substance use that can be predicted to some degree.

12. **Answer: E.** Alcohol intoxication is a good short-term predictor of violence.

13. **Answer: D.** In an adult patient deemed to be incompetent, the doctor can proceed to treat the patient if treatment is in the patient's best interests.

14. **Answer: B.** Most offenders with mental disorders do not commit offenses directly related to the symptoms. They are more often likely to commit petty offenses and can be treated by a general psychiatrist. The majority of such offenders do not have a personality disorder, though a higher percentage than average do. They should receive treatment rather than punishment.

15. **Answer: B.** The presence of personality disorder, alcohol and drug use, mental retardation, schizophrenia, and depression are all associated with criminal behavior.

16. **Answer: D.** Shoplifting and other kinds of theft are the most common offenses committed by women.

17. **Answer: C.** Sexual offenses are overrepresented in people with mental retardation. This may be because of their ignorance or unawareness of social mores or taboos and because of the high likelihood of their being caught. People with mental retardation are also more likely to indulge in arson. The majority of delinquent youth are not mentally retarded, and criminals are not necessarily of low intelligence.

18. **Answer: E.** Pathological jealousy is the most common psychiatric disorder associated with homicide that is followed by suicide. Killing of an elderly spouse in poor health, killing of a child, and multiple murders by a depressed, paranoid, or intoxicated person are also seen. Twenty to twenty-five percent of all jealous men who killed their spouses also committed suicide.

19. **Answer: B.** To be fit to plead, defendants need not understand that what they did was wrong. They only need to understand the charges.

20. **Answer: D.** A history of violence in the past is the most powerful indicator of violence in the future. Lack of regret, morbid jealousy, and alcohol and drug abuse are also predictors of violence.

21. **Answer: D.** The competence to make a will, called testamentary capacity, requires that patients know the nature and extent of their property, the fact that they're making a bequest, and the identities of their natural beneficiaries. The property need not be given to the natural beneficiaries.

22. **Answer: A.** Autonomy is the patient's right to self-determination. Beneficence is the duty of the physician to act in the best interests of the patient.

23. **Answer: B.** The most common role of a psychiatrist in court is that of an expert witness.

24. Answer: B. In its Model Penal Code, the American Law Institute (ALI) recommended that "persons are not responsible for criminal conduct if, at the time of such conduct, as a result of mental disease or defect, they lacked substantial capacity either to appreciate the criminality of their conduct or to confirm their conduct to the requirement of the law."

25. Answer: C. Durable power of attorney permits the advance selection of a substitute decision maker who can act without the necessity of court proceedings when the signatory becomes incompetent through illness or dementia.

Chapter 9

SUBSTANCE USE

QUESTIONS

1. Which of the following is one of the diagnostic criteria for substance dependence?
- **A.** Absence from work
- **B.** Use of the substance in hazardous situations
- **C.** Substance-related legal problems
- **D.** Withdrawal symptoms
- **E.** Neglect of children because of substance use

2. Which of the following is true?
- **A.** Withdrawal symptoms are needed for a diagnosis of dependence.
- **B.** Withdrawal is seen only when the substance used is stopped.
- **C.** The signs and symptoms of withdrawal are the same for all drugs.
- **D.** The severity of withdrawal is not related to the amount of substance used.
- **E.** The severity of withdrawal is related to the duration and pattern of use.

3. Which of the following is associated with use of illicit drugs?
- **A.** High socioeconomic status
- **B.** Low availability of drugs
- **C.** High crime rate
- **D.** Low unemployment
- **E.** Good schools

4. Which of the following is a risk factor for alcoholism?
- **A.** Female sex
- **B.** Identical twin with alcoholism
- **C.** Adoptive father with alcoholism
- **D.** Family history of schizophrenia
- **E.** Family history of ADHD

5. In women, which of the following is the most common comorbid condition seen with drug abuse and dependence?

    A. Antisocial personality disorder

    B. Phobic disorder

    C. Alcohol abuse or dependence

    D. Major depression

    E. Dysthymia

6. What is the most common comorbid psychiatric disorder in prisoners with addictive disorders?

    A. Antisocial personality disorder

    B. Schizophrenia

    C. Depression

    D. Bipolar disorder

    E. Phobic disorder

7. Alcoholism is associated with all of the following personality types *except*

    A. Low self-directedness

    B. High novelty seeking

    C. High harm avoidance

    D. Low reward dependence

    E. Low cooperativeness

8. Severe alcohol withdrawal is associated with all the following medical complications *except*

    A. Magnesium deficiency

    B. Wernicke's encephalopathy

    C. Hypertension

    D. Hyperglycemia

    E. Seizures

9. Which of the following is a good first-line drug for alcohol detoxification?

    A. Chlorpromazine

    B. Chlordiazepoxide

    C. Carbamazepine

    D. Clonidine

    E. Barbiturates

10. When depression and anxiety are prominent before detoxification, which of the following is true?

    A. Treatment with an antidepressant should be started.

    B. Their presence indicates the need for inpatient detoxification.

    C. Their presence predicts dropout from detoxification.

    D. Symptoms usually disappear in about 3 to 4 weeks.

    E. A DSM-IV Axis I diagnosis should be made immediately.

11. Which of the following does not predict a risk of suicide in patients with alcoholism?

    A. Comorbid depression

    B. Severity of alcoholism

    C. Parental alcoholism

    D. Early age of onset of drinking

    E. Previous self-harm

12. Which of the following is not useful in the assessment of a patient with alcoholism?

    A. CAGE

    B. AUDIT

    C. CAMCOG

    D. MCV

    E. CDT

13. Which of the following is a stage in the theory of change?

    A. Revision

    B. Contemplation

    C. Realism

    D. Denial

    E. Shock

14. Which of the following is a feature of Cloninger's type 1 alcoholism?

    A. Early onset

    B. Incidence in both men and women

    C. Impulsivity

    D. Antisocial personality traits

    E. Positive family history

15. Which of the following is the origin of motivation-enhancing techniques in treating substance abuse?
- **A.** Cognitive-behavioral therapy
- **B.** Operant conditioning
- **C.** Psychodynamic theories
- **D.** Milan school of family therapy
- **E.** Theory of change

16. Which of the following is associated with withdrawal from alcohol?
- **A.** Elevated dopaminergic function
- **B.** Reduced dopaminergic function
- **C.** Increased GABA activity
- **D.** Decreased glutaminergic activity
- **E.** Increased serotonin function

17. Which of the following receptors is postulated to be essential for the development of opiate dependence?
- **A.** Kappa
- **B.** Delta
- **C.** Mu
- **D.** Serotonin
- **E.** Dopamine

18. Which of the following receptors associated with ion channel activities is inhibited by alcohol?
- **A.** 5-HT3
- **B.** Glutamate
- **C.** GABA-A
- **D.** Acetylcholine

19. You are asked to see a 42-year-old male patient on a surgical ward who had a major operation 2 days ago and is now exhibiting bizarre behavior. He expresses fears that aliens are coming to take him away and appears to be responding to hallucinations. On examination he is tremulous and sweating but appears oriented and denies any hallucinations. His laboratory workup is subnormal with increased MCV and GGT. What is the most likely cause of his symptoms?

   A. Alcohol withdrawal
   B. Schizophrenia
   C. Severe depression
   D. Delirium tremens
   E. Alcoholic hallucinosis

20. Which of the following is *not* true of delirium tremens?

   A. If untreated, it has a high mortality rate.
   B. Hallucinations may involve the patient's occupation.
   C. Aphasia is common.
   D. Patients are highly suggestible.
   E. The delusions are fragmented and unsystematized.

21. Which of the following is a characteristic feature of alcohol dependence?

   A. Rapid reinstatement after abstinence
   B. Absenteeism on Fridays
   C. Tendency to exaggerate drinking
   D. Drinking only in the company of others
   E. Ability to control drinking when interpersonal problems increase

22. Which of the following is *not* true of alcohol withdrawal?

   A. It is associated with increased autonomic activity.
   B. Mild cases can be treated at home.
   C. Severity of symptoms peaks on the day that the drinking stops.
   D. Benzodiazepines are effective in suppressing hallucinations.
   E. Home detoxification is contraindicated if patient has a history of seizure disorder.

23. Alcohol dependence is associated with
- **A.** Maternal separation in childhood
- **B.** Family history of depression
- **C.** Paranoid personality disorder
- **D.** Family history of alcoholism
- **E.** Alcohol dehydrogenase deficiency

24. Alcohol withdrawal is associated with all the following *except*
- **A.** Affect-laden dreams
- **B.** Absence seizures
- **C.** Coarse tremors
- **D.** Auditory hallucinations
- **E.** Hypersomnolence

25. Which of the following is *not* a complication of alcohol abuse?
- **A.** Decreased serum testosterone
- **B.** Carcinoma esophagus
- **C.** Hypertension
- **D.** Cardiomyopathy
- **E.** Parkinson's disease

26. Which of the following is an effect of alcohol on sleep?
- **A.** Increased sleep latency
- **B.** Decreased sleep fragmentation
- **C.** Decreased episodes of waking
- **D.** Decreased REM sleep
- **E.** Increased stage IV sleep

27. Methyl alcohol poisoning can cause all of the following *except*
- **A.** Blindness
- **B.** Metabolic alkalosis
- **C.** Convulsions
- **D.** Vomiting
- **E.** Death

28. All of the following arouse a suspicion of alcohol dependence *except*
  A. Unexplained absence from work
  B. Smell of alcohol on breath
  C. Hypnogogic hallucination
  D. Morning nausea
  E. Morning tremors

29. Which of the following is true of Korsakoff syndrome?
  A. Disorientation is usually present.
  B. Confabulation is essential for diagnosis.
  C. Immediate memory is affected.
  D. It can be caused by continuous vomiting.
  E. Clouding of consciousness is a characteristic feature.

30. Which of the following is not seen in chronic alcoholism?
  A. Hypoglycemia
  B. Hemochromatosis
  C. Campbell de Morgan spots
  D. Marchiafava-Bignami syndrome
  E. Optic atrophy

31. Alcohol dependence is more common in
  A. African Americans than in Whites
  B. Jews than in non-Jews
  C. Married persons than in unmarried
  D. Middle-class persons than in persons of other socioeconomic classes
  E. Doctors than in the general population

32. Which of the following symptoms favors a diagnosis of amphetamine-induced psychotic disorder rather than schizophrenia?
  A. Predominance of auditory hallucinations
  B. Inappropriate affect
  C. Little or no evidence of disordered thinking
  D. Marked affective flattening
  E. Alogia

33. Which of the following is true regarding alcoholic hallucinosis?
   A. It's caused by thiamine deficiency.
   B. Some patients progress to develop schizophrenia.
   C. Auditory hallucinations are generally pleasant.
   D. Patients are confused and disoriented.
   E. Hallucinations are usually in the third person.

34. What is the primary goal of treatment for most alcoholics?
   A. Increased productivity
   B. Increased self-awareness
   C. Increased relationships
   D. Total abstinence
   E. Participation in AA

35. All of the following are features of alcohol withdrawal tremors *except*
   A. Abducens nerve palsy
   B. Visual hallucinations
   C. Disorientation
   D. Tremors
   E. Tachycardias

36. A 45-year-old man who drinks a quart of whisky a day reports feelings of hopelessness, suicidal thoughts, sleeplessness, and weight loss. What is the most appropriate diagnosis?
   A. Major depression
   B. Adjustment disorder
   C. Alcohol withdrawal
   D. Dysthymia
   E. Alcohol-induced mood disorder

37. Complications in pregnancy of an opiate-addicted mother include all of the following *except*
   A. Low birth weight
   B. Cleft palate in the fetus
   C. Intrauterine death
   D. Abruptio placentae
   E. Neonatal opioid withdrawal

38. Which of the following is true about LSD?
    A. It results in hypotension and falls.
    B. Pinpoint pupils are a reliable indicator of LSD use.
    C. It can cause neuroleptic malignant syndrome.
    D. Hallucinations are usually tactile.

39. Which of the following is not a complication of amphetamine use?
    A. Hypotension
    B. Weight loss
    C. Depression
    D. Paranoid psychosis

40. How do amphetamines cause euphoriant effects?
    A. By decreasing synaptic dopamine concentration
    B. By increasing 5 HT concentration
    C. By increasing dopamine concentration
    D. By increasing noradrenaline concentration
    E. By binding to the mu receptors

41. Which of the following is not seen in heroin withdrawal?
    A. Rhinorrhea
    B. Muscle cramps
    C. Miosis
    D. Diarrhea

42. Withdrawal seizures are not associated with
    A. Heroin
    B. Meprobamate
    C. Phenobarbital
    D. Diazepam
    E. Alcohol

43. A 40-year-old woman presents to the ER with confusion and drowsiness. She is ataxic and her speech is slurred. She has lateral nystagmus with normal pupils. Respirations are shallow. Shortly after, she has respiratory arrest and grand mal seizure. The family reports that she has been taking sleeping pills for a long time. What is the most likely cause for her presentation?

    A. Antidepressant overdose

    B. Anticholinergic overdose

    C. Barbiturate overdose

    D. Benzodiazepine withdrawal

    E. Opiate overdose

44. All of the following are physiologic effects of cocaine use *except*

    A. Vasoconstriction

    B. Tachycardia

    C. Pupillary constriction

    D. Hypertension

    E. Decreased appetite

45. Which of the following is not an early symptom of withdrawal from barbiturates?

    A. Coarse tremor

    B. Nystagmus

    C. Hypertension

    D. Seizures

    E. Anxiety

46. When compared to withdrawal from heroin, withdrawal from methadone is more likely to be

    A. Delayed

    B. Susceptible to delirium

    C. Painful

    D. Of shorter duration

    E. Dangerous

47. Which of the following substances causes the highest number of deaths?

    A. Alcohol

    B. Cocaine

    C. Nicotine

    D. Marijuana

    E. Heroin

48. Which of the following is caused by cocaine toxicity?

  A. Bradycardia

  B. Hypothermia

  C. Hypersomnia

  D. Hypotension

  E. Intracranial hemorrhage

49. Why is methadone used as a substitute for heroin in the treatment of heroin dependence?

  A. It reduces addiction to other drugs.

  B. It has less potential to cause dependence than heroin.

  C. It prevents psychotic symptoms.

  D. It blocks mu opioid receptors in the brain.

  E. It suppresses opioid withdrawal symptoms for a longer time.

50. A 26-year-old patient without any cardiac risk factors suffers a myocardial infarction. What substance is most likely to be the cause?

  A. PCP

  B. Sedative

  C. Hallucinogen

  D. Stimulant

  E. Alcohol

51. Hallucinations, elevated blood pressure, and minimal pain when skin folds are squeezed are most likely to be associated with

  A. Amphetamines

  B. PCP

  C. LSD

  D. Marijuana

  E. Alcohol

52. On which of the following does PCP have an antagonistic effect?

  A. Glycine

  B. GABA

  C. Dopamine

  D. Serotonin

  E. Glutamate

53. What neurotransmitter is associated with benzodiazepine withdrawal?
- **A.** Acetylcholine
- **B.** GABA
- **C.** Norepinephrine
- **D.** Serotonin
- **E.** Dopamine

54. Which of the following is true about opiate use?
- **A.** The majority of people who use opiates for nonmedical reasons develop opiate dependence.
- **B.** Opiate addicts score high on "sensation-seeking" behavior.
- **C.** The majority of opiate-addicted individuals carry a lifetime diagnosis of a psychiatric disorder.
- **D.** Schizophrenia is the most common comorbid psychiatric disorder.

55. Which of the following substances is the most commonly used by persons with schizophrenia?
- **A.** Cocaine
- **B.** Marijuana
- **C.** Benzodiazepine
- **D.** Alcohol
- **E.** Nicotine

56. Which of the following mediates the effects of cocaine?
- **A.** Norepinephrine
- **B.** Acetylcholine
- **C.** Dopamine
- **D.** Serotonin
- **E.** GABA

57. Which of the following is true about heroin addiction?
- **A.** Inspection of the person's limbs reliably excludes intravenous use.
- **B.** HIV testing is mandatory.
- **C.** Endocarditis is a common complication.
- **D.** Urinary testing confirms the amount of drug consumed.
- **E.** Withdrawal symptoms are rarely life threatening.

58. A patient with alcohol dependence is ataxic, confused, and had a seizure after admission to a substance abuse clinic a day ago. He has no history of seizures. What is the most appropriate parenteral drug for this patient?

    A. Lorazepam

    B. Phenytoin

    C. Thiamine

    D. Folate

    E. Valproic acid

59. Which of the following triads of symptoms best describes Wernicke's encephalopathy?

    A. Hallucinations, ataxia, and peripheral neuropathy

    B. Hallucinations, confabulation, and peripheral neuropathy

    C. Hallucinations, ataxia, and tremors

    D. Ophthalmoplegia, seizures, and confusion

    E. Ophthalmoplegia, ataxia, and global confusion

60. Which of the following is a feature of alcoholic blackouts?

    A. Loosening of associations

    B. Reaction to a traumatic event

    C. Confabulation

    D. Anterograde amnesia following intoxication

    E. Retrograde amnesia following intoxication

61. All of the following are physical features seen in alcoholism *except*

    A. Arcus senilis

    B. Palmar erythema

    C. Peripheral neuropathy

    D. Café au lait spots

    E. Spider nevi

62. In which of the following is degeneration of the dorsal nucleus of the thalamus mamillary bodies found?

    A. Alzheimer disease

    B. Wilson disease

    C. Binswanger disease

    D. Creutzfeldt-Jakob disease

    E. Wernicke-Korsakoff syndrome

63. Which of the following is not seen in caffeine withdrawal?
- **A.** Depression
- **B.** Hallucinations
- **C.** Headache
- **D.** Insomnia
- **E.** Nervousness

64. Which of the following is most useful in differentiating between schizophrenia and alcohol withdrawal delirium?
- **A.** Agitation
- **B.** Hallucinations
- **C.** Affect
- **D.** Level of consciousness
- **E.** Paranoid delusions

65. Which of the following is true about disulfiram?
- **A.** It is contraindicated in people on antidepressants.
- **B.** Treatment with it should not be started on an outpatient.
- **C.** Its effects may persist for several days after it is discontinued.
- **D.** It should routinely be given to all alcoholics.
- **E.** It requires large quantities of alcohol to produce a reaction.

66. Which of the following is not a cause of delirium and confusion in the elderly?
- **A.** Depressive disorder
- **B.** Electrolyte imbalance
- **C.** Urinary retention
- **D.** Constipation
- **E.** Medication toxicity

67. What should be the first step in management of a young adult with marital problems, depression, and alcohol dependence?
- **A.** Couple therapy
- **B.** Antidepressant therapy
- **C.** Insight-oriented psychotherapy
- **D.** Treatment with disulfiram
- **E.** Detoxification and encouragement of abstinence

68. Which of the following is not a feature of fetal alcohol syndrome?
- A. Renal defects
- B. Cardiac defects
- C. Severe mental retardation
- D. Growth retardation
- E. Facial dysmorphism

69. Which of the following is a psychological manifestation of sedative abstinence?
- A. Sweating
- B. Lethargy
- C. Shakiness
- D. Impaired memory
- E. Tremors

70. Which of the following is not a feature of Korsakoff psychosis?
- A. Normal consciousness
- B. Disturbance of affect
- C. Disturbance of volition
- D. Distress about memory impairment
- E. Abulia

71. What is the half-life of LAAM?
- A. 8 hours
- B. 24–36 hours
- C. 48 hours
- D. 72–96 hours

72. How long should alcohol be avoided following cessation of disulfiram?
- A. 24 hours
- B. 3 days
- C. 7 days
- D. 1 month
- E. 3 months

73. Which of the following is true of caffeinism?
- A. Withdrawal symptoms start after 48 hours.
- B. Withdrawal symptoms can last up to 1 week.
- C. Caffeine has a half-life of 12 hours.
- D. Withdrawal symptoms can be life threatening.
- E. Muscle relaxation occurs.

ANSWERS

1. **Answer: D.** The diagnostic criteria for substance dependence require a presence of three or more of the following in a 12-month period: tolerance, withdrawal, use of substance in larger amounts and for longer periods than intended, persistent desire to control use or unsuccessful efforts to control use, spending a great deal of time in obtaining the substance, impairment of social occupational or recreational activities, and use of the substance despite knowledge that it is harmful.

2. **Answer: E.** The severity of withdrawal symptoms is related to the duration and pattern of use. It is also related to the amount of substance used. The signs and symptoms vary for different drugs and may emerge even on reduction of the dose. Withdrawal symptoms are one of the criteria to diagnose dependence, but are not essential.

3. **Answer: C.** Use of illicit substances is associated with low socioeconomic class, high availability of the substance, high unemployment, poor inner-city schools, and a high crime rate.

4. **Answer: B.** Males are at increased risk of developing alcoholism. The rate of alcohol problems increases with the number of alcoholic relatives, the severity of their illness, and the closeness of their genetic relationship to the person. There is an enhanced risk of alcoholism in the offspring of alcoholic parents, even when the children are separated from the biological parents. The risk is not enhanced by being raised by an alcoholic adoptive family. A family history of ADHD or schizophrenia is not a risk factor for alcoholism although patients with this disorder and PTSD, social anxiety, etc. may use alcohol to excess sometimes as a means of self-medication.

5. **Answer: C.** Antisocial personality disorder, phobic disorder, major depression, dysthymia, social phobia, and PTSD are all comorbid with drugs of abuse. However, alcohol dependence and abuse is the most likely comorbidity to be seen with drug abuse and dependence.

6. **Answer: A.** Antisocial personality disorder is a most common comorbid condition seen in prisoners with substance abuse.

7. **Answer: C.** Alcoholism is associated with low self-directedness, high novelty seeking (impulsivity), low reward dependence (aloofness), low cooperativeness, and low harm avoidance (risk-taking). Novelty seeking predicts early-onset alcoholism, criminality, and other substance use.

8. **Answer: D.** Alcohol withdrawal is sometimes associated with hypoglycemia. It can also cause withdrawal seizures, delirium, tremors, insomnia, vomiting, hallucinations, agitation, anxiety, and autonomic hyperactivity. Magnesium deficiency, Wernicke's encephalopathy, and hypertension may also be seen as sequelae of heavy drinking and even withdrawal.

9. **Answer: B.** Various benzodiazepines, including lorazepam, chlordiazepoxide, or diazepam, can be used to enable patients to withdraw from alcohol over a period of 4 to 7 days. Antipsychotics like haloperidol can be used in severe withdrawal. Carbamazepine, clonidine, and beta-blockers are also used. However, most clinicians prefer to use benzodiazepines as first-line agents.

10. **Answer: D.** Depressive symptoms are present in about 40–80% of people with heavy alcohol intake. However, after about 3 to 4 weeks of abstinence, only about 5–10% of patients continue to have depressive symptoms, even without any treatment. Hence, such patients should not be diagnosed with major depression without a fair period of abstinence. The presence of depression does not indicate the need for inpatient detoxification, nor does it predict dropout from detoxification.

11. **Answer: B.** Civility of alcoholism has not been shown to be predictive of suicide in patients with alcoholism (Berglund & Ojehagen 1998). The other factors mentioned are known risk factors.

12. **Answer: C.** CAMCOG is used in the assessment of dementia in the elderly. CAGE is a four-item questionnaire to screen for a problem with alcohol use. AUDIT (Alcohol Use Disorders Identification Test) is a standardized questionnaire regarding quantity and frequency of drinking. MCV (mean corpuscular volume) is increased in patients with alcoholism. CDT (carbohydrate-deficient transferrin) is a reasonably sensitive and specific marker of heavy drinking and may be used in monitoring abstinence during treatment.

13. **Answer: B.** Assessing the patient's motivation for change using the motivational interview (Miller & Rollinck 1991) involves gaining an understanding of the patient's reasons for seeking treatment. The stages may be classified along a continuum from precontemplation to contemplation to determination to action to maintenance.

14. **Answer: B.** Cloninger classified alcoholics into two distinct subtypes: type 1, or milieu limited alcoholism, and type 2, or male-limited alcoholism. Type 1 affects both male and females and has onset after age 25. Persons with this type of alcoholism do not have a strong family history of alcoholism or criminality and rarely engage in fights or are arrested while drinking. Type 2 alcoholism occurs only in men and is characterized by an inability to abstain from alcohol and heavy consumption rates. Dependence begins before the age of 25 and is associated with recurrent medical and social consequences of alcoholism as well as a personal and family history of criminality.

15. Answer: E. Motivation-enhancing techniques (Miller & Rollinck) have their origins in the theories of change.

16. Answer: B. Withdrawal symptoms from alcohol are associated with reduced dopaminergic function. They are also associated with reduced GABA, increased glutaminergic function, and reduced 5-HT3 function.

17. Answer: C. The three major types of opioid receptors are mu, kappa, and delta. Most of the opioid drugs are mu agonists. They produce analgesia, altered mood, decreased anxiety, respiratory depression, and suppression of cough. Most of the new agonists are full agonists and produce maximal response in opioid responsive types. When any mu agonist is used chronically, tolerance and physical dependence develop.

18. Answer: B. Alcohol enhances ion channel activities associated with nicotinic acetylcholine, serotonin 5-HT3, and GABA type A receptors, whereas it inhibits ion channel activities associated with glutamate receptors and voltage-gated calcium channels.

19. Answer: D. The symptoms described are strongly suggestive of delirium tremens. Such symptoms can arise in patients being admitted to the hospital for an operation and hence abstaining from alcohol. The clinical features are clouding of consciousness, difficulty sustaining attention, disorientation, autonomic hyperactivity with tachycardia, excess sweating, and lability of blood pressure. Patients also have fleeting delusions and hallucinations. The symptoms should resolve with adequate treatment.

20. Answer: C. Aphasia is not seen in delirium tremens. Patients are highly suggestible. Hallucinations may include any modality but typically are visual or auditory and are persecutory. Delusions are usually fragmented and unsystematized, unlike those of schizophrenia. The condition has a high mortality rate (15–20%) if untreated.

21. Answer: A. Rapid reinstatement to previous levels of tolerance after a period of abstinence is a feature of dependence. Absenteeism on Mondays is typically associated with alcoholism. Patients tend to minimize their drinking. Patients with alcoholism typically tend to drink alone. They also have an inability to control their drinking in the presence of increasing personal problems.

22. Answer: C. Severe alcohol withdrawal may be characterized by a wide variety of symptoms, including autonomic instability. The symptoms peak 2 to 3 days after cessation of drinking. Mild cases may be treated at home. Patients with a history of seizure disorder should be treated in hospital because of the risk of reemergence of seizures. Hallucinations are seen in withdrawal, and the use of benzodiazepines to suppress withdrawal can help with the suppression of hallucinations.

23. Answer: D. A family history of alcoholism is strongly associated with development of alcoholism in the proband. The closer the affected relative genetically and the greater the number of affected relatives, the higher the risk of alcoholism.

24. Answer: B. Alcohol withdrawal is typically associated with tonic-clonic seizures. It does not cause petit mal seizures. Coarse tremors, auditory hallucinations, paranoid delusions, visual hallucinations, hypersomnolence, and insomnia may also be seen.

25. Answer: E. Long-term use of alcohol can affect a number of systems in the body and can cause blackouts, peripheral neuropathy, cerebellar degeneration, liver damage (including fatty liver and cirrhosis), carcinoma esophagus, pancreatitis, hypertension, hypercholesterolemia, alcoholic cardiomyopathy, reduced serum testosterone, and cancer of the liver and stomach. It does not cause Parkinson's disease per se.

26. Answer: D. Alcohol consumed in the evening decreases sleep latency. It also causes a decrease in REM sleep and stage IV (deep) sleep. It causes more sleep fragmentation and more and longer episodes of awakening.

27. Answer: B. Methyl alcohol consumption results in increased serum osmolality, severe anion gap metabolic acidosis, tachypnoea, confusion, convulsions, blindness, vomiting, and death.

28. Answer: C. Hypnagogic hallucination is a phenomenon that occurs in normal persons as they fall asleep. Unexplained absence from work, smell of alcohol on the breath, morning nausea, and tremors all arouse a suspicion of alcohol dependence.

29. Answer: D. Korsakoff syndrome is characterized by anterograde and retrograde amnesia and impairment in visuospatial, abstract, and other types of learning. The level of recent memory is out of proportion to the global level of cognitive impairment. Immediate memory is usually preserved. Confabulation may be seen. The patient has a clear consciousness. In addition to alcohol use, prolonged severe vomiting can cause Korsakoff syndrome.

30. Answer: C.

31. Answer: E. Alcohol dependence is more common in doctors than the general population. It is more common in Whites than African Americans and Chinese and more common in non-Jews than in Jews. Jews have the highest proportion who consumes alcohol but the lowest number of persons with alcohol problems. Other groups, such as the Irish, have higher rates of severe alcohol problems and high rates of absenteeism. Unmarried persons and members of lower social economic groups are also more likely to abuse alcohol.

32. **Answer: C.** Amphetamine-induced psychotic disorder can at times be indistinguishable from schizophrenia. The hallmark of amphetamine-induced psychotic disorder is paranoia. It is also characterized by the predominance of visual hallucinations, appropriate affect, hyperactivity, hypersexuality, confusion and incoherence, little or no evidence of thought disorder, and lack of affective flattening and alogia.

33. **Answer: B.** About 3% of patients have psychotic symptoms in the context of heavy drinking. In a very small number of patients, the symptoms may persist on cessation of alcohol use and later meet the criteria for schizophrenia. Auditory hallucinations in alcoholic hallucinosis are derogatory and in the second person. All this occurs on a background of clear consciousness.

34. **Answer: D.** Although increased productivity, self-awareness, better relationships, and participation in AA are all goals of treatment, total abstinence is the primary goal of most alcoholics.

35. **Answer: A.** Alcohol withdrawal does not cause abducens nerve palsy. All the other symptoms are well-known features of withdrawal.

36. **Answer: E.** About 80% of persons who are currently drinking heavily report mood symptoms mimicking those of a depressive disorder. DSM-IV labels the symptoms as an alcohol-induced mood disorder in the context of heavy and repetitive use of any brain depressant, including alcohol.

37. **Answer: B.** Opiate use in pregnancy is associated with decreased fetal growth and low birth weight but not with any teratogenic effects. It can also cause intrauterine death and abruptio placentae, and the infant may have withdrawal symptoms.

38. **Answer: C.** The onset of action of LSD occurs within 1 hour, peaks within 2 to 4 hours, and lasts 8 to 12 hours. The sympathomometic effects include tremors, tachycardia, hypertension, hyperthermia, sweating, blurring of vision, and mydriasis. Death can also occur. A syndrome similar to neuroleptic malignant syndrome can also occur with LSD. Hallucinations are usually visual, although auditory and tactile hallucinations are sometimes seen. Emotions may be unusually intense and change abruptly and often.

39. **Answer: A.** Amphetamine use can cause hypertension and result in intracranial hemorrhage, arrhythmias, and acute cardiac failure. It also can cause psychotic symptoms and mood symptoms including mania and depression on withdrawal. Amphetamines and cocaine can also cause anxiety disorders and symptoms similar to obsessive-compulsive disorder. High doses over a prolonged period cause impotence. Amphetamines also cause insomnia and sleep deprivation.

40. **Answer: C.** Cocaine and amphetamines cause euphoriant effects by increasing dopamine concentrations. They increase synaptic dopamine levels by inhibiting the activity of dopamine transporters. Cocaine and amphetamines increase extracellular dopamine levels in the striatum; euphoria is related to the occupancy of dopamine transporters by cocaine and amphetamines.

41. **Answer: C.** Miosis is associated with opiate use and intoxication. Withdrawal results in mydriasis. All of the other features mentioned are seen in withdrawal.

42. **Answer: A.** Withdrawal from heroin is very distressing but not life threatening. It does not result in seizures. Withdrawal from diazepam, alcohol, phenobarbitone, or meprobamate can cause seizures.

43. **Answer: D.** The symptoms suggest withdrawal symptoms from a benzodiazepine following the cessation of use.

44. **Answer: C.** Cocaine use causes pupillary dilatation.

45. **Answer: C.** Physiologic dependence on barbiturates may result from a daily dose of 4 mg of pentobarbital for 3 months. Discontinuation results in anxiety, insomnia, anorexia, coarse tremors, muscle weakness, myoclonic jerks, orthostatic hypotension, vomiting, EEG changes, and seizures. At higher doses, delirium and disorientation, visual hallucinations, and frightening dreams may develop.

46. **Answer: A.** Withdrawal symptoms from methadone and levo-alpha-acetyl-methadol (LAAM) may be delayed for 1 to 3 days following the last dose, and peak symptoms may not occur until the third to eighth day. The symptoms may persist for several weeks because of the longer half-life of methadone as compared to heroin. With morphine and heroin, symptoms start as early as 8 to 12 hours after discontinuation of the drugs, peak at about 48 hours, and run their course in 7 to 10 days.

47. **Answer: C.** The substance that causes the highest number of deaths is nicotine. Smoking is also a risk factor for lung cancer, cardiovascular disease, COPD, and low birth weight.

48. **Answer: E.** Cocaine intoxication and abuse can result in effects on a number of organ systems, including hypertension, intracranial hemorrhage, tachycardias and arrhythmias, MI, myocarditis, shock, sudden death, seizures, subarachnoid hemorrhage, cerebral infarction, pneumothorax, respiratory arrest, hyperthermia, abortion, and infections like AIDS, infective endocarditis, and hepatitis B.

49. **Answer: D.** Methadone acts by blocking the mu opioid receptors in the brain. It thus reduces addiction to other drugs, but that is not the prime reason for its use in dependence. It is also addictive and does not have any effect on psychosis. Because of its long half-life, it only needs to be given once a day.

50. **Answer: D.** Stimulants like amphetamines and cocaine increase the risk of cardiovascular events, including intracranial hemorrhage, arrhythmias, MI, myocarditis, shock, and sudden death.

50. **Answer: A.** Amphetamines can result in hallucinations, hypertension, and altered pain sensation. The excess of dopamine accounts for the elevated threshold for self-stimulation and pain.

51. **Answer: C.** Alcohol has various effects on the central nervous system, including amnesia. The condition of alcohol-induced persisting amnestic disorder is a result of a severe deficiency of thiamine. This results in Wernicke's encephalopathy and Korsakoff syndrome. Long-term use can also result in alcohol-induced dementia.

52. **Answer: A.** Drugs that bind to PCP receptors also block N-methyl-D-aspartate (NMDA) activated channels. NMDA receptors process binding sites for glutamate and glycine. Glutamate is released from presynaptic nerve endings in a pulsatile manner and rapidly deactivated. The local glycine concentration sets the tonic levels of NMDA excitability, thus determining the degree to which presynaptic glutamate release leads to postsynaptic excitation.

53. **Answer: B.** Benzodiazepine withdrawal is mediated by GABA receptors. Withdrawal symptoms consist of disturbances of mood and cognition, disturbances of sleep, physical signs and symptoms, and perceptual disturbances. Symptoms appear within 24 hours and peak at about 48 hours. Symptoms of abrupt discontinuation of benzodiazepines with long half-lives may not peak until 2 weeks.

54. **Answer: C.** According to the National Comorbidity Survey, 7.5% of individuals who used opioids for nonmedical purposes and 23% of individuals who used heroin eventually developed opioid dependence. Opiate addicts tend to score low on "sensation seeking" and tend to avoid excess internal and external stimulation. Eighty to ninety percent of addicted persons carry a lifetime diagnosis of a psychiatric disorder. Major depressive disorder and antisocial personality disorder are the two most common psychiatric disorders.

55. **Answer: E.** Nicotine is the substance most commonly used by schizophrenics.

56. **Answer: C.** Amphetamines and cocaine act by increasing the release of dopamine.

57. Answer: E. Withdrawal symptoms from heroin, although extremely distressing, are rarely life threatening. Inspection of the limbs, although useful in determining intravenous drug use, is not reliable. HIV testing is not mandatory and the patients have to consent to it like other patients. Endocarditis, although sometimes present, is not common. Urine testing can detect the presence of opiates but is not useful to quantify the amount used.

58. Answer: C. This patient is likely to have Wernicke's encephalopathy, which is secondary to deficiency of thiamine, which is associated with long-term drinking. Many of the symptoms can be reversed fairly rapidly with parenteral thiamine.

59. Answer: E. Wernicke's encephalopathy is characterized by ophthalmoplegia, ataxia, and confusion. There may be sixth nerve palsy.

60. Answer: D. Alcoholic blackouts are characterized by anterograde amnesia. This occurs with a blood alcohol concentration in the range of 200–300 mg per dl.

61. Answer: D. Café au lait spots are seen in neurofibromatosis. Spider nevi and palmar erythemia can be seen in liver diseases resulting from alcohol use. Arcus senilis and peripheral neuropathy are also seen in alcoholism.

62. Answer: E. The neuropathology of Wernicke-Korsakoff syndrome consists of neuronal loss, microhemorrhage, and gliosis in the paraventricular and periaqueductal gray matter. The medial dorsal nucleus of the thalamus, mamillary bodies, mamillothalamic tract, and anterior thalamus may also be affected.

63. Answer: B. Caffeine withdrawal begins 20–24 hours after the last use of caffeine. The symptoms reach their maximal intensity within 48 hours and resolve in 2 to 7 days. Headache is the most common feature. Other symptoms include sleepiness, reduced concentration, anxiety, insomnia, irritability, muscle aches, and yawning. Hallucinations are not characteristic.

64. Answer: D. Patients with alcohol withdrawal delirium typically have impaired consciousness, whereas patients with schizophrenia have symptoms on a background of clear consciousness. Hallucinations, affective disturbance, agitation, and delusions may be present in both conditions.

65. Answer: C. Disulfiram is an aldehyde dehydrogenase inhibitor that causes the accumulation of acetaldehyde after ethanol consumption. This can result in severe reaction with respiratory depression, cardiovascular collapse, arrhythmias, coma, cerebral edema, convulsions, and death. Its effects persist for more than 6 days following cessation of use of alcohol. It is not contraindicated with antidepressants and may be given to patients with good support systems as an outpatient. All patients are not suitable and even small amounts of alcohol can precipitate a reaction.

66. Answer: A. Depressive disorder by definition occurs on a background of clear consciousness. A variety of causes can precipitate delirium and confusion in the elderly.

67. Answer: E. A wide variety of sequelae can result from alcohol use, including depression and marital problems. Many of these resolve with cessation of alcohol use. Hence, detoxification and abstinence are the first step before other issues are dealt with.

68. Answer: C. Fetal alcohol syndrome is associated with facial dysmorphism with epicanthic folds, microcephaly, underdeveloped philtrum, and thin upper lip. Renal defects include renal hypoplasia and bladder diverticuli. Cardiac defects include atrial and ventricular septal defects. Mental retardation is usually mild when present and may be accompanied by behavioral difficulties including hyperactivity.

69. Answer: D. Impaired memory is a psychological manifestation. All the others are somatic or physical manifestations.

70. Answer: D. Patients with Korsakoff syndrome may have disturbance of affect, volition, abulia, and confabulation on a background of clear consciousness. Patients are seldom distressed by the memory impairment or even aware of it.

71. Answer: D. LAAM has a long half-life of 72 to 96 hours and is hence given three times a week.

72. Answer: C. Following cessation of disulfiram, the restoration of alcohol dehydrogenase depends on de novo enzyme synthesis, which can take about 1 week.

73. Answer: B. Withdrawal symptoms from stopping caffeine use can last up to 1 week. They begin within about 12 to 24 hours. Symptoms are not life threatening, and muscle tension is a feature. Caffeine has a half-life of 3 to 6 hours.

Chapter 10

EATING DISORDERS AND SEXUAL DISORDERS

QUESTIONS

1. Which of the following is true regarding bulimia nervosa?
   A. Individuals with bulimia have enlargement of the parotid gland.
   B. There is an increased frequency of depression in people with bulimia nervosa.
   C. Persons with bulimia nervosa have a 30% prevalence of substance abuse or dependence.
   D. Persons with bulimia nervosa exhibit mildly elevated levels of serum amylase.
   E. All of the above

2. Patients with bulimia nervosa are characterized by scars on the knuckles of their hands from constantly putting their hands into their mouths to induce vomiting. What is this sign called?
   A. Russell's sign
   B. Feingold's sign
   C. McCain's sign
   D. None of the above

3. An 18-year-old girl presents to the student guidance clinic at her school. She reports that she has a problem with eating. She describes eating too much and faster than usual in episodes that she is unable to control. She usually does this when not in the presence of others. She does not report any purging behavior. What is the name for the disorder she describes?

    A. Bulimia nervosa

    B. Impulse control disorder

    C. Binge eating disorder

    D. None of the above

4. Which of the following is *not* true for anorexia nervosa?

    A. It is more common in females.

    B. It is more prevalent in developing countries.

    C. Patients have a body weight less than 85% of that expected.

    D. Patients have an intense fear of gaining weight.

    E. In postmenarchal women, there is an absence of at least three consecutive menstrual cycles.

5. For which of the following are hormone levels decreased in patients with anorexia nervosa?

    A. GnRH

    B. FSH

    C. LH

    D. Estrogen

    E. All of the above

6. Which of the following medical complications is seen with anorexia nervosa?

    A. Leucopenia

    B. Hypokalemic alkalosis

    C. Lanugo

    D. Fatty degeneration of the liver

    E. All of the above

7. Patients with bulimia nervosa sometimes develop cardiac myopathy. What is the most common cause?

    A. Electrolyte disturbances

    B. Starvation

    C. Loss of cardiac muscle

    D. Toxicity from ipecac

    E. All of the above

8. Which of the following is not a good prognostic indicator for anorexia nervosa?
- A. Early age of onset
- B. Late age of onset
- C. No purging behavior
- D. No previous hospitalization for the illness
- E. Parents who are cooperative and willing to come for family therapy

9. What is considered the first line of treatment for bulimia nervosa?
- A. Family therapy
- B. Interpersonal therapy
- C. Pharmacotherapy
- D. Cognitive-behavioral therapy
- E. Brief psychoanalytic therapy

10. Which of the following is true regarding the epidemiology of eating disorders?
- A. The incidence has been consistently increasing over the last 50 years.
- B. It is more prevalent in Western cultures.
- C. Bulimia nervosa has a prevalence rate of 1%.
- D. Anorexia nervosa has a mortality rate of around 5–15%.
- E. All of the above

11. Patients suffering from anorexia nervosa have a high incidence of which of the following psychiatric conditions?
- A. Obsessive-compulsive disorder
- B. Major depression
- C. Social phobia
- D. Decreased sexual interest
- E. All of the above

12. What percentage of patients with anorexia eventually develops symptoms of bulimia?
- A. 10%
- B. 30%
- C. 40%
- D. 50%
- E. 70%

13. What is the most commonly abused substance in bulimia nervosa patients?
   A. Amphetamines
   B. Alcohol
   C. Opioids
   D. Benzodiazepines
   E. None of the above

14. Which of the following medications has been found useful in the treatment of anorexia nervosa?
   A. Fluoxetine
   B. Sertraline
   C. Chlorpromazine
   D. Cyprohepatidine
   E. All of the above

15. Which is the most common age of onset of anorexia nervosa?
   A. Between 14 and 15
   B. 18
   C. Both between 14 and 15 and at age 18 (a bimodal peak)
   D. 12–13
   E. None of the above

16. A 31-year-old man reports that he has to use women's undergarments to get sexually aroused. He admits to spending an inordinate time searching for and acquiring these garments. This has led to significant distress to him. On questioning he reports that he is not sexually attracted to males and that his sexual fantasies always involve females. What condition does this person have?
   A. Fetishism
   B. Transvestic fetishism
   C. Frotteurism
   D. Gender identity disorder
   E. None of the above

17. A 38-year-old divorced man presents to the outpatient clinic. He reports that the only way he can attain sexual arousal and gratification is by dressing in women's clothes. He also reports that even his fantasies involve cross-dressing. He admits that his wife has frequently caught him wearing her clothes and that was one of the reasons she divorced him. What condition does this person have?

   A. Gender identity disorder
   B. Transvestic fetishism
   C. Exhibitionism
   D. Fetishism
   E. None of the above

18. Which of the following is characteristic of gender identity disorder?

   A. The person's repeated desire to be, or insistence that he or she is, of the opposite sex
   B. Persistent fantasies of being the other sex
   C. Intense desire to participate in the past experiences of the other sex
   D. Preference for playmates of the other sex during childhood
   E. All of the above

19. A 27-year-old prisoner serving time in a correctional facility for a sexual offense is seen by a psychiatrist. He reports that he gets intense sexual arousal from rubbing his genital area against the bodies of members of the opposite sex. What is the condition he describes called?

   A. Exhibitionism
   B. Frotteurism
   C. Fetishism
   D. Sadism
   E. None of the above

20. Which of the following is true regarding pedophilia?

   A. The person with this disorder has recurrent sexually arousing fantasies, urges, or behavior involving sexual activity with a prepubescent child or children.
   B. This behavior leads to frequent social and legal problems.
   C. For a diagnosis of pedophilia, the perpetrator should be at least 16 years old and 5 years older than the child or children involved in the sexual activity.
   D. There are two forms of pedophilia: exclusive and nonexclusive.
   E. All of the above

21. Which of the following is true about sexual masochism?

A. The masochistic person has recurrent intense sexually arousing fantasies, urges, or behaviors involving the act of being humiliated, beaten, bound, or made to suffer in other ways.

B. It can involve being pinned and pierced.

C. Hypoxyphilia can lead to accidental death.

D. It can involve having the wish to be treated as an infant and dressed in diapers.

E. All of the above

22. What is klismaphilia?

A. Use of enemas to get sexual arousal

B. Sexual arousal by defecating on a partner

C. Concentrating sexual activity on one part of the body and excluding the rest of the body

D. Scatalogia

E. None of the above

23. Which of the following is used to treat sexual offenders?

A. Medroxyprogesterone

B. Fluoxetine

C. Cognitive-behavioral therapy

D. Leuprolide

E. All of the above

24. Which of the following substances of abuse can lead to sexual dysfunction?

A. Alcohol

B. Cocaine

C. Opioids

D. Amphetamines

E. All of the above

25. Which of the following is true regarding the epidemiology of homosexuality in United States?

A. Homosexual orientation is reported by 2.8% of men surveyed.

B. Homosexual orientation is reported by 1.4% of women surveyed.

C. Nine percent of men surveyed report having had at least one homosexual experience as an adult.

D. Five percent of women surveyed report having had at least one homosexual experience as an adult.

E. All of the above

26. When did the American Psychiatric Association remove homosexuality from the list of mental disorders?

    A. 1953

    B. 1963

    C. 1973

    D. 1983

    E. 1993

ANSWERS

1. **Answer: E.** The majority of the patients with bulimia nervosa remain within the normal weight range. Bulimia is associated with an increased incidence of depression, anxiety, and substance abuse. Enlargement of the parotid gland is common in bulimics and is associated with elevated serum amylase. Repeated vomiting can lead to erosion of the teeth by constant exposure of the enamel to gastric juices.

2. **Answer: A.** Patients with bulimia nervosa frequently induce vomiting by putting their fingers in their throats. This leads to scarring and calluses over the knuckles of the hand, which is known as Russell's sign.

3. **Answer: C.** Binge eating disorders are characterized by frequent episodes of binging (eating in a short time, say a 2-hour period, a large amount of food that is more than most people can or will eat). During these episodes patients have a sense of lack of control over eating and they report that they are unable to stop eating. According to the diagnostic criteria, episodes occur at least 2 days a week for 6 months and are not associated with purging behavior.

4. **Answer: B.** Persons with anorexia nervosa characteristically refuse to maintain body weight above the low normal for age and height. They have an intense fear of gaining weight or becoming fat. The body weight is kept at less than 85% of the weight that is considered normal for age and height. Body mass index is usually less than 17.5. Eating disorders in general are more prevalent among females and in Western cultures.

5. **Answer: E.** Amenorrhea, which is defined as absence of three consecutive menstrual cycles, is one of the pathognomonic features of females suffering from anorexia nervosa. It is due to the decreased secretion of gonadotropin-releasing hormone (GnRH). Decreased secretion of GnRH also leads to decreased secretion of FSH, LH, and estrogen.

6. **Answer: E.** The following medical complications are associated with anorexia nervosa: leucopenia, hypokalemic alkalosis, electrolyte disturbances, cardiac arrhythmia, loss of cardiac muscle, fatty degeneration of the liver, elevated serum cholesterol levels, and amenorrhea. Lanugo is the fine, babylike hair present all over the body of anorexics.

7. **Answer: D.** Patients with bulimia ingest ipecac to induce vomiting. Ipecac toxicity can lead to cardiomyopathy.

8. Answer: B. The following are considered good prognostic indicators in eating disorder patients: early age of onset (before 18), no previous hospitalization for the illness, and no purging behavior. Presence of parents who are willing to come for family therapy is also considered a good prognostic indicator.

9. Answer: D. Cognitive-behavioral therapy (CBT) is considered the first-line treatment for bulimia nervosa. It has been shown that at least 40% to 50% of patients receiving CBT abstain from binge eating and purging at the end of 16 to 20 weeks of the therapy. Antidepressants have also been used in the treatment of bulimia. The dosage is the same as that used for treatment of depression.

10. Answer: E. The incidence of bulimia nervosa and anorexia nervosa has been shown to be increasing in the last 50 years. Both these disorders are more prevalent in Western cultures. The female-to-male ratio in eating disorders ranges from 10:1 to 20:1. Bulimia has a prevalence of 1%. Anorexics have a mortality rate of 5–15%. Bulimics have a lower mortality rate, 0–3%.

11. Answer: E. Patients suffering from anorexia nervosa have been shown to have a high comorbidity of major depression, obsessive-compulsive disorder, social anxiety, and decreased sexual interest. Patients with comorbid obsessive-compulsive disorder develop that disorder after the onset of anorexia.

12. Answer: D. It has been shown that half of the patients with anorexia nervosa eventually develop signs of bulimia.

13. Answer: B. Substance abuse is common in patients with bulimia nervosa. Alcohol is the most commonly abused substance in this group of patients. Patients with bulimia are also known to abuse amphetamines to reduce their appetites.

14. Answer: E. Treatment of anorexia nervosa involves a multidisciplinary approach including medical management of the complications, psychoeducation, cognitive-behavioral therapy, and pharmacotherapy. The best use of medications is as an adjunct to psychoeducation and CBT. The medications that have been found useful in the treatment of anorexia nervosa are chlorpromazine, fluoxetine, and cyprohepatidine.

15. Answer: C. Anorexia nervosa has two peak times of onset. The first is between ages of 14 and 15. The second peak is at 18 years of age. However, anorexia has also been reported in prepubescent females and postmenopausal females.

16. Answer: A. Fetishism involves the use of nonliving objects (fetishes) to attain sexual arousal and gratification. It usually involves focusing on items like women's lingerie, shoes, stockings, or gloves. The fetish is strongly preferred or required for sexual gratification. The disorder usually does not involve cross-dressing.

17. Answer: B. Transvestic fetishism involves cross-dressing. This is more prevalent in males. The person dresses in the clothes of the opposite sex to attain sexual arousal. The person is almost always heterosexual and over the past 6 months has had recurrent fantasies or sexual urges and behavior involving cross-dressing.

18. Answer: E. Gender identity disorder is characterized by a person's strong and persistent desire to belong to the other sex or insistence that he or she belongs to the other sex. Men with this disorder have a preference for female attire, and women have a strong preference for male attire. The person also reports having persistent discomfort with his or her sex.

19. Answer: B. Frotteurism involves sexual arousal by rubbing the genital areas against or by fondling a nonconsenting person. For a diagnosis according to DSM-IV, this behavior has to be present consistently for 6 months. Peak onset occurs in young men between 15 to 25 years of age; incidence declines in the population older than 25.

20. Answer: E. Pedophilia is characterized by recurrent fantasies, urges, and behaviors involving sexual activity with a prepubescent child or children. The perpetrator is at least 16 years of age and 5 years older than the victim. Pedophilia is either of the exclusive type, in which the person is attracted only to children, or the nonexclusive type.

21. Answer: E. Sexual masochism involves attaining sexual arousal and gratification by being humiliated, beaten, bound, or made to suffer in other ways. Among the methods used are self-mutilation, blindfolding, paddling, spanking, whipping, being urinated or defecated upon, and forced cross-dressing. Infantilism involves the desire to be treated as an infant and dressed in diapers. Hypoxyphilia involves sexual arousal by deprivation of oxygen by noose, ligature, plastic bag, or nitrites. Hypoxyphilia can lead to accidental death.

22. Answer: A. Klismaphilia is the use of enemas to achieve sexual arousal. Coprophilia, interest in feces, in some individuals is associated with attaining sexual pleasure by defecating on a partner. Partialism involves concentrating sexual activity on one part of the body and excluding other parts totally. Telephone scatalogia involves making obscene telephone calls to attain sexual arousal.

23. Answer: E. Medroxyprogesterone and leuprolide can be used to reduce sexual drive. SSRIs can also reduce craving for sexual expression. Sexual offenders do not have the skills necessary for maintaining a regular sexual relationship. Cognitive-behavioral therapy is useful in treating sexual offenders.

24. Answer: E. For a diagnosis of substance-induced sexual function to be made, the dysfunction should occur during or within 1 month following substance indication. There should also be evidence from history, physical examination, and laboratory findings that the substance caused the sexual dysfunction. The following substances are known to cause sexual dysfunction: alcohol, amphetamines, cocaine, opioids, sedatives, hypnotics, and anxiolytics.

25. Answer: E. In a study conducted by University of Chicago, 2.8% of the men and 1.4% of the women who were surveyed reported homosexual orientation; 9% of men and 5% of women reported that they had at least one homosexual experience as an adult.

26. Answer: C. It was in 1973 that the American Psychiatric Association removed homosexuality from the Diagnostic and Statistical Manual (DSM).

Chapter 11
MENTAL RETARDATION

QUESTIONS

1. Which of the following criteria is required for a diagnosis of mental retardation to be made?
   A. Onset before age 16
   B. Onset before age 18
   C. Deficit in at least one area of adaptive functioning
   D. IQ below 90
   E. Absence of a mental illness

2. What is the mental age of an adult with moderate mental retardation?
   A. 3 years or less
   B. 6 years or less
   C. 9 years or less
   D. 12 years or less
   E. 15 years or less

3. Which of the following is true about mild mental retardation?
   A. It is diagnosed in persons with IQ less than 70 but more than 55.
   B. Persons with this condition can only perform simple elementary tasks.
   C. Most persons with this condition live in supported supervised care settings.
   D. Persons with mild retardation constitute about 3–4% of those classified as mentally retarded.
   E. Persons with this condition never learn to read or write.

4. Which of the following conditions has an increased prevalence in persons with mental retardation?

    A. Visual impairment

    B. Speech impediment

    C. Hearing difficulty

    D. Cerebral palsy

    E. All of the above

5. What proportion of persons with severe mental condition have a seizure disorder?

    A. 5%

    B. 15%

    C. 25%

    D. 33%

    E. 75%

6. What is the single most common cause of mental retardation?

    A. Fragile-X syndrome

    B. Down syndrome

    C. CNS trauma

    D. Edward syndrome

    E. Alcoholism in the mother

7. Which of the following is not a feature of Down syndrome?

    A. Hypothyroidism

    B. Atlantoaxial instability

    C. Long, thin hands

    D. Early dementia

    E. Oblique palpebral fissures

8. Which of the following is not seen in fragile-X syndrome?

    A. Large head

    B. Short stature

    C. Hyperextensible joints

    D. Macro-orchidism

    E. Catlike cry

9. Which of the following is a characteristic feature of Prader-Willi syndrome?
   A. Anorexia
   B. Compulsive eating behavior
   C. Tall stature
   D. Hypertonic muscles
   E. Large hands and feet

10. Which of the following is not a feature of Rett disorder?
   A. Deterioration in communication skills
   B. Autistic traits
   C. Characteristic hand movements
   D. Equal prevalence in males and females
   E. Increased incidence of seizure disorder

11. Which of the following is a characteristic feature of Lesch-Nyhan syndrome?
   A. Macrocephaly
   B. Micrognathia
   C. Self-mutilation
   D. Compulsive overeating
   E. Café au lait spots

12. Severe mental retardation is seen in which of the following conditions?
   A. Wilson disease
   B. Prader-Willi syndrome
   C. Klinefelter syndrome
   D. Thalassemia
   E. Turner syndrome

13. Which of the following is not a feature of Asperger syndrome?
   A. Stilted speech
   B. Eccentric lifestyle
   C. Above average intelligence
   D. Unusual speech
   E. Restricted interests and behaviors

14. Which of the following conditions is less common in patients with mental retardation than in the general population?
- **A.** Anxiety
- **B.** Behavioral problems
- **C.** Schizophrenia
- **D.** Anorexia nervosa
- **E.** Epilepsy

15. Which of the following is *not* true regarding seizure disorder in patients with mental retardation?
- **A.** It is difficult to control.
- **B.** It frequently causes schizophreniform psychosis.
- **C.** It causes intellectual deterioration.
- **D.** It usually requires more than one drug for adequate control.
- **E.** It rarely results in violence.

16. Which of the following may cause loss of skills in a person with Down syndrome?
- **A.** Depression
- **B.** Hypothyroidism
- **C.** Dementia
- **D.** Hearing loss
- **E.** All of the above

17. Which of the following is true regarding children with mental retardation?
- **A.** They are at the same risk of being abused as children with normal intelligence.
- **B.** They can be harmed by sex education.
- **C.** They cannot benefit from psychotherapy.
- **D.** They may not disclose whether they have been abused.
- **E.** They should be discouraged from relating their abusive experiences.

18. Which of the following is not a feature of sexual abuse in children with mental retardation?
- **A.** It can increase disruptive behavior.
- **B.** It can result in stereotyped behaviors.
- **C.** It presents in the same way as in children without mental retardation.
- **D.** It can result in regression of abilities.
- **E.** It can result in sophisticated sexualized behaviors.

19. All of the following are depressive features in persons with mental retardation *except*

A. Increased self-injury

B. Diurnal behavioral changes

C. Talking to self and laughing

D. Crying

E. Appetite disturbance

20. Which of the following is true regarding the interview of patients with mental retardation?

A. The interview should begin with leading questions.

B. Yes/no questions should be used.

C. Diagnostic overshadowing is a useful technique.

D. Use of pen and paper is helpful.

E. The interview should be terminated in as short a time as possible.

21. In the treatment of aggression and behavior problems in patients with mental retardation, all of the following are true *except*

A. A multidisciplinary approach is the most useful.

B. Treatment may be provided in an inpatient or outpatient setting.

C. Pharmacotherapy should be avoided.

D. Simultaneous introduction of two treatment modalities should be avoided.

E. Treatment depends on the underlying etiology.

22. Which of the following is true of Asperger syndrome?

A. Onset is after age 3 years.

B. Nonverbal deficits are more common than verbal deficits.

C. Relatives have an increased risk of schizophrenia.

D. Motor coordination problems may be seen.

E. Speech acquisition is normal.

23. Which of the following statements is true regarding Asperger syndrome?

A. It can easily be differentiated from autism.

B. It is less common than classic autism.

C. It has a major genetic component.

D. It resolves in adulthood.

E. It is associated with delayed cognitive development.

24. What is the approximate proportion of persons with Down syndrome who have neurofibrillary tangles in the brain by the age of 50?

    A. 5%

    B. 35%

    C. 50%

    D. 75%

    E. 100%

25. What is the most common reason for psychiatric consultation in patients with mental retardation?

    A. Anxiety

    B. Aggression

    C. Depression

    D. Psychosis

ANSWERS

1. **Answer: B.** Mental retardation is characterized by significantly subaverage intellectual functioning, with IQ approximately 70 or below, onset before age 18 years, and concurrent deficits in or impairment of functioning. The essential feature of mental retardation is significantly below-average general intellectual functioning that is accompanied by significant limitations in adaptive functioning in at least two of the following skill areas: communication, self-care, home living, social interpersonal skills, use of community resources, self-direction, functional academic skills, work, leisure, health, and safety.

2. **Answer: C.** Persons with mental retardation that is categorized by DSM-IV as moderate have the mental age of a 9-year-old; persons with Down syndrome function at this level. Moderate mental retardation constitutes about 10% of cases of mental retardation. Most individuals with this level of mental retardation acquire communication skills during early childhood years. They profit from vocational training and, with moderate supervision, can attend to their own personal care. They can also benefit from training in social and occupational skills and may learn to travel independently in familiar places. During adolescence their difficulties in recognizing social conventions may interfere with peer relationships. In their adult years the majority are able to perform unskilled or semiskilled work under supervision in sheltered workshops or in the general workforce. They adapt well to life in the community, usually in supervised settings.

3. **Answer: A.** Persons with mild mental retardation have an IQ of 55 to 70. Eighty-five percent of persons with mental retardation are in this category. They typically develop social and communication skills during the preschool years, have minimal sensorimotor impairment, and often are not distinguishable from children without mental retardation until a later age. By their late teens, they can acquire academic skills up to approximately the sixth grade level. During their adult years they usually achieve social and vocational skills adequate for minimum self-support but may need supervision, guidance, and assistance especially when under unusual social or economics stress. With appropriate supports, individuals with mild mental retardation can usually live successfully in the community either independently or in supervised settings.

4. **Answer: E.** All of the conditions mentioned have an increased prevalence in those with mental retardation. In addition, psychiatric conditions like ADHD, anxiety disorders, and psychosis are also more common than in the general population.

5. **Answer: D.** The prevalence of seizure disorder in those with mental retardation varies with the severity of mental retardation. The prevalence is 15–20% in persons with mild mental retardation, whereas it ranges from 30% to as high as 50% in those with severe retardation.

6. **Answer: B.** Down syndrome is the most common cause of mental retardation. The risk increases with increasing maternal age. Fragile X is the most common inherited cause of mental retardation.

7. **Answer: C.** Down syndrome is characterized by short stature, round skull, brachycephaly, epicanthic folds, Brushfield spots, single palmar crease, high arched palate, protruded tongue, syndactyly, short hands, and atlantoaxial instability. Patients are also prone to develop dementia in their 40s.

8. **Answer: E.** Catlike cry is not a feature of fragile-X syndrome but, rather, a feature of cri-du-chat syndrome, which is caused by deletion of the short arm of chromosome 5. Fragile-X syndrome accounts for half of all the X-linked cases of mental retardation. The genetic abnormalities that characterize this syndrome are caused by abnormal repetition of the trinucleotide CGG at a fragile site on the X chromosome. Persons with fragile-X syndrome have a shorter than average height, macro-orchidism, large head, a high, arched palate, hyperextensible joints, flat feet, inguinal and hiatus hernia, enlarged aortic root, and mitral valve prolapse. Epilepsy may be seen in 25% of individuals.

9. **Answer: B.** The main features of Prader-Willi syndrome are hypotonia, hypogonadism, hypomentia, and obesity. The majority of children have mild to moderate mental retardation. They develop hyperphagia between the ages of 1 and 4. They also manifest developmental delay and hypogenitalism. Other features are small hands and feet, cleft palate, incurved foot, congenital dislocation of the hip, scoliosis, heart disease, and deafness.

10. **Answer: D.** Rett syndrome is seen in females exclusively. A normally developing child begins to slow or regress in her development within the first year or two of life and develops unusual characteristic or stereotyped hand movements. Loss of developmental skill occurs, and head growth decelerates. As individuals with Rett syndrome approach adolescence, they have increased spasticity, scoliosis, bruxism, hyperventilation, apnea, and seizures.

11. **Answer: C.** Eighty-five percent of persons with Lesch-Nyhan syndrome exhibit self-injurious behavior. Lesch-Nyhan syndrome is an X-linked recessive condition. Infants with Lesch-Nyhan syndrome develop hypertonia, spasticity, ataxia, and choreoathetosis. Most children who are affected have severe mental retardation, and half of them develop seizures. Microcephaly and macrognathia may be present. They also show physical and verbal aggression.

12. Answer: B. Some children with Prader-Willi syndrome have severe mental retardation, although the majority of children affected have mild to moderate mental retardation. The other conditions mentioned are not typically associated with severe mental retardation.

13. Answer: C. The essential features of Asperger syndrome are severe and sustained impairment of social interaction and the development of restricted, repetitive patterns of behavior, interests, and activities. In the early development of a child with Asperger syndrome there is no significant delay in acquisition of spoken or receptive language or in cognitive development or self-help skills. Children with Asperger syndrome often exhibit an eccentric social lifestyle, as opposed to the passive, aloof style in autism. Certain aspects of communication may become deviant over time; for example, poor prosody, unusual rate of speech, and other deviances may be shown. Cognitive functions may be characterized by areas of relative strength (auditory and verbal skills and rote learning) and areas of weakness (visuo-motor and visuoperceptual skills).

14. Answer: D. Anorexia nervosa is not commonly seen in persons with mental retardation.

15. Answer: B. Seizure disorder with mental retardation does not frequently cause schizophreniform psychosis. Seizure disorder is common in persons with mental retardation. It is difficult to control and may require treatment with more than one medication. Over time, the seizures can accelerate the person's intellectual deterioration. The seizures per se rarely result in violence.

16. Answer: E. Various conditions can present as loss of skills in persons with mental retardation, including depression, psychosis, anxiety, dementia, and physical conditions, including hypothyroidism, pain, and hearing and visual loss.

17. Answer: D. Children with mental retardation may not disclose sexual abuse because of the inability to verbalize, lack of understanding, or fear. They are at high risk of sexual abuse. People with mental retardation do benefit from psychotherapy and should not be discouraged from relating their abusive experiences.

18. Answer: C. Sexual abuse of children with mental retardation can present as increase in disruptive behavior, stereotyped movements, depression, or anxiety. It can also result in regression of abilities or sophisticated or new sexualized behaviors.

19. Answer: C. Depression in people with mental retardation may present with increase in self-injury, diurnal behavioral changes, crying, increased tearfulness, psychomotor retardation, self-absorption, loss of interest in usual activities, and disturbance of sleep and appetite. Depressive moods may not be verbalized. Talking to self and laughing is more likely to suggest psychosis.

20. Answer: D. Special interviewing techniques may need to be used for persons with mental retardation. The interview should begin with open questions. Questions of either/or variety are particularly helpful. The use of pen and paper by the patient to write or draw is helpful. Interviewees should be given a longer than usual time because of their mental retardation and should not be hurried through the interview.

21. Answer: C. Pharmacotherapy *does* have a very useful role in the treatment of aggressive behavior. A multidisciplinary approach is best. A combination of pharmacotherapy and behavioral intervention is often the most helpful. Treatment should be based on a search for underlying causes. It can be done with the patient as an inpatient or an outpatient basis.

22. Answer: D. Some patients with Asperger syndrome are clumsy and have problems with motor coordination. Verbal deficits are more common than nonverbal deficits. Relatives are not at increased risk of schizophrenia.

23. Answer: C. Asperger syndrome has a major genetic component. It is difficult to distinguish from autism and is more prevalent than classic autism. It continues into adulthood and is not associated with cognitive impairment.

24. Answer: E. Almost everyone with Down syndrome has neurofibrillary tangles by the age of 50.

25. Answer: B. Aggression is the most common reason that psychiatric consultation is sought for individuals among the mentally retarded population. The other conditions mentioned are also more common in the mentally retarded population than in the general population.

Chapter 12

SLEEP DISORDERS

QUESTIONS

1. The following are true about night terrors *except*
   A. Episodes occur during stage 2 sleep.
   B. It is a dissociative state.
   C. Violent behavior may occur.
   D. Family history is rarely seen.
   E. The person with night terrors usually has no recollection of the events.

2. Which of the following is true regarding somnambulism?
   A. It occurs toward early morning.
   B. It is never familial.
   C. It occurs during stage 3 and stage 4 sleep.
   D. Criminal activity is common.
   E. It is most common between the ages of 5 and 12 years.

3. Which of the following is true regarding nightmares?
   A. Incidence is most common between the ages of 10 and 12 years.
   B. They occur during REM sleep.
   C. Nightmares can be caused by anxiety.
   D. The person experiencing nightmares has no recollection of the dreams.
   E. Persons subject to nightmares commonly sleepwalk after the nightmares.

4. Which of the following is true regarding narcolepsy?
   A. It begins in middle age.
   B. It is more prevalent among women than men.
   C. There is commonly a family history of narcolepsy.
   D. It is associated with HLA DR2.
   E. It is not commonly associated with cataplexy.

5. Which of the following is used to diagnose narcolepsy?
   A. Multiple Sleep Latency Test
   B. Dexamethasone suppression test
   C. NPT
   D. Waking the patient
   E. Observing the patient's response to ECT

6. Which of the following medications has been found to be particularly effective for treating insomnia associated with depression?
   A. Sertraline
   B. Mirtazepine
   C. Trazodone
   D. Venlafaxine
   E. Escitalopram

7. Which of the following is a characteristic feature of REM sleep?
   A. Loss of muscle tone
   B. K complexes
   C. Sleep spindles
   D. Alpha activity on EEG
   E. Onset 30 minutes after sleep onset

8. All the following are true about sleep in depression *except*
   A. Slow-wave sleep is increased.
   B. REM sleep rebound occurs after stopping treatment.
   C. Antidepressants disturb REM sleep.
   D. There is shortened REM latency.
   E. REM activity in the first half of the night is increased.

9. All of the following are true of stage 2 sleep *except*
   A. It accounts for 24% of total sleep.
   B. K complexes occur.
   C. Benzodiazepines promote this stage of sleep.
   D. Sleep spindles occur.
   E. Delta waves occur.

10. All of the following are true about psychophysiologic insomnia *except*

A. The condition typically begins in early adulthood.

B. Stress precipitates psychophysiologic insomnia.

C. Persons with this condition do not have any obvious psychiatry disorder.

D. This condition accounts for 50% of cases seen at a sleep center.

E. There is a possible genetic contribution.

ANSWERS

1. **Answer: A.** Night terrors occur in stage 4 sleep (deep sleep). Peak incidence is between 4 and 7 years of age. The child wakes up from sleep in a terrified state, does not respond when spoken to, and does not appear to see objects or people. Instead the child appears to be hallucinating and may be talking to and looking at people or things that are not actually present. This behavior may continue for up to 15 minutes, during which time the child does not respond to comforting. Eventually, the child goes back to sleep, and upon awaking, has no recollection of the events.

2. **Answer: C.** Somnambulism, or sleepwalking, typically occurs between the ages of 8 and 14 years. It occurs in stage 3 or 4 of sleep. The child arises calmly from bed with a blank facial expression and cannot be awakened without difficulty. Criminal activity is uncommon. The condition may be familial.

3. **Answer: B.** Nightmares occur during REM sleep. They are unlike night terrors in that the child can be awakened and has a clear recollection of the events. Daytime anxieties and frightening television programs may be contributory.

4. **Answer: D.** Narcolepsy is associated with HLA DR2 in up to 99% of cases. Onset is typically in the early 20s, and it affects men and women equally. Very rarely is there a family history of narcolepsy in a narcoleptic patient. Cataplexy is seen in up to 90% of patients with narcolepsy.

5. **Answer: A.** Diagnosis can be confirmed by means of the Multiple Sleep Latency Test. Narcolepsy is a tetrad of features: hypersomnolence is found in 100% of cases, cataplexy in 90%, sleep paralysis in 40%, and hypnogogic hallucinations in 30%. At least 50% of persons with narcolepsy also have a major affective disorder or personality problems. Honda et al. (1983) described the association between narcolepsy and HLA DR2, which they found to be positive in 99% of patients. First-degree relatives have a 40-fold higher chance of having the illness than the general population. Sleep attacks are irresistible and usually occur in boring situations. Diagnosis is usually delayed, and the quality of life in these patients is very poor. Treatment includes psychostimulants (methylphenidate and amphetamine) and sedatives (if paradoxically disrupted nocturnal sleep occurs). Cataplexy is treated with tricyclic antidepressants.

6. **Answer: C.** Almost all the antidepressants suppress REM sleep to some extent. Most of the antidepressants help sleep disturbances secondary to depression. Trazodone has been found to be particularly effective in treatment of sleep disturbances associated with depression.

7. Answer: A. Loss of muscle tone is a characteristic feature of REM (rapid eye movement) sleep, also known as paradoxical sleep, which typically starts 90 to 120 minutes after the onset of sleep and then alternates with periods of non-REM sleep in the sleep cycle. It is during REM sleep that most dreaming occurs. K complexes and sleep spindles are characteristic of stage 2 sleep. Early REM onset is seen in depression. REM sleep within a few minutes of sleep onset is suggestive of narcolepsy. Alpha activity is not seen in REM sleep.

8. Answer: A. In depression, patients complain of lack of sleep, early morning awakening, and not feeling refreshed by sleep. Sleep studies show shortened REM latency, increase in REM sleep, and decreased slow-wave deep sleep. Most of the antidepressants suppress REM sleep.

9. Answer: A. Stage 2 is a physiologic stage of sleep that typically accounts for 40% to 50% of the total sleep time. Benzodiazepines promote stage 2 at the expense of stages 3 and 4. Stage 2 is characterized by sleep spindles and K complexes.

10. Answer: D. Psychophysiologic insomnia accounts for about 15% of the cases seen at any sleep center. It typically starts in the early 20s and may persist for decades. Stress seems to precipitate it and the insomnia persists long after the stressor is overcome. Persons with psychophysiologic insomnia do not have any obvious psychiatric disorders. Their anxiety is mainly associated with their preoccupation about the insomnia and not about other areas of life. First-degree relatives of persons with this sleep disturbance also have sleep problems, which suggests a possible genetic contribution.

Chapter 13

PERSONALITY DISORDERS

QUESTIONS

1. A 55-year-old woman lives on her own. She wears odd clothes and pokes around in her neighbors' garbage cans. She claims to have psychic powers but does not report hearing voices. What is the most likely diagnosis for her condition?

    A. Schizoid personality disorder

    B. Schizotypal personality disorder

    C. Asperger syndrome

    D. Avoidant personality disorder

2. Which of the following is true about personality disorders?

    A. They rarely cause subjective distress.

    B. They mellow with age.

    C. They respond well to treatment.

    D. They cause little or no impairment in functioning.

3. Which of the following is true of borderline personality disorder?

    A. It is less common than antisocial personality disorder.

    B. The majority of persons with this disorder are female.

    C. The rate of suicide in persons with borderline personality disorder is the same as that of the general population.

    D. Antidepressants are the treatment of choice.

4. Which of the following is common in the childhood history of patients with borderline personality disorder?

    A. Shyness

    B. Psychosis

    C. Conduct disorder

    D. Sexual abuse

    E. Magical and odd beliefs

5. A 25-year-old woman begins to see a therapist because of loneliness and feelings of being unloved and unwanted with some mild depressive symptoms. She flirts constantly with the therapist and is hurt when the therapist does not reciprocate. Which of the following disorders is she is most likely to have?

    A. Antisocial personality disorder

    B. Borderline personality disorder

    C. Schizotypal personality disorder

    D. Obsessive-compulsive personality disorder

    E. Histrionic personality disorder

6. Which of the following is characteristic of persons with paranoid personality disorder?

    A. Obsession

    B. Psychotic behavior

    C. Litigiousness

    D. Anxiety

7. With which of the following personality disorders is social phobia most likely to be confused?

    A. Avoidant

    B. Dependent

    C. Schizoid

    D. Paranoid

8. Which of the following is true regarding factitious disorder?

    A. The goal of the person exhibiting the symptoms is to avoid unpleasant consequences at work.

    B. It is easily diagnosed.

    C. It is the same as malingering.

    D. The goal of the person exhibiting the symptoms is to assume the sick role.

9. Which of the following is true regarding narcissistic personality disorder?

    A. Narcissistic traits are common in adolescents.

    B. It is more common in females.

    C. Individuals with narcissistic personality disorder have very high self-esteem.

    D. Individuals with this disorder are good at empathizing with others.

10. For which of the following purposes is the Thematic Apperception Test (TAT) most useful?

    A. As an aid in the differential diagnosis

    B. In assessment of motivational variables

    C. In assessment of a patient's intellectual level

    D. In assessment of the risk of suicide in a patient

ANSWERS

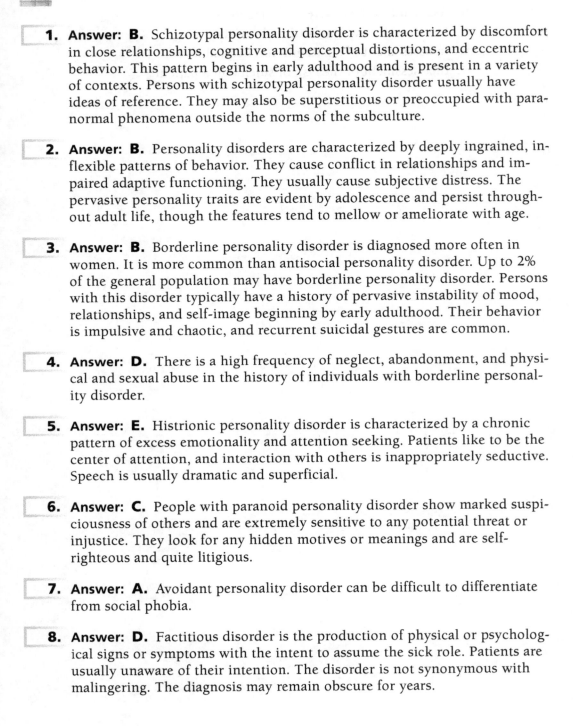

1. **Answer: B.** Schizotypal personality disorder is characterized by discomfort in close relationships, cognitive and perceptual distortions, and eccentric behavior. This pattern begins in early adulthood and is present in a variety of contexts. Persons with schizotypal personality disorder usually have ideas of reference. They may also be superstitious or preoccupied with paranormal phenomena outside the norms of the subculture.

2. **Answer: B.** Personality disorders are characterized by deeply ingrained, inflexible patterns of behavior. They cause conflict in relationships and impaired adaptive functioning. They usually cause subjective distress. The pervasive personality traits are evident by adolescence and persist throughout adult life, though the features tend to mellow or ameliorate with age.

3. **Answer: B.** Borderline personality disorder is diagnosed more often in women. It is more common than antisocial personality disorder. Up to 2% of the general population may have borderline personality disorder. Persons with this disorder typically have a history of pervasive instability of mood, relationships, and self-image beginning by early adulthood. Their behavior is impulsive and chaotic, and recurrent suicidal gestures are common.

4. **Answer: D.** There is a high frequency of neglect, abandonment, and physical and sexual abuse in the history of individuals with borderline personality disorder.

5. **Answer: E.** Histrionic personality disorder is characterized by a chronic pattern of excess emotionality and attention seeking. Patients like to be the center of attention, and interaction with others is inappropriately seductive. Speech is usually dramatic and superficial.

6. **Answer: C.** People with paranoid personality disorder show marked suspiciousness of others and are extremely sensitive to any potential threat or injustice. They look for any hidden motives or meanings and are self-righteous and quite litigious.

7. **Answer: A.** Avoidant personality disorder can be difficult to differentiate from social phobia.

8. **Answer: D.** Factitious disorder is the production of physical or psychological signs or symptoms with the intent to assume the sick role. Patients are usually unaware of their intention. The disorder is not synonymous with malingering. The diagnosis may remain obscure for years.

9. Answer: A. Narcissistic traits are common in adolescence, but most individuals do not progress to develop a personality disorder. Narcissistic personality disorder is characterized by a pervasive pattern of grandiosity, need for admiration, and lack of empathy. The prevalence is less than 1% of the general population. Persons with this disorder have a very vulnerable sense of self, and criticism leaves them unfeeling degraded and shallow.

10. Answer: B. The Thematic Apperception Test (TAT) is most useful in assessing motivational variables. It provides a case study exploration of a person's personality.

Chapter 14

PSYCHOPHARMACOLOGY

QUESTIONS

1. All of the following are true *except*
   A. Gastric emptying is delayed by MAOIs.
   B. Food increases the absorption of diazepam.
   C. Drugs must be ionized to be absorbed by passive diffusion.
   D. In an acid pH, basic drugs will be poorly absorbed.
   E. Rectal administration avoids first-pass metabolism.

2. Which of the following is true about receptors?
   A. 5-HT2A antagonists improve REM sleep.
   B. 5-HT1A antagonists are anxiolytic.
   C. Most antipsychotics are D2 antagonists.
   D. D2 receptors are found in the limbic system.
   E. Alpha-2 adrenergic antagonists can cause reduced norepinephrine release.

3. What is the term for the process of hepatic extraction of orally administered drugs before they reach systemic circulation?
   A. Clearance
   B. Elimination rate constant
   C. First-pass effect
   D. Half-life
   E. Steady state

4. Which of the following is true about lipophilic drugs?
   A. They are slowly absorbed.
   B. They have a large volume of distribution.
   C. They have a low first-pass aspect.
   D. They cross the blood–brain barrier very slowly.
   E. They are incompletely absorbed.

5. Which of the following can inhibit the cytochrome P-450 system?
- **A.** Alcohol
- **B.** Smoking
- **C.** Anticonvulsants
- **D.** SSRIs
- **E.** Barbiturates

6. All of the following can cause an increase in the plasma drug concentration of tricyclic antidepressants *except*
- **A.** SSRIs
- **B.** Carbamazepine
- **C.** Disulfiram
- **D.** Methadone
- **E.** Methylphenidate

7. All of the following in combination with MAOIs can cause serotonin syndrome *except*
- **A.** L-tryptophan
- **B.** Fluoxetine
- **C.** Clomipramine
- **D.** Tyramine
- **E.** St. John's wort

8. Which of the following is not a lipophilic drug?
- **A.** Lithium
- **B.** Haloperidol
- **C.** Nortryptiline
- **D.** Propranolol
- **E.** Diazepam

9. All of the following are precursors of monoamines *except*
- **A.** 5-hydroxytryptophan
- **B.** Dihydroxyphenyl alanine
- **C.** 5-hydroxydopamine
- **D.** 5-hydroxytryptamine
- **E.** L-tryptophan

10. Which of the following is not a function mediated by serotonin?

    A. Aggressive behavior

    B. Sleep

    C. Problem-solving behavior

    D. Weight gain

    E. Sexual behavior

11. Which of the following is a precursor of norepinephrine?

    A. Serotonin

    B. Epinephrine

    C. Acetylcholine

    D. Dopamine

12. With which of the following is cholestatic jaundice most commonly seen?

    A. Lithium

    B. Chlordiazepoxide

    C. Chlorpromazine

    D. Fluoxetine

    E. Amitryptiline

13. Which of the following mediates hypotension following chlorpromazine use?

    A. Depression of the respiratory center

    B. Ionotropic effect on heart

    C. Alpha-adrenergic blocking effect

    D. H1 (histamine) blocking effect

    E. Alpha-adrenergic agonist effect

14. Which of the following drugs is useful as an antiemetic?

    A. Naloxone

    B. Tetracycline

    C. Caffeine

    D. Epinephrine

    E. Chlorpromazine

15. The elimination of which of the following benzodiazepines is not influenced by liver disease?

   A. Midazolam

   B. Alprazolam

   C. Chlordiazepoxide

   D. Lorazepam

   E. Diazepam

16. At which of the following receptors do benzodiazepines act?

   A. GABA-B receptor

   B. 5-HT1A receptor

   C. GABA-A receptor

   D. D2 (Dopamine)

   E. Chloride channels

17. What was the first benzodiazepine to be used in treatment of patients?

   A. Diazepam

   B. Lorazepam

   C. Temazepam

   D. Chlordiazepoxide

   E. Nitrazepam

18. Which of the following is true about diazepam?

   A. Peak plasma concentrations are reached in 2 to 3 hours.

   B. Intramuscular absorption is faster than oral.

   C. It is highly lipid-soluble.

   D. It is about 50–60% protein bound in the body.

   E. It does not cross the placenta.

19. What is the primary site of metabolism of diazepam?

   A. Kidneys

   B. Liver

   C. Small intestine

   D. Spleen

   E. Body fat

20. Which of the following is not a side effect of benzodiazepines?
   A. Ataxia
   B. Nightmares
   C. Drowsiness
   D. Amnesia
   E. Restlessness

21. Which of the following is not seen with benzodiazepine use?
   A. Induction of hepatic microsomal enzymes
   B. Leucopenia
   C. Esinophilia
   D. Change in plasma cortisol
   E. Respiratory depression

22. Which of the following is true regarding benzodiazepines?
   A. Chlordiazepoxide has a longer half-life than diazepam.
   B. Diazepam is more lipid-soluble than lorazepam.
   C. Lorazepam is more extensively distributed in the body than diazepam.
   D. Temazepam produces active metabolites.

23. Which of the following has the shortest half-life?
   A. Alprazolam
   B. Oxazepam
   C. Temazepam
   D. Flurazepam
   E. Lorazepam

24. Which of the following has active metabolites?
   A. Oxazepam
   B. Chlordiazepoxide
   C. Temazepam
   D. Triazolam
   E. Lorazepam

25. Which of the following is not a symptom of benzodiazepine withdrawal?
    A. Hallucinations
    B. Tremor
    C. Depression
    D. Tinnitus
    E. Depersonalization

26. Which of the following may raise plasma concentrations of benzodiazepines?
    A. Barbiturates
    B. Cimetidine
    C. Phenytoin
    D. Carbamazepine
    E. Rifampicin

27. Which of the following features is not seen in children born to mothers taking benzodiazepines?
    A. Cleft lip
    B. Cleft palate
    C. Respiratory depression
    D. Absent arms and legs
    E. Withdrawal symptoms

28. Which of the following is a feature of the sleep pattern upon benzodiazepine withdrawal?
    A. Decrease in REM sleep
    B. Decreased sleep latency
    C. REM sleep rebound
    D. Increased stage 4 sleep
    E. Suppression of NREM sleep

29. How long does it take for tolerance to benzodiazepines to develop?
    A. 2 days
    B. 2–3 weeks
    C. 1–2 months
    D. 4–6 months
    E. At least 6 months

30. To which of the following can a person taking benzodiazepines have cross-tolerance?

    A. Antipsychotics

    B. SSRIs

    C. MAOIs

    D. Alcohol

    E. Noradrenergic reuptake inhibitors

31. Which of the following is true regarding drug dependence in patients on benzodiazepines?

    A. It is associated with drugs with long half-life.

    B. It is associated with the short duration of treatment.

    C. It is more likely in patients with passive and dependent personality traits.

    D. Symptoms begin 1 to 2 weeks after stopping the drug.

    E. Symptoms usually resolve within a week.

32. With which of the following is lithium administration during pregnancy associated?

    A. Ebstein's anomaly

    B. Depression in the infant

    C. Neural tube defects

    D. Hyperglycemia in the newborn

33. Which of the following drugs can produce ataxia at therapeutic doses?

    A. Imipramine

    B. Carbamazepine

    C. Pimozide

    D. Chlorpromazine

    E. Fluoxetine

34. The presence of benzodiazepine withdrawal as opposed to anxiety is suggested by all of the following *except*

    A. Hyperawareness of senses

    B. Abnormal sense of body movement

    C. Dysphoria

    D. Poor sleep with excess worry

    E. Metallic taste in the mouth

35. Which of the following is an effect of benzodiazepines in therapeutic dosage?
   A. They block the reuptake of amines.
   B. They prevent stress-induced increase in brain metabolism.
   C. They depress the cardiovascular system.
   D. They inhibit monoamine oxidase.
   E. They affect the reticular activating system.

36. Which of the following is not a side effect of benzodiazepines?
   A. Ataxia
   B. Confusional state
   C. Acute dystonia
   D. Aggression
   E. Drowsiness

37. Which of the following is false regarding benzodiazepines?
   A. They potentiate GABA.
   B. They may have hangover effects.
   C. They modulate chloride channel flow.
   D. They are used to abort seizures.
   E. Their effects are antagonized by naloxone.

38. All of the following drugs can cause tremors *except*
   A. Amitriptyline
   B. Diazepam
   C. Lithium
   D. Haloperidol
   E. Phenelzine

39. Which of the following is true about tricyclic antidepressants?
   A. They are safer than ECT in patients with a history of myocardial infarction.
   B. They should be avoided in patients with early cataract.
   C. They cause weight loss.
   D. They potentiate the pressor effect of norepinephrine.
   E. Concurrent antipsychotic administration can attenuate their actions.

40. All of the following are side effects of tricyclic antidepressants *except*
   A. Blurred vision
   B. Tachycardia
   C. Tremors
   D. Impotence
   E. Diarrhea

41. Which of the following is a side effect of tricyclic antidepressants?
   A. Cataract
   B. Hypertension
   C. Hypothyroidism
   D. Xerostomia
   E. Gastric ulcers

42. Which of the following drugs has a therapeutic window?
   A. Amitriptyline
   B. Nortryptiline
   C. Protryptiline
   D. Imipramine
   E. Clomipramine

43. Which of the following is false regarding tricyclic overdose?
   A. Gastric aspiration is helpful.
   B. Antiarrhythmia drugs should be used routinely.
   C. Cardiac monitoring is important.
   D. Convulsions can occur.
   E. Desipramine is the most lethal tricyclic antidepressant.

44. Which of the following is not a contraindication for the use of tricyclic antidepressants?
   A. Narrow-angle glaucoma
   B. Heart block
   C. Previous myocardial infarction 2 years ago
   D. Prostate hypertrophy
   E. Cardiac arrhythmias

45. Which of the following tricyclics is a secondary amine?
    A. Clomipramine
    B. Desipramine
    C. Amitriptyline
    D. Doxepine
    E. Imipramine

46. Which of the following is an effect of using tricyclic antidepressants?
    A. Increase in postsynaptic 5-HT2 activity
    B. Increased cAMP activity
    C. Down-regulation of beta-adrenergic receptors
    D. Increased sensitization of presynaptic 5-HT1A receptors
    E. Blockade of histamine H2 receptors

47. For which condition is the relation strongest between blood concentration monitoring and response to tricyclic antidepressants?
    A. Dysthymia
    B. Minor depression
    C. Depression in outpatients with depression
    D. Depression in inpatients with melancholic depression
    E. Adjustment disorder

48. Which of the following has the most anticholinergic effects?
    A. Clomipramine
    B. Amitriptyline
    C. Nortryptiline
    D. Desipramine
    E. Amoxapine

49. Which of the following is most effective in treating chronic pain?
    A. Citalopram
    B. Fluoxetine
    C. Imipramine
    D. Amitriptyline
    E. Clomipramine

50. Which of the following drugs has the least effect on blood pressure?

    A. Amitriptyline

    B. Clomipramine

    C. Nortryptiline

    D. Imipramine

    E. Desipramine

51. Which tricyclic is most lethal in overdose?

    A. Amitriptyline

    B. Clomipramine

    C. Nortryptiline

    D. Imipramine

    E. Desipramine

52. What is the most effective therapeutic plasma concentration for nortryptiline?

    A. 150–200 ng per ml

    B. 200–250 ng per ml

    C. 50–150 ng per ml

    D. 115–150 ng per ml

    E. 25–50 ng per ml

53. A 46-year-old woman has experienced depressed mood for the past 2 months. However, her appetite has increased, and so has her weight. She reports sleeping up to 15 hours per day. She also has mood reactivity. To which drug is her condition most likely to respond?

    A. Fluoxetine

    B. Phenelzine

    C. Imipramine

    D. Paroxetine

    E. Amitriptyline

54. The antidepressant action of MAOI is mediated through all of the following mechanisms *except*

    A. Down-regulation of beta-adrenergic receptors

    B. Down-regulation of 5-HT2 receptors

    C. Down-regulation of alpha-2 receptors

    D. Inhibition of MAO-A

    E. Inhibition of MAO-B

55. The inability of the patient's body to deaminate which of the following causes the hypertensive crisis seen with MAOIs.

    A. Tryptophan

    B. Leucine

    C. Tyramine

    D. Tyrosine

    E. Tranylcypromine

56. All of the following can cause a hypertensive crisis when taken with MAOIs *except*

    A. Cheese

    B. Banana

    C. Red wine

    D. Yeast extracts

    E. Aged meats

57. A 45-year-old patient who has been receiving treatment with phenelzine for a long time presents with confusion, agitation, and elated mood. On examination, she is sweating and her body temperature is elevated. Her partner reports that she has recently started a new medication for migraines. What does this clinical picture resemble?

    A. Rhabdomyolysis

    B. Neuroleptic malignant syndrome

    C. Respiratory infection

    D. Cheese reaction

    E. Serotonin syndrome

58. When switching from an SSRI to an MAOI, a "washout" period of 2 weeks is recommended for all of the following *except*

    A. Citalopram

    B. Paroxetine

    C. Clomipramine

    D. Fluoxetine

    E. Sertraline

59. All of the following are side effects of MAOIs *except*

    A. Mania

    B. Blurred vision

    C. Seizures

    D. Peripheral neuropathy

    E. Alopecia

60. MAOIs can interact with all of the following *except*

    A. Cough medicines

    B. NSAIDs

    C. Opiates

    D. Clomipramine

    E. Levodopa

61. Which of the following is a contraindication to the use of MAOIs?

    A. Congestive cardiac failure

    B. Concurrent use of tricyclic antidepressants

    C. Pheochromocytoma

    D. Asthma

    E. Concurrent use of calcium antagonists

62. Which of the following is true about mirtazepine?

    A. It does not affect histamine receptors.

    B. It blocks alpha-2 auto receptors.

    C. It has an alerting effect.

    D. It reduces appetite.

    E. It has no effect on the blood.

63. Which of the following is not a side effect of nefazodone?

    A. Somnolence

    B. Hypotension

    C. Nausea

    D. Priapism

    E. Dry mouth

64. Phenelzine has been shown to be more effective than placebo in the treatment of all of the following *except*

    A. Atypical depression

    B. Psychotic depression

    C. Animal phobia

    D. Social phobia

    E. Agoraphobia

65. Which of the following is safe when taken with tranylcypromine?

    A. Pethidine

    B. Quinidine

    C. Methyldopa

    D. Acetaminophen

    E. Ephedrine

66. Which of the following SSRIs has the shortest half-life?

    A. Fluoxetine

    B. Paroxetine

    C. Fluvoxamine

    D. Sertraline

    E. Citalopram

67. How long does it take citalopram to achieve a steady-state plasma level?

    A. 24 hours

    B. 3 days

    C. 7 days

    D. 10 days

    E. 21 days

68. Which of the following is true about SSRIs?

    A. They reach peak levels within 1 hour of ingestion.

    B. Long-term use results in reduced 5-HT function.

    C. Fluoxetine has a half-life of about 2 days.

    D. They should be avoided in patients with cardiac disease.

69. All of the following are side effects of SSRIs *except*

    A. Diarrhea

    B. Constipation

    C. Loss of appetite

    D. Cardiac arrhythmias

    E. Tremors

70. Which of the following is a side effect of SSRIs?

    A. Hypertension

    B. Anorgasmia

    C. Tachycardias

    D. Alopecia

    E. Dry mouth

71. All of the following can be caused by SSRIs *except*
- **A.** Nausea
- **B.** Convulsions
- **C.** Agitation
- **D.** Akathisia
- **E.** Premature ejaculation

72. Which of the following is true about SSRIs?
- **A.** Switching from SSRI to MAOIs has no risks.
- **B.** Fluoxetine has less effect on P-450 enzymes than citalopram.
- **C.** Fluoxetine increases the risk of spontaneous abortion.
- **D.** There is very little data on SSRIs and breastfeeding.
- **E.** Sertraline is the most lethal SSRI in overdose.

73. Which of the following is most likely to cause discontinuation syndrome?
- **A.** Fluoxetine
- **B.** Citalopram
- **C.** Paroxetine
- **D.** Sertraline
- **E.** Fluvoxamine

74. Which of the following pharmacologic differences is important in choosing among different SSRIs?
- **A.** Affinity for sigma opioid receptors
- **B.** Potency in inhibiting 5-HT reuptake
- **C.** Selectivity in inhibiting 5-HT reuptake
- **D.** Potency on dopamine receptors
- **E.** Inhibition of hepatic cytochrome P-450 isoenzyme

75. What is the most common adverse reaction reported with SSRIs?
- **A.** Headache
- **B.** Nausea
- **C.** Diarrhea
- **D.** Tremor
- **E.** Dizziness

76. Which SSRI is most likely to cause delayed ejaculation?
  A. Fluoxetine
  B. Citalopram
  C. Paroxetine
  D. Sertraline
  E. Fluvoxamine

77. Abrupt discontinuation of which of the following SSRIs is *least* likely to cause a discontinuation reaction?
  A. Fluoxetine
  B. Citalopram
  C. Paroxetine
  D. Sertraline
  E. Fluvoxamine

78. At which of the following receptors does trazodone act?
  A. Histamine (H1) receptors
  B. Muscarinic receptors
  C. Alpha-adrenergic receptors
  D. Dopamine receptors
  E. Norepinephrine receptors

79. Which of the following is not a side effect of trazodone?
  A. Priapism
  B. Orthostatic hypotension
  C. Drowsiness
  D. Seizures
  E. Headaches

80. Which of the following is true regarding methadone?
  A. It has to be given twice a day.
  B. It can be given once a week.
  C. Its use results in reduction of criminal activity.
  D. It enhances the euphoriant effects of heroin.
  E. It acts at different receptors to heroin.

81. Which of the following is a side effect of methadone?
   A. Hypertension
   B. Diarrhea
   C. Tachycardia
   D. Respiratory depression
   E. Midriasis

82. What is the most common finding on postmortem examination in people who have died after initiation of methadone treatment?
   A. Myocardial death
   B. Chronic persistent hepatitis
   C. Brain hemorrhage
   D. Pulmonary embolism
   E. GI bleeding

83. Which of the following is associated with LAAM?
   A. Respiratory depression
   B. Renal failure
   C. Cardiac failure
   D. Prolonged QT interval
   E. Hypertension

84. The dose of methadone needs to be higher in patients on all of the following medications *except*
   A. Phenytoin
   B. Carbamazepine
   C. Rifampicin
   D. Phenobarbitone
   E. Erythromycin

85. Where is lithium primarily excreted?
   A. Lungs
   B. Kidneys
   C. Sweat
   D. Feces
   E. Liver

86. Which of the following has been shown to decrease mortality in bipolar disorder?
   A. Divalproex sodium
   B. Carbamazepine
   C. Lithium
   D. Olanzapine
   E. Fluoxetine

87. Which of the following is a good prognostic factor for response to lithium in bipolar disorder?
   A. Rapid-cycling mania
   B. Mixed mania
   C. Episode pattern of depression, mania, euthymia
   D. Episode pattern of mania, depression, euthymia
   E. Comorbid substance use

88. Lithium is used in the treatment of all of the following conditions *except*
   A. Bipolar I disorder
   B. Bipolar II disorder
   C. Depressive disorder
   D. Obsessive-compulsive disorder
   E. Schizoaffective disorder

89. All of the following are neurologic side effects of lithium *except*
   A. Tremor
   B. Aphasia
   C. Changes on the ECG
   D. Seizures
   E. Peripheral neuropathy

90. Which of the following is an indication of lithium toxicity?
   A. Hypothyroidism
   B. Weight gain
   C. Polyuria
   D. Psoriasis
   E. Coarse tremor

91.   What is the treatment for severe lithium intoxication?

   A. Gastric lavage
   B. Activated charcoal
   C. Hemodialysis
   D. Polystyrene sulfonate resin
   E. Correction of dehydration

92.   Which of the following is not a cardiovascular side effect of lithium?

   A. T-wave changes in the ECG
   B. Heart block
   C. Impaired sinus node function
   D. Hypertension
   E. Syncopal episodes

93.   Which of the following does not predispose to lithium toxicity?

   A. Thiazide diuretic
   B. ACE inhibitor
   C. Impaired renal function
   D. Electrolyte imbalance
   E. High-salt diet

94.   Which of the following is not a side effect of lithium?

   A. Hypothyroidism
   B. Weight gain
   C. Hyperparathyroidism
   D. Neutropenia
   E. Erectile dysfunction

95.   Which of the following anti-inflammatory drugs is safe in combination with lithium?

   A. Indomethacin
   B. Diclofenac Na
   C. Aspirin
   D. Naproxen
   E. Piroxicam

96. Orthostatic hypotension is caused by blockade of which of the following receptors?
- A. Alpha-1
- B. 5-HT1
- C. H1
- D. Alpha-2
- E. D3 (Dopamine-3)

97. Which of the following is false regarding the management of lithium overdose?
- A. Emesis or lavage may be used.
- B. Mannitol or urea may be used to increase lithium excretion.
- C. NaCl should be avoided.
- D. Hemodialysis may be needed if patient does not respond to supportive measures.

98. Which of the following factors predicts a good response to carbamazepine in bipolar affective disorder?
- A. History of good response to lithium
- B. Strong family history of bipolar disorder
- C. Bipolar I disorder
- D. Rapid-cycling mania
- E. Unstable episode frequency

99. Carbamazepine can cause all of the following side effects *except*
- A. Sedation
- B. Marked cognitive decline
- C. Ataxia
- D. Diplopia
- E. Peripheral neuropathy

100. Which of the following is not a side effect of carbamazepine?
- A. Thrombocytopenia
- B. Hypernatremia
- C. Elevated LFTs
- D. Water intoxication
- E. Lowering of cholesterol

101. Carbamazepine is contraindicated in all of the following situations *except*
- A. Concurrent therapy with SSRIs
- B. Concurrent therapy with MAOIs
- C. History of bone marrow suppression
- D. Narrow-angle glaucoma
- E. Hypersensitivity to amitriptyline

102. Which of the following can increase the plasma concentration of carbamazepine?
- A. Cimetidine
- B. Erythromycin
- C. Fluoxetine
- D. Phenytoin
- E. Lamotrigine

103. Valproate exerts its effects mainly by acting on which of the following receptors?
- A. 5-HT
- B. Dopamine
- C. Sodium channels
- D. GABA
- E. NMDA

104. Predictors of good response to valproate include all of the following *except*
- A. Rapid-cycling mania
- B. Pure mania
- C. Dysphoric mania
- D. Comorbid substance abuse
- E. Panic attacks

105. Valproate is indicated in all of the following patients *except*
- A. A 32-year-old woman with bipolar I and partial response to lithium
- B. A 42-year-old man with rapid-cycling mania
- C. A 68-year-old man with bipolar disorder complicated by head trauma
- D. A 28-year-old man with bipolar disorder and history of seizure disorders
- E. A 36-year-old man with bipolar I and good response to lithium

106. Which of the following is not a side effect of valproate?

    A. Dyspepsia

    B. Dysarthria

    C. Thrombocytosis

    D. Ataxia

    E. Weight gain

107. Valproate decreases the serum concentration of which of the following drugs?

    A. Amitriptyline

    B. Phenytoin

    C. Fluoxetine

    D. Phenobarbital

    E. Diazepam

108. Which of the following is not a side effect of valproate?

    A. Acute pancreatitis

    B. Hepatic toxicity

    C. Jaundice

    D. Renal failure

    E. Weight gain

109. Sexual dysfunction with paroxetine can be treated by switching the patient to

    A. Sertraline

    B. Clomipramine

    C. Bupropion

    D. Amitriptyline

110. Which of the following drugs in therapeutic dosage may cause ataxia?

    A. Chlorpromazine

    B. Risperidone

    C. Lithium

    D. Imipramine

    E. Carbamazepine

111.   Which of the following is true regarding lithium in the body?
  A. It is not ionized.
  B. It is excreted through the kidneys.
  C. It is lipid-soluble.
  D. It is not absorbed from the gut.
  E. It cannot be detected in the saliva.

112.   All of the following classes of drugs cause weight gain *except*
  A. Lithium
  B. Benzodiazepines
  C. Tricyclic antidepressants
  D. Atypical antipsychotics
  E. Valproate

113.   Which of the following is not a side effect of lamotrigine?
  A. Headache
  B. Diplopia
  C. Steven Johnson syndrome
  D. Blurred vision
  E. Weight gain

114.   Which of the following is not a side effect of topiramate?
  A. Confusion
  B. Psychomotor slowing
  C. Weight loss
  D. Weight gain
  E. Fatigue

115.   Which of the following is *not* true regarding venlafaxine?
  A. It is a SNRI.
  B. It lacks anticholinergic efforts.
  C. It can lower the seizure threshold.
  D. It can be given safely with MAOIs.
  E. It can cause hypertension.

116.   Which of the following is a side effect of SSRIs?
    A. Excessive daytime sleepiness
    B. Akathisia
    C. Acute dystonia
    D. Tardive dyskinesia

117.   All of the following associations between antipsychotics and the classes to which they belong are correct *except*
    A. Haloperidol–butyrophenone
    B. Chlorpromazine–phenothiazine
    C. Olanzapine–benzisoxazole
    D. Clozapine–dibenzodiazipine
    E. Trifluoperazine–phenothiazine

118.   Which of the following is a side effect of conventional antipsychotic drugs?
    A. Psoriasis
    B. Hypertension
    C. Diarrhea
    D. Impotence
    E. Hypersalivation

119.   Which of the following is not a side effect of antipsychotic drugs?
    A. Prolonged QT interval
    B. Leukocytosis
    C. Retinal pigmentation
    D. Weight gain
    E. Torsades de pointes

120.   Which of the following is not a recognized side effect of chlorpromazine?
    A. Hypotension
    B. Galactorrhea
    C. Impotence
    D. Hypothyroidism
    E. Cardiac arrhythmias

121. Which of the following is not a side effect of haloperidol?
   A. Tardive dyskinesia
   B. Hypertension in combination with MAOIs
   C. Acute dystonia
   D. Cholestatic jaundice
   E. Akathisia

122. Which of the following is not a side effect of trifluoperazine?
   A. Dystonia
   B. Myoclonus
   C. Oculogyric crisis
   D. Spastic paraplegia
   E. Acute restlessness

123. Which of the following is a feature of neuroleptic malignant syndrome?
   A. Decreased white blood cells
   B. High mortality if untreated
   C. Higher incidence in female patients than male patients
   D. Higher incidence in elderly patients
   E. Hypothermia

124. Which of the following drugs does not induce liver enzymes?
   A. Haloperidol
   B. MAOIs
   C. Chlorpromazine
   D. Barbiturates
   E. Carbamazepine

125. Which of the following is a side effect of chlorpromazine?
   A. Hemolytic anemia
   B. Teratogenicity
   C. Hypertension
   D. Hypothermia

126. Which of the following drugs is excreted more rapidly in urine of high pH?
   A. Amphetamine
   B. Pethidine
   C. Phenobarbitone
   D. Imipramine

127. How does haloperidol differ from chlorpromazine?
   A. Haloperidol does not have antiemetic effects.
   B. Haloperidol has no anticholinergic effects.
   C. Haloperidol is more likely to cause postural hypotension.
   D. Haloperidol is less likely to cause urinary retention.
   E. Haloperidol does not cause ejaculatory failure.

128. Which of the following should be used with caution in patients with acute-angle glaucoma?
   A. Pyridostigmine
   B. Thioridazine
   C. Tetrabenazine
   D. Baclofen
   E. Diazepam

129. Which of the following is a feature of neuroleptic malignant syndrome?
   A. Preserved level of consciousness
   B. Gradual onset
   C. Leucopenia
   D. Hyperthermia
   E. Hypotonia

130. Which of the following is a feature of drug-induced tardive dyskinesia?
   A. It is more common in male patients.
   B. It is present during sleep.
   C. It is worse on stopping antipsychotics.
   D. Benztropine is an effective treatment.
   E. Movements are painful.

131. All of the following are risk factors for the development of tardive dyskinesia *except*

    A. Affective disorders

    B. Brain injury

    C. Increasing age

    D. Longer duration of treatment

    E. Male sex

132. Which of the following is *not* true about risperidone?

    A. It has a high affinity for 5-HT2A receptors.

    B. It causes hyperprolactinemia at high doses.

    C. It causes weight gain.

    D. It causes extrapyramidal side effects.

    E. It does not cause neuroleptic malignant syndrome.

133. Which of the following is true regarding olanzapine?

    A. It is not an effective antimanic agent.

    B. It causes high levels of extrapyramidal side effects.

    C. It can cause marked sedation.

    D. It causes negligible weight gain.

    E. It causes agranulocytosis.

134. Which of the following is false regarding quetiapine?

    A. It causes less weight gain than clozapine.

    B. It does not cause extrapyramidal side effects.

    C. It can cause constipation.

    D. It has a high affinity for muscarinic receptors.

    E. It has lower affinity for all receptors than clozapine.

135. Which of the following statements is true regarding clozapine?

    A. It acts mainly on D1 receptors.

    B. It has selective striatal D2 blockade.

    C. It has a high affinity for D4 receptors.

    D. It has no action on alpha-2 adrenergic receptors.

    E. It has minimal action on 5-HT2 receptors.

136. All of the following are side effects of clozapine *except*

   A. Bradycardia
   B. Weight gain
   C. Hypersalivation
   D. Seizures
   E. Agranulocytosis

137. Which of the following antipsychotic drugs has the greatest propensity to cause seizures?

   A. Risperidone
   B. Olanzapine
   C. Clozapine
   D. Quetiapine
   E. Aripiprazole

138. Which of the following is true regarding clozapine and agranulocytosis?

   A. Two to four percent of patients being treated with clozapine develop agranulocytosis.
   B. The risk of agranulocytosis increases with the duration of treatment with clozapine.
   C. Men are at greater risk than women.
   D. The dosage of clozapine should be reduced when WBC falls below 2,000 cells per mm^3.
   E. The risk of agranulocytosis increases with age.

139. Chronic barbiturate intoxication causes all of the following *except*

   A. Dysarthria
   B. Nystagmus
   C. Decreased frontal fast activity on EEG
   D. Withdrawal delirium
   E. Brisk tendon reflexes

140. Which of the following is true about the use of SSRIs in premenstrual dysphoric disorder?

   A. It cannot be combined with hormonal treatments.
   B. They are poorly tolerated.
   C. They inhibit ovulation.
   D. They have fewer side effects when used in menstrual syndrome.
   E. They can be used exclusively in the luteal phase.

141. All of the following reduce libido *except*

    A. Carbamazepine

    B. Imipramine

    C. Diazepam

    D. Haloperidol

    E. Olanzapine

142. Which of the following can be caused by use of drugs with anticholinergic properties?

    A. Pupillary constriction

    B. Urinary retention

    C. Diarrhea

    D. Excessive salivation

143. Which of the following is true regarding aripiprazole?

    A. It is a partial agonist at dopamine receptors.

    B. It reduces dopamine synthesis and release by stimulating presynaptic autoreceptors.

    C. It is a partial agonist at 5-HT1A receptor.

    D. All of the above

    E. None of the above

144. How many deaths are attributed to the use of mechanical restraints in the United States each year?

    A. 0–10

    B. 200–400

    C. 500–800

    D. 50–150

    E. >1,000

145. Which of the following is considered an advantage of using a combination of haloperidol and lorazepam intramuscularly in agitated patients?

    A. It reduces agitation more rapidly.

    B. It requires fewer injections to achieve control of behavior.

    C. There is decreased incidence of EPS.

    D. There is a reduced need for concomitant anticholinergic treatment.

    E. All of the above

146. Which of the following is not a characteristic of an ideal parenteral antipsychotic?

    A. Rapid onset of therapeutic effect

    B. Profound sedation

    C. Low risk of hypotension

    D. Low risk of EPS

147. Which of the following is true regarding cognitive function in patients with schizophrenia?

    A. Eighty-five percent of patients with schizophrenia show some degree of cognitive impairment.

    B. Cognitive function deteriorates very fast during the prodromal period of 1 to 2 years preceding the development of frank signs and symptoms of schizophrenia.

    C. Conventional antipsychotics lead to further deterioration of the cognitive functions.

    D. Cognitive impairment is a predictor of poor outcome.

    E. All of the above

148. Which of the following is considered a feature of metabolic syndrome?

    A. Abdominal obesity

    B. Elevated triglycerides

    C. Low HDL levels

    D. Blood pressure higher than 135/85 mm Hg

    E. All of the above

149. In pharmacodynamic terms, how is the therapeutic index defined?

    A. The dose at which 50% of patients experience a specific toxic effect

    B. The dose at which 50% of patients have a specified therapeutic effect

    C. The ratio of the median toxic dose to the median effective dose

    D. None of the above

150. Which of the following can be used for the treatment of sexual dysfunction associated with antipsychotics?
  A. Neostigmine
  B. Yohimbine
  C. Bethanecol
  D. Cyproheptadine
  E. All of the above

151. Which of the following is an inducer of CYP 2D6 enzyme?
  A. Carbamazepine
  B. Fluoxetine
  C. Paroxetine
  D. All of the above
  E. None of the above

152. Which of the following inhibits the CYP 3A4 isoenzyme?
  A. Nefazodone
  B. Paroxetine
  C. Sertraline
  D. Fluvoxamine
  E. All of the above

153. Which of the following medicines when coadministered with lithium leads to decrease in lithium levels?
  A. Acetazolamide
  B. Furosemide
  C. Indomethacin
  D. Thiazide
  E. None of the above

154. Which of the following can lead to increased tricyclic drug concentration when coadministered with tricyclic antidepressants?
  A. Methadone
  B. Cimetidine
  C. SSRIs
  D. Methylphenidate
  E. All of the above

155. Which of the following when coadministered with MAOIs can lead to serotonin syndrome?
  A. SSRIs
  B. L-tryptophan
  C. Buspirone
  D. St. John's wort
  E. All of the above

156. Which of the following when coadministered with carbamazepine can lead to a decrease in carbamazepine levels?
  A. Fluoxetine
  B. Lamotrigine
  C. Erythromycin
  D. Allopurinol
  E. Phenytoin

157. Which of the following when coadministered with haloperidol leads to a decrease in haloperidol levels?
  A. Carbamazepine
  B. Phenobarbital
  C. Nicotine
  D. All of the above
  E. None of the above

158. Which of the following medications can lead to extrapyramidal side effects?
  A. Perphenazine
  B. Prochlorperazine
  C. Metoclopramide
  D. All of the above
  E. None of the above

159. What percentage of D2 receptor must an antipsychotic drug occupy to cause extrapyramidal side effects?
  A. More than 50%
  B. More than 60%
  C. More than 65%
  D. More than 70%
  E. More than 80%

160. How long after neuroleptic malignant syndrome develops can a rechallenge with an antipsychotic be done?

   A. Never
   B. After 1 year
   C. After 6 weeks
   D. After 1 month
   E. After 2 weeks

161. Which of the following is *not* true regarding neuroleptic malignant syndrome?

   A. It has a prevalence rate of 0.02–2.4% in patients exposed to antipsychotics.
   B. It has a mortality rate of around 10–20%.
   C. The mortality is much higher with depot antipsychotic preparation.
   D. Leucopenia is a feature of NMS.
   E. Atypical antipsychotics can also lead to NMS.

162. What percentage of people with acute dystonia developed dystonia within 3 days?

   A. More than 70%
   B. More than 40%
   C. More than 50%
   D. More than 80%
   E. More than 90%

163. Which of the following isoenzymes is involved in the metabolism of carbamazepine?

   A. CYP 1A2
   B. CYP 3A4
   C. CYP 2D6
   D. None of the above
   E. All of the above

164. Which of the following is not a side effect associated with valproate?

   A. Hair loss
   B. Hirsutism
   C. Polycystic ovaries
   D. Thrombocytopenia
   E. Agranulocytosis

165. Which of the following is true regarding treatment with low-potency typical antipsychotics to control agitation in patients with dementia?

    A. There is an increased incidence of hypotension.

    B. Low-potency antipsychotics could lead to worsening of cognitive functions.

    C. There is an increased incidence of sedation.

    D. All of the above

    E. None of the above

166. Use of which of the following over-the-counter medications is not advisable in a sexually active 22-year-old female college student?

    A. Acetaminophen

    B. Motrin

    C. Loratidine

    D. St. John's wort

167. Which of the following liver enzymes should be regularly monitored for the first 16 weeks when the patient is taking tacrine?

    A. AST

    B. ALT

    C. Gamma GT

    D. Alkaline phosphatase

168. A 32-year-old patient is being treated with 450 mg of clozapine for chronic paranoid schizophrenia. The patient missed his appointment with his psychiatrist on Friday, although he got his WBC count done the previous day. He presented to the ER with relapse of symptoms. He was admitted since he was very agitated. He was started back on clozapine at the same dose. The next morning he was found unconscious near his bed with a bump on the head. Which of the following could have led to this clinical situation?

    A. Starting the patient on clozapine

    B. Starting the patient on same dose of clozapine

    C. Not starting the patient on benztropine

    D. None of the above

169. Which of the following provocative tests cannot be used for panic disorder?

    A. Lactate infusion

    B. Carbon dioxide inhalation

    C. Caffeine infusion

    D. Alcohol infusion

170. Which of the following statements is *not* true regarding stimulants?

    A. Methylphenidate acts in the CNS mainly by inhibiting the reuptake of dopamine.

    B. Amphetamine acts by inhibiting the uptake of dopamine.

    C. Cocaine acts by leading to the release of dopamine in the CNS.

    D. Amphetamine intoxication leads to pupillary dilation.

171. What percentage of the THC from inhaled cannabis smoke penetrates the blood–brain barrier?

    A. 100%

    B. Less than 1%

    C. 50%

    D. 10%

172. The symptoms of a 19-year-old woman who was diagnosed with bipolar disorder have been stabilized by treatment with lithium. She presents to the OB/GYN physician for a routine checkup. Her urine pregnancy test comes up positive. What is the most common teratogenic heart condition associated with taking lithium during the first trimester of pregnancy?

    A. Atrial septal defect

    B. Ventricular septal defect

    C. Anomaly of tricuspid valve

    D. Anomaly of mitral valve

173. Who among the following was awarded the Nobel Prize for medicine for his work in psychosurgery?

    A. Cerletti

    B. Moniz

    C. Vaughn

    D. Delay

174. Which of the following antipsychotics in dosages in excess of 100 mg/day can lead to retinitis pigmentosa?

    A. Chlorpromazine

    B. Perphenazine

    C. Thioridazine

    D. None of the above

175. Which of the following is not a side effect associated with chlorpromazine?
   A. Photosensitivity reactions
   B. Slate gray discoloration of skin exposed to sunlight
   C. Granular deposits in anterior lens and posterior cornea with long-term use
   D. Retinal pigmentation with long-term use

ANSWERS

1. Answer: C. Drugs do not need to be ionized to be absorbed by passive diffusion. Gastric emptying is delayed by MAOIs as well as by tricyclic antidepressants. Food inhibits absorption of most drugs. Diazepam is one of the few drugs whose absorption is increased in the presence of food. First-pass metabolism in the liver occurs with orally administered drugs; rectal and intravenous administration avoids this metabolism in the liver.

2. Answer: D. D2 receptors are found in the limbic system. 5-HT2A antagonists improve slow-wave sleep. Partial 5-HT1A agonists such as buspirone have anxiolytic properties. Most antipsychotic drugs are D2 antagonists not agonists. Choice E is wrong because alpha-2 adrenergic antagonists increase the release of norepinephrine.

3. Answer: C. First-pass effect is the process of hepatic metabolism of orally administered drugs; it can be avoided by intravenous administration. Clearance is a measure of the drugs' elimination from the body. Elimination rate constant is the percentage of drug in the body eliminated per unit time. Half-life is the time required for the concentration in the plasma to fall by one-half. Steady state is the drug concentration achieved when the amount administered per unit time equals the amount eliminated per unit time

4. Answer: B. Lipophilic drugs have a large volume of distribution. They are rapidly and completely absorbed, have a first-pass effect, and rapidly cross the blood–brain barrier.

5. Answer: D. All of the drugs mentioned, except SSRIs, stimulate the P-450 system.

6. Answer: B. Carbamazepine is an inducer of liver enzymes and hence causes a decrease in the levels of tricyclic antidepressants. All of the other drugs mentioned inhibit the liver enzymes and hence cause an increase in the level of tricyclic antidepressants in the blood.

7. Answer: D. Tyramine in combination with MAOIs causes hypertensive crisis and not a serotonin syndrome. L-tryptophan, fluoxetine, and clomipramine all can cause serotonin syndrome; administering any of them in combination with MAOIs is contraindicated. There are isolated case reports of St. John's wort causing serotonin syndrome in combination with MAOIs; it is best to avoid the combination.

8. Answer: A. Lithium is not lipophilic; all the other drugs mentioned are. Lithium is a chemical element used in the form of the salt lithium carbonate in psychopharmacology. It is rapidly and completely absorbed. It has low protein-binding properties and no metabolites.

9. **Answer: D.** Serotonin is also called 5-hydroxytryptamine.

10. **Answer: C.** Aggressive behavior, sleep, weight gain, and sexual behavior are all mediated to some extent by serotonin. Problem-solving behavior is not.

11. **Answer: D.** Norepinephrine is synthesized from tyrosine. Tyrosine is oxidized to dihydroxyphenylalanine (L-DOPA). L-DOPA undergoes decarboxylation into dopamine. It further undergoes B-oxidation into norepinephrine.

12. **Answer: C.** Cholestatic jaundice is most commonly seen with phenothiazines, particularly chlorpromazine. This condition may persist for several months after cessation of chlorpromazine. Eventual recovery without cirrhosis is usual. Neither lithium nor benzodiazepines cause cholestatic jaundice. Tricyclic antidepressants can occasionally lead to abnormal results in liver function tests. SSRIs can also lead to abnormal results in liver-function tests.

13. **Answer: C.** Hypotension following administration of chlorpromazine is due to its alpha-adrenergic blocking effect. H1 receptors are responsible for sedation. Chlorpromazine can decrease cardiac contractility as well as prolonged atrial and ventricular conduction time. It also induces ECG abnormalities like prolongation of QT and PR intervals and depression of ST segments.

14. **Answer: E.** Many of the phenothiazines, such as chlorpromazine, have antiemetic properties. This is probably due to dopamine blockade at the chronoreceptor trigger zone in the floor of the fourth ventricle and an anticholinergic action on the emetic center in the brainstem.

15. **Answer: D.** Some drugs, like lorazepam and temazepam undergo only the phase of metabolism of benzodiazepines called phase II. Drugs that undergo phase I metabolism, such as the other drugs mentioned, are more subject to the effects of age, liver disease, or enzyme-inducing drugs. Phase I involves hydroxylation, deamination, or N-dealkylation and often results in the production of an active metabolite. In phase II, drugs or their metabolites undergo acetylation or conjugation and functional groups are added to the molecule.

16. **Answer: C.** When a benzodiazepine binds to the benzodiazepine receptor, it augments the effects of GABA via an allosteric interaction between the benzodiazepine receptor and the GABA-A receptor. Benzodiazepines enhance chloride inflow and the inhibitory effects of GABA. They do not have effects on chloride channels by themselves. They do not act on 5-HT1A or D2 receptors. GABA-B receptors are not involved in mediating the effects of benzodiazepines or barbiturates.

17. **Answer: D.** The first benzodiazepine to be used in patients was chlordiazepoxide, in 1960; the second was diazepam, in 1962.

18. Answer: C. Diazepam is highly lipid-soluble and diffuses rapidly into the central nervous system. It is 90–95% protein-bound and is stored in body fat and brain tissue. It crosses the placenta and also is found in breast milk. Peak plasma levels are reached in 30 to 90 minutes. The elimination half-life is between 30 and 100 hours.

19. Answer: B. Most benzodiazepines are metabolized primarily in the liver.

20. Answer: B. Nightmares are not a side effect of benzodiazepines but instead are seen on withdrawal of benzodiazepines. Withdrawal causes an increase in REM sleep, which results in dreaming, nightmares, and nocturnal awakenings. Ataxia is especially common in the elderly. Sedation and drowsiness are prominent side effects of most benzodiazepines. Anterograde amnesia is also seen and sometimes used therapeutically, for example in anesthesia induction. Paradoxical restlessness and behavioral disinhibition are seen in some patients.

21. Answer: A. Benzodiazepines, unlike barbiturates and alcohol, do not induce hepatic microsomal enzymes. Leucopenia and eosinophilia can be seen, though rarely. Benzodiazepines also cause changes in plasma cortisol. Respiratory depression is mainly seen with intravenous use.

22. Answer: B. Diazepam is more lipid-soluble and extensively distributed than lorazepam. The half-life of chlordiazepoxide is 6 to 20 hours, whereas that of diazepam is 30 to 100 hours. Temazepam and lorazepam do not produce active metabolites.

23. Answer: D. Flurazepam has a half-life of 2 hours. Alprazolam, oxazepam, temazepam, and lorazepam all have half-lives of 6 to 20 hours.

24. Answer: B. Only chlordiazepoxide has active metabolites (demethylchlordiazepoxide, demoxepam, and nordiazepam). The others do not.

25. Answer: A. Tremor, depression, tinnitus, depersonalization, insomnia, fatigue, sweating, concentration difficulties, increased sensory perception, and a sensation of movement or abnormal sway are features of benzodiazepine withdrawal. Psychotic symptoms are not classically seen.

26. Answer: B. Cimetidine inhibits hepatic enzymes and hence raises the level of many drugs, including benzodiazepines. The other drugs listed are enzyme inducers and hence increase metabolism.

27. Answer: D. Absent arms and legs is a teratogenic effect of thalidomide. Cleft lip and palate, respiratory depression, and withdrawal symptoms have been reported in children born to mothers taking benzodiazepines, but in general, their use in pregnancy is relatively safe if clinical issues outweigh the risks.

28. **Answer: C.** Benzodiazepines suppress REM sleep and stage 4 sleep. With chronic use, tolerance develops to this effect and after 2 weeks of continuous use, the total amount of REM sleep returns to normal. On withdrawal, the normal physiologic drive to induce REM sleep is unmasked and thus a rebound REM occurs.

29. **Answer: B.** Tolerance is defined as the need to use larger doses to achieve the same effects with repeated administration. Tolerance to the sedative effects may begin within days and is usually pronounced by 2 to 3 weeks. Tolerance to the anticonvulsant effects also occurs rapidly, and hence benzodiazepines cannot be used in seizure prophylaxis.

30. **Answer: D.** Cross-tolerance occurs with other benzodiazepines, barbiturates, and alcohol, probably because of the proximity of their sites of action at the GABA benzodiazepine complex.

31. **Answer: C.** People with passive and dependent personality traits are more likely to develop withdrawal symptoms. Withdrawal symptoms are more prominent with longer duration of treatment and with the use of substances with a short half-life. Symptoms emerge within a few days of discontinuation of medication and may last for as long as 1 to 2 weeks.

32. **Answer: A.** Lithium administration during pregnancy is associated with Ebstein's anomaly. Anticonvulsants cause fetal craniofacial and neural tube defects.

33. **Answer: B.** Carbamazepine can produce ataxia at therapeutic doses. Imipramine, pimozide, chlorpromazine, and fluoxetine do not typically produce ataxia.

34. **Answer: D.** Poor sleep and excess worry can be features of benzodiazepine withdrawal but are more likely to be symptoms of anxiety. Hyperawareness of senses, abnormal body sensations, dysphoria, and metallic taste in the mouth are all symptoms of benzodiazepine withdrawal.

35. **Answer: E.** Wakefulness and sleep are mediated by the reticular activating system and other midbrain structures, particularly the locus caeruleus. Benzodiazepines act by modulating these parts of the brain. They do not block the reuptake of amines, nor do they inhibit monoamine oxidase. They have minimal effects on the cardiovascular system.

36. **Answer: C.** Acute dystonia is a side effect of conventional antipsychotic agents. Benzodiazepines do not cause dystonia and may occasionally be useful to relieve it. Ataxia, drowsiness, and paradoxical aggression may be seen with the use of benzodiazepines. On occasion, a confusional state may be seen, especially in the elderly.

37. Answer: E. The effects of benzodiazepines are antagonized by flumazenil, which is a benzodiazepine receptor antagonist. Benzodiazepines act on the GABA-A receptor. They produce hangover effects depending on the dose and half-life of the drug. They increase the flow of chloride ions into the neurons, which results in hyperpolarization of the cells. They are used to abort seizures; however, they cannot be used as prophylaxis for seizures because tolerance develops rapidly.

38. Answer: B. All of the products listed except diazepam can cause tremors. Diazepam is used to treat tremors.

39. Answer: D. Tricyclic antidepressants potentiate the pressor effects of norepinephrine. It has been suggested that tricyclic antidepressants given to patients who, following a myocardial infarction, may increase the risk of sudden death. They should be avoided in patients with glaucoma not cataract. Concurrent administration of antipsychotic drugs actually increases the effect of the tricyclic antidepressants and antipsychotics.

40. Answer: E. Tricyclic antidepressants have anticholinergic side effects, including dry mouth, urinary hesitancy, delirium, and constipation not diarrhea. Paralytic ileus may occasionally occur. Desipramine and nortryptiline have lower incidence of anticholinergic side effects.

41. Answer: D. Xerostomia or dry mouth is an anticholinergic side effect of tricyclic antidepressants. They can worsen glaucoma, cause hypotension, and result in the healing of gastric ulcers because of their anticholinergic effects. They do not have effects on the thyroid.

42. Answer: B. Nortryptiline is the only tricyclic antidepressant that has consistently been shown to have an effective therapeutic window. The levels of some other tricyclics can be measured, but their usefulness is doubtful.

43. Answer: B. Antiarrhythmia drugs are not used routinely following an overdose. Cardiotoxicity is the most common cause of death. Seizures and CNS depression can occur. The greatest number of deaths has occurred with amitriptyline, but the highest fatality rate is for desipramine.

44. Answer: C. A previous myocardial infarction 2 years ago does not automatically constitute a contraindication to the use of tricyclics. Glaucoma, heart block, prostatic hypertrophy, and cardiac arrhythmias can all be worsened by tricyclic antidepressants, which are therefore contraindicated.

45. Answer: B. Desipramine, nortryptiline, and protryptiline are secondary amines. Amitriptyline, clomipramine, doxepine, imipramine, and trimipramine are tertiary amines. Amoxapine and maprotiline are tetracyclics.

46. Answer: C. One of the primary efforts of tricyclic antidepressants is the down-regulation of beta-adrenergic receptors with continued use. There is a decrease in 5-HT2 activity and cyclic AMP activity. There is blockade of histamine H1 receptors not H2 receptors.

47. Answer: D. The strongest correlation between blood concentration monitoring and response to tricyclic antidepressants is seen in patients with severe depression with melancholic features.

48. Answer: B. Amitriptyline has the most anticholinergic effects; desipramine has the least effect. Nortryptiline has the least effect on orthostatic hypotension.

49. Answer: D. Amitriptyline is the most effective antidepressant to treat chronic pain.

50. Answer: C. Nortryptiline has the least effect on orthostatic hypotension. It is most likely in patients who have preexisting orthostatic hypotension, and the elderly are particularly vulnerable.

51. Answer: E. Desipramine is the most lethal tricyclic in overdose; however, most tricyclic overdose deaths occur with amitryptiline.

52. Answer: C. Therapeutic window is an optimal range of plasma concentration for a drug. The utility of this is most established for nortryptiline and is between 50–150 ng per ml.

53. Answer: B. The patient here presents with features of atypical depression. This has been shown to respond best to MAOIs.

54. Answer: E. Changes in several presynaptic and postsynaptic receptors follow the increase in concentration of the amines and neurotransmitters caused by MAOIs. Down regulation of beta, alpha-adrenergic, 5-HT2, and tryptamine receptors occurs after long-term administration of MAOIs. Monoamine oxidase has two isoenzyme forms, MAO-A and MAO-B. They metabolize different neurotransmitters. Serotonin and norepinephrine are preferred substrates for the A form, dopamine is a substrate for both A and B, and phenylethylamine is metabolized by the B isoenzyme. MAOIs primary inhibit MAO-A.

55. Answer: C. Tyramine, as substrate of MAO is present in certain fermented foodstuffs like red wine, cheese, yeast extracts, pickled fish, etc. Patients being treated with MAO inhibitors are unable to deaminate tyramine, normally broken down by MAO-A in the gut. This results in the displacement of intracellular stores of norepinephrine and can cause a pressor response resulting in hypertensive crisis or "cheese reaction."

56. Answer: B. Banana does not cause a hypertensive crisis with MAOIs, although the skin of a banana can.

57. Answer: E. The symptoms described are typical of serotonin syndrome. The drug that the patient started taking recently for her migraines is sumatriptan. The combination of phenelzine and sumatriptan can cause serotonin syndrome. This syndrome can also occur if phenelzine is combined with SSRIs. Hence, when switching from MAOIs to SSRIs and tricyclics or vice versa, a minimum of 2 weeks "washout" period is required for drug clearance.

58. Answer: D. When switching from SSRI to MAOI, a washout period of 5 weeks is recommended for fluoxetine because of its long half-life.

59. Answer: E. Alopecia is not a side effect of MAOIs. MAOIs can precipitate manic episodes in patients with a history of bipolar disorder. They can cause blurred vision. They also lower the seizure threshold. A peripheral neuropathy resulting from pyridoxine deficiency can occur with phenelzine. A discontinuation syndrome may be seen on sudden cessation of MAOIs.

60. Answer: B. MAOIs do not interact with NSAIDs. Cough medicines, nasal decongestants, bronchodilators, appetite suppressants, and levodopa (L-dopa) can lead to a sympathomimetic crisis in conjunction with MAOIs. Clomipramine can cause serotonin syndrome. MAOIs potentiate the pharmacologic action of opiates. Their coadministration can lead to a severe toxic syndrome characterized by excitement, muscular rigidity, hyperpyrexia, flushing, hypotension, respiratory depression, and coma.

61. Answer: C. A pheochromocytoma that secretes catecholamines would augment a sympathomimetic crisis. Concurrent use of tricyclic antidepressants is safe if it is monitored closely. MAOIs can be used in cardiac failure. They can also be used in asthma. Some of the hypertensive reactions may be treated with nifedipine, but they must be monitored because hypotension is a known side effect of MAOIs.

62. Answer: B. Mirtazapine acts by blocking presynaptic alpha-2 adrenergic autoreceptors, leading to an increase in the release of norepinephrine. Mirtazapine is also a potent antagonist of H1 receptors, which explains its somnolence-inducing effects. Mirtazapine reduces REM sleep, increases REM sleep latency, and improves deep sleep. It also causes increased appetite and weight gain. There are also reports of agranulocytosis with mirtazapine.

63. Answer: D. Priapism is not associated with nefazodone. It is associated with trazodone. All of the other mentioned effects can be caused by nefazodone.

64. Answer: C. Animal phobias typically respond to behavioral therapies.

65. Answer: D. Of the drugs listed in the answer choices, only acetaminophen has no reaction when used in combination with MAOIs.

66. Answer: C. The half-life of fluvoxamine is about 15 hours. Fluoxetine has a half-life of about 4 to 6 days. Paroxetine about 21 hours, sertraline about 26 hours, and citalopram has a half-life of 35 hours.

67. Answer: C. Citalopram takes about 7 days to achieve steady state. Fluoxetine takes about 28 days, fluvoxamine about 5 to 7 days, paroxetine about 5 to 10 days, and sertraline about 7 days.

68. Answer: B. Long-term use of SSRIs results in reduced 5-HT2 functions. The time to peak plasma levels varies from 4 hours for citalopram to 6 to 8 hours for fluoxetine. SSRIs are safe in patients with a history of cardiac disease.

69. Answer: D. SSRIs are the safest antidepressants in patients with cardiac disease. They do not cause arrhythmias. They can cause diarrhea or constipation. They also have variable effects on the appetite. They can cause tremors.

70. Answer: B. Anorgasmia, delayed ejaculation, and impotence have been reported with SSRIs. In fact some SSRIs may be used in the treatment of premature ejaculation. SSRIs do not have significant effects on blood pressure. They can cause clinically insignificant slowing of the heart rate. They do not cause alopecia or dry mouth.

71. Answer: E. SSRIs do not cause premature ejaculation. They cause delayed ejaculation. They are, however, responsible for nausea, convulsions, agitation, akathisia, dystonia, orolingual dyskinesia, and worsening of neuroleptic-induced parkinsonism.

72. Answer: D. Sertraline is the most lethal SSRI in overdose. A washout period of 2 weeks should be observed for all SSRIs when switching to MAOIs except for fluoxetine, for which a 4-week washout period should be observed.

73. Answer: C. Paroxetine is most frequently associated with discontinuation on abrupt cessation. It is hence recommended that it be gradually tapered and withdrawn.

74. Answer: E. The main difference that would be important in choosing among the different SSRIs would be their action on the P-450 isoenzyme. The other considerations would be less important because the clinical implications would be lower. Citalopram is the most selective inhibitor of 5-HT reuptake and paroxetine the most potent. In contrast to the tricyclic antidepressants, they have very little affinity for different types of adrenoceptor, muscarinic, and dopamine receptors.

75. Answer: B. The most common adverse effects reported with SSRIs are gastrointestinal in nature, with nausea being the most common.

76. Answer: C. All SSRIs can cause delayed ejaculations, and fluoxetine, paroxetine, and sertraline have been studied as a treatment for premature ejaculation. However paroxetine is most likely to cause delayed ejaculation.

77. Answer: A. Abrupt discontinuation of fluoxetine is least likely to cause a discontinuation syndrome by virtue of its long half-life.

78. Answer: C. Trazodone has antagonistic actions at peripheral alpha-adrenergic receptors. This blockade accounts for adverse effects like orthostatic hypertension, dry mouth, and priapism. Trazodone also has significant antagonistic activity at 5-HT2A receptors. Chronic administration of trazodone down regulates 5-HT2 receptors causing a decrease in the number of receptor binding sites in the central nervous system. Trazodone has very little affinity for muscarinic, histamine, dopamine, and norepinephrine receptors.

79. Answer: D. Trazodone is not known to lower the seizure threshold.

80. Answer: C. Methadone has been shown to reduce illicit drug use and criminality and increase employment in a number of studies. Methadone is typically given once a day. It blocks the euphoriant effects of heroin and acts as pure agonists at the mu-receptors.

81. Answer: D. Methadone can cause respiratory depression. It causes hypotension, constipation, bradycardia, miosis, and hypothermia.

82. Answer: B. Risk of overdose is greatest during induction into maintenance treatment, prior to the development of tolerance. Death typically occurs 2 to 6 days after initiation of treatment. Chronic persistent hepatitis is often found in post-mortem examination suggesting that decreased methadone elimination may contribute to overdose in causing death.

83. Answer: D. LAAM is associated with prolonged QT interval.

84. Answer: E. Erythromycin inhibits hepatic enzymes. All of the other mentioned drugs are hepatic enzyme inducers. The rate of metabolism increases, which would necessitate an increase in the dose.

85. Answer: B. Lithium is not bound to plasma protein, is not metabolized, and is excreted unchanged solely by the kidney. It passes freely through the glomerular membrane. This is independent of serum concentration. Renal lithium clearance is relatively constant for each individual, but is proportional to glomerular filtration as measured by creatinine clearance. If creatinine clearance decreases lithium excretion will be reduced and serum lithium levels will rise. Sodium is required for renal lithium excretion. When sodium is depleted, lithium renal clearance is reduced, risking toxic serum levels of lithium.

86. Answer: C. Lithium is the only drug that has been shown to decrease mortality in patients with bipolar disorder. Clozapine has been shown to reduce mortality in patients with schizophrenia.

87. Answer: D. An episode pattern of mania-depression-euthymia is associated with good response to treatment. Rapid cycling and mixed states respond better to carbamazepine and valproate. Comorbid substance use and atypical bipolar illness do not respond well to lithium. Other good prognostic factors are a good previous response to lithium, pure bipolar illness, and a family history of bipolar disorders. Poor prognostic factors include paranoid features and poor social support.

88. Answer: D. Lithium is not used in the treatment of obsessive-compulsive disorder. It can be used in bipolar disorder, depression, schizoaffective disorder, and aggression and mood swings in patients with mental retardation.

89. Answer: B. Lithium can cause dysarthria, especially in toxic doses. It does not, however, cause aphasia. Lithium causes a fine tremor. It may be alleviated by beta-blockers like propranolol. It can cause T-wave flattening and inversion on the ECG in about 30% of patients. This is benign and reversible. Lithium can also cause peripheral neuropathy.

90. Answer: E. The presence of coarse tremors is highly suggestive of lithium toxicity. Other signs of toxicity are vomiting, diarrhea, dysarthria, ataxia, lassitude, restlessness, agitation, and seizures. Hemodialysis is the most effective treatment for lithium toxicity. Hypothyroidism, weight gain, polyuria, and exacerbation of psoriasis are side effects seen at therapeutic doses.

91. Answer: C. Treatment of lithium toxicity involves supportive measures. Frequent determinations of lithium levels are useful to monitor progress. If renal function is unimpaired, it is normally only necessary to increase fluid intake. Increasing lithium renal excretion by saline infusion or osmotic diuresis can also be helpful. In severe intoxication, the most effective treatment is hemodialysis.

92. Answer: D. Lithium does not cause hypertension. It causes all the other cardiac changes mentioned.

93. Answer: E. Lithium intoxication can be precipitated by dehydration, reduced renal clearance, or by drug interactions, such as with thiazide diuretics. Renal lithium elimination will be impaired by medical illness associated with pyrexia, vomiting, or diarrhea and reduced sodium intake. Adequate sodium levels are necessary for sodium excretion. In severe sodium deficiency states, lithium begins to be reabsorbed from the distal portions of the tubules. This elevates serum lithium levels, which in turn inhibit sodium reabsorption by inhibiting aldosterone.

94. Answer: D. Lithium can cause leukocytosis, which has no clinical relevance. Lithium can cause hypothyroidism and hyperthyroidism although hypothyroidism is more common. It can result in raised serum parathormone levels. The resulting elevation in serum calcium and parathyroid hormone is usually transient. It can cause erectile dysfunction.

95. Answer: C. Aspirin, acetaminophen, and sulindac are safe with lithium. Nonsteroidal anti-inflammatory drugs (NSAIDs) inhibit prostaglandin synthesis, which may reduce renal clearance of lithium and thus elevate plasma levels of lithium. This effect has been reported for indomethacin, ibuprofen, phenylbutazone, diclofenac, and piroxicam. Careful monitoring is needed for patients on lithium when they are started on NSAIDs, especially those who rely on prostaglandins to maintain optimal renal function, like the elderly and those in cardiac failure.

96. Answer: A. Orthostatic hypertension is caused by blockade of alpha-1 adrenergic receptors. The elderly are at particular risk for development of orthostatic hypotension. Treatment includes drinking at least 2 liters of fluid per day, adding salt to food, reassessing the dosages of any antihypertensive medication, and wearing support hose.

97. Answer: C. Sodium chloride may be needed in lithium toxicity if it is due to sodium depletion.

98. Answer: D. Carbamazepine is indicated for mixed mania and rapid-cycling bipolar disorder. Good response to lithium, family history of bipolar affective disorder, and bipolar I disorder are predictors of good response to lithium.

99. Answer: B. Carbamazepine causes dizziness, diplopia, ataxia, sedation, confusion, dry mouth, hyponatraemia, abnormal liver function tests, rashes, leucopenia, thrombocytopenia, agranulocytosis, and aplastic anemia. It does not cause marked cognitive decline.

100. **Answer: B.** Carbamazepine is associated with hyponatremia and sometimes causes water intoxication. The retention of water and dilutional hyponatremia is opposite to the effect of lithium and is an alternative to lithium for patients with severe diabetes insipidus. Patients on high doses of carbamazepine and the elderly are more prone to hyponatremia. Thrombocytopenia and leucopenia are recognized side effects of carbamazepine. If these symptoms appear, the drug needs to be discontinued. Carbamazepine can increase total cholesterol, but this is largely by increasing HDL and hence is unlikely to have deleterious consequences on the cardiovascular system.

101. **Answer: A.** Carbamazepine is contraindicated in patients with a history of bone marrow suppression, narrow-angle glaucoma, or hypersensitivity to tricyclic compounds. It should also be avoided in patients on MAOIs. A 2-week lag period should be observed between stopping an MAOI and starting carbamazepine.

102. **Answer: D.** Administration of phenytoin, phenobarbital, theophyllines, or valproate concurrently with carbamazepine can cause decreased carbamazepine plasma concentrations. All the other drugs mentioned increase carbamazepine plasma concentration.

103. **Answer: D.** Valproate inhibits the catabolism of GABA, decreases GABA turnover, increases GABA type B receptor density, and increases the release of GABA. It hence acts primarily by potentiation of central nervous system GABA function.

104. **Answer: B.** Pure mania is a predictor of good response to lithium. All the other conditions have been shown to be predictors of good response to valproate.

105. **Answer: E.** In a healthy young male with bipolar disorder and good response to lithium, it is best to continue with lithium. Patients with partial response to lithium might respond well to valproate, likewise for rapid-cycling mania. Comorbid head trauma and seizure disorder would also predict a good response to valproate.

106. **Answer: C.** Valproate causes thrombocytopenia not thrombocytosis. This is usually reversible. It also causes platelet dysfunction, coagulation disturbances, and agranulocytosis, though these are rare.

107. **Answer: B.** The serum concentration of phenytoin is decreased by valproate. Amitriptyline and fluoxetine may increase valproate concentrations. Valproate increases the serum concentration of phenobarbital and causes increased sedation. Serum concentration of diazepam is increased by valproate. These effects are mainly due to competition at protein binding sites.

108. Answer: D. Valproate does not typically cause renal failure. It does however cause acute pancreatitis and weight gain. Valproate associated hepatotoxicity is an idiosyncratic reaction and is not related to the dosage. The risk factors for hepatotoxicity are young age, use of multiple antiepileptic drugs, and the presence of developmental delay or a metabolic disorder.

109. Answer: C. Sexual dysfunction with SSRIs is one of the most commonly seen side effects with this class of drugs. The management may involve switching from the SSRI to nefazodone or bupropion, either of which is much less likely to cause sexual dysfunction.

110. Answer: E. Carbamazepine can cause ataxia at therapeutic doses. The other drugs can cause ataxia, but only at high or toxic doses.

111. Answer: B. Lithium can be detected in the saliva and is excreted through the kidneys. It is found in the ionized form, is absorbed from the gastrointestinal tract, is not bound to protein, and is not lipid-soluble.

112. Answer: B. Benzodiazepines do not cause weight gain. All the other classes of drugs mentioned have the propensity to cause weight gain.

113. Answer: E. Lamotrigine is weight neutral. It can cause all of the other mentioned effects.

114. Answer: D. Topiramate is unique among most anticonvulsants as it causes weight loss. Because of this side effect, it could, in theory, be combined with other anticonvulsants to counteract weight gain. Its side effects include psychomotor slowing, difficulty with concentration, speech and language problems, somnolence, fatigue, memory problems, irritability, and depression.

115. Answer: D. Concurrent therapy with MAOIs is contraindicated when venlafaxine is being administered, and a washout period of 2 weeks should be maintained between the two agents. Venlafaxine is a selective serotonin and noradrenergic reuptake inhibitor. It has no affinity for cholinergic, histaminergic, and opioid receptors. It can lower the seizure threshold. Treatment with venlafaxine is associated with sustained hypertension, especially in patients treated with more than 300 mg per day.

116. Answer: C. Some SSRIs, especially fluoxetine, are associated with an increase in psychomotor activation including akathisia, especially in the first 2 to 3 weeks of use. Most SSRIs have a very low propensity to cause sedation. They do not cause acute dystonia or tardive dyskinesia.

117. Answer: C. Risperidone is a benzisoxazole. Olanzapine is a thienobenzodiazepine. All the other associations are correct.

118. Answer: D. Typical antipsychotics can cause erectile dysfunction. They do not cause psoriasis, but they can cause discoloration of the skin in body parts exposed to sunlight. They cause postural hypertension, constipation, and dry mouth.

119. Answer: B. Many older antipsychotic drugs can cause leucopenia, thrombocytopenia, and pancytopenia, although patients' blood counts usually return to normal. On the EEG, the drugs cause prorogation of the QT and PR intervals, blunting of T waves, and depression of the ST segment. They also can cause torsades de pointes. High doses of thioridazine can cause retinal pigmentation. Patients on long-term treatment with chlorpromazine can develop granular deposits in the anterior lens and posterior cornea. Many of the antipsychotics are associated with significant weight gain.

120. Answer: D. The main endocrine effect of chlorpromazine is elevation of prolactin levels, which can result in galactorrhea. They cause erectile dysfunction, retrograde ejaculation, and loss of libido. They also cause postural hypotension. Cardiac arrhythmias are especially associated with thioridazine.

121. Answer: E. Haloperidol does not cause hypertension in combination with MAOIs. High potency antipsychotics such as haloperidol have minimal effects on the cardiovascular system. Haloperidol can, however, cause akathisia, cholestatic jaundice, and tardive dyskinesia and is particularly implicated in the causation of acute dystonia.

122. Answer: D. By itself, trifluoperazine does not cause paraplegia. Like most typical antipsychotics, it can cause dystonia, myoclonus, oculogyric crisis, and restlessness.

123. Answer: B. Neuroleptic malignant syndrome is a potentially fatal complication caused by antipsychotic drugs. Its features include hyperthermia, muscle rigidity, autonomic instability, fluctuating consciousness, leucocytosis, myoglobinuria, and acute renal failure. It may have a mortality rate of 20–30% if untreated. It is twice as common in male patients than in female patients and is more likely to occur in younger patients.

124. Answer: B. MAOIs do not induce hepatic enzymes. All the other drugs mentioned can.

125. Answer: D. Chlorpromazine can cause hypothermia. Thioridazine causes retinal pigmentation. Chlorpromazine can cause granular deposits in the anterior lens and posterior cornea. They do not cause hemolytic anemia although rarely they can cause leucopenia and thrombocytopenia. There is very little evidence to suggest any association between prenatal exposure to an antipsychotic and increased incidence of congenital malformations. Chlorpromazine causes postural hypotension not hypertension.

126. Answer: C. Phenobarbitone is excreted in alkaline urine.

127. Answer: D. Because haloperidol is a high-potency antipsychotic with low anticholinergic potency, it is less likely than chlorpromazine to cause urinary retention. It does have some anticholinergic effects as well as antiemetic effects. Chlorpromazine is more likely than haloperidol to cause postural hypotension. It also can cause ejaculatory failure.

128. Answer: B. Thioridazine and other low-potency antipsychotics can worsen glaucoma and hence should be used with caution. The other drugs listed either have no effects or are used in the treatment of glaucoma.

129. Answer: D. Hyperthermia is a feature of neurotic malignant syndrome. The onset is usually sudden and it results in hypertonicity of muscles.

130. Answer: C. Tardive dyskinesia is a movement disorder that develops following long-term treatment with antipsychotics. It consists of involuntary movements of the mouth and tongue and choreoathetoid movements of fingers, toes, and trunk. When dosages of antipsychotics are decreased or discontinued, abnormal movements may worsen. Antiparkinsonian medications may worsen the movements. The movements are not painful and in many cases they are not distressing to the patient and are more often noticed by others. They disappear during sleep.

131. Answer: E. Tardive dyskinesia is more common in female patients. The prevalence increases with age and is higher in patients with a strong affective component to their illness and in those with brain injury. Longer duration of treatment and the dosage of antipsychotics are other risk factors.

132. Answer: E. Risperidone-induced cases of neuroleptic malignant syndrome have been reported in the literature. Risperidone does have a high affinity for 5-HT2A receptors in addition to D2 antagonism. It also has high affinity for alpha-1 and alpha-2 receptors but low affinity for beta and muscarinic receptors. It can raise plasma prolactin levels, particularly at higher doses. Another dose-related effect is the development of extrapyramidal side effects. It is also associated with weight gain, although not as much as is olanzapine.

133. Answer: C. Olanzapine has antagonistic effects at 5-HT2A, D1, D2, M1, H1, 5-HT2C, 5-HT3, 5-HT6, and alpha-1 receptors. It is a stronger antagonist of 5-HT than dopamine. Its has higher M and H receptor antagonism than risperidone and ziprasidone. Its side effect profile includes weight gain, somnolence, orthostatic hypotension, rare extrapyramidal side effects, and development of diabetes mellitus. No hematologic changes have been reported. It is an effective antimanic agent, and its use in the maintenance therapy of bipolar disorder is being evaluated.

134. **Answer: D.** Quetiapine has a high affinity for 5-HT2, H1, alpha-1, and alpha-2 receptors, moderate affinity for D2 receptors, and low affinity for D1 receptors. It has very low affinity for M1 and D4 receptors. It has a much lower receptor blockade profile than other antipsychotics, including clozapine. It has no extrapyramidal adverse effects and causes only transient elevations in serum prolactin levels. Other side effects include constipation, dry mouth, somnolence, and postural hypotension.

135. **Answer: C.** Clozapine has a tenfold higher affinity for D4 receptors than other antipsychotics. It has a relatively low affinity for D2 receptors and a high affinity for 5-HT2 receptors. It causes a strong alpha-1 and alpha-2 receptor blockade. Clozapine has selective preference for the mesolimbic dopamine system as opposed to the striatal dopamine blockade by conventional antipsychotics.

136. **Answer: A.** The most common cardiovascular side effect of clozapine is tachycardia and hypotension not bradycardia; tachycardia is a direct effect of the vagolytic properties of clozapine. Rarely, clozapine can cause hypertension. Clozapine has marked effects on weight, which may be because of strong affinity of the 5-HT1 and H1 receptors for the drug. Hypersalivation is another distressing side effect of clozapine seen in one-third to one-half of persons being treated with clozapine. It also lowers the seizure threshold and can precipitate seizures. Valproate is the preferred drug to treat clozapine-induced seizures. Agranulocytosis is seen in 1–2% of patients on clozapine and is the most well-known and potentially fatal side effect of clozapine.

137. **Answer: C.** Clozapine has the greatest propensity to precipitate seizures. The risk of seizures increases with dosages of more than 500 mg per day. A preexisting seizure disorder or head trauma is a risk factor. The risks can be lowered by monitoring clozapine concentration, ordering an EEG before raising the dosage to more than 600 mg per day, and lowering the dosage after a seizure has occurred.

138. **Answer: E.** Agranulocytosis develops in 1–2% of patients on clozapine, and the risk increases with age. The risk is highest in the first 3 months of treatment. Risk is higher in females. White blood cell monitoring should be done weekly for the first 6 months and then every other week. Any fever or sign of infection is an indication for a white blood cell count. If the patient has a WBC count below 2,000 or a granulocyte count below 1,000, clozapine should be discontinued. Other hematologic changes with clozapine are eosinophilia, leucopenia, neutropenia, and thrombocytopenia.

139. **Answer: C.** Chronic barbiturate intoxication causes increased frontal fast activity on EEG. It can cause dysarthria, nightmares, delirium, and brisk tendon reflexes.

140. Answer: E. SSRIs can be used exclusively in the luteal phase in the treatment of premenstrual syndrome. They can be combined with other hormonal treatments. They are well tolerated. They do not inhibit ovulation, and the side effect profile is the same irrespective of the condition for which they are used.

141. Answer: C. Benzodiazepines are not known to reduce libido. The other drugs, including antipsychotics and antidepressants, can suppress the libido.

142. Answer: B. Drugs with anticholinergic properties cause mydriasis, cycloplegia, urinary retention, and increased urinary tract infections and constipation.

143. Answer: D. Aripiprazole, which was approved by FDA in 2002, is a novel antipsychotic. It is a partial agonist at the dopamine receptors. So it acts as a dopamine agonist at the hypodopaminergic areas and as a dopamine antagonist at the hyperdopaminergic areas. Partial agonist activity at the 5-HT1A receptor also contributes to the overall efficacy of aripiprazole as an antipsychotic.

144. Answer: D. It has been estimated that around 8.5% of all the psychiatric patients require mechanical restraints for agitation. Because the use of mechanical restraints has been associated with around 50 to 150 deaths per year, it is advisable to try other types of interventions such as verbal, behavioral, or environmental interventions and pharmacologic interventions before resorting to mechanical restraints.

145. Answer: E. The haloperidol and lorazepam injection can be administered using the same syringe. The combination helps to calm agitated patients more quickly. Therefore the patients require far fewer injections. There is a reduced incidence of extrapyramidal side effects with the combination, and there is less need for concomitant treatment with cholinergic drugs.

146. Answer: B. An ideal parenteral antipsychotic should achieve the clinical effect without sedating the patient. The following are considered as features of an ideal parenteral antipsychotic: quick onset of therapeutic effect, calming without sedation, low risk of EPS, low risk of hypotension, and low risk of cognitive impairment.

147. Answer: E. Around 85% of the patients with schizophrenia exhibit cognitive impairment to a certain extent. Cognitive functions show a rapid decline during the prodromal period. Patients treated with conventional antipsychotic medications show a further decline in cognitive functions. Impaired cognitive function is considered a poor prognostic indicator.

148. Answer: E. According to the definition of metabolic syndrome, the patients should have three of the following five features for a diagnosis to be made: abdominal obesity obesity (men >40 inches; women >35 inches), elevated triglycerides (>150 mg/dl), low HDL (men <40; women <50), elevated blood pressure (>130/85 mm Hg), and elevated fasting blood glucose (>110 mg/dl).

149. Answer: C. Median effective dose is the dose at which 50% of the patients have a specified therapeutic effect. The median toxic dose is the dose at which half of the patients have the specified therapeutic effect. Therapeutic index is the ratio of median toxic dose to median effective dose.

150. Answer: E. Taking neostigmine 30 mg orally before sexual intercourse helps patients with ejaculatory dysfunction. Bethanechol and yohimbine can be used for impaired erectile dysfunction, as can Viagra, Cialis, and Levitra. Cyproheptadine can be given to females with orgasmic dysfunction.

151. Answer: A. Carbamazepine is an inducer of CYP 2D6 isoenzyme, whereas fluoxetine and paroxetine are inhibitors.

152. Answer: E. All of the following drugs can inhibit CYP 3A4 isoenzyme: fluoxetine, fluvoxamine, paroxetine, and sertraline. This effect leads to cardiotoxic effects when these medicines are combined with nonsedating antihistamines like terfenadine and astemizole. But they can be used with later developed antihistamines like cetrizine and loratidine. Fluvoxamine also leads to inhibition of CYP 1A2 isoenzyme.

153. Answer: A. Acetazolamide when coadministered with lithium leads to a decrease in lithium concentration, whereas the thiazides, indomethacin, and furosemide lead to an increase in lithium levels. Acetazolamide, a carbonic anhydrase inhibitor, leads to decreased lithium concentrations because it increases clearance of lithium. Theophylline also leads to a decreased lithium concentration when coadministered. Most NSAIDs, when coadministered with lithium, lead to decreased clearance of lithium and lead to increased concentrations.

154. Answer: E. All of the following drugs can lead to an increase in tricyclic drug levels when coadministered: SSRIs, cimetidine, quinidine, disulfiram, methylphenidate, and methadone. When tricyclic antidepressants are coadministered with SSRIs and cimetidine, the dosage of the tricyclics should be lowered.

155. Answer: E. All the SSRIs when combined with MAOIs can lead to serotonin syndrome. The other medications that can lead to serotonin syndrome when combined with MAOIs include L-tryptophan, St. John's wort, and buspirone.

156. Answer: E. Phenytoin and valproate lead to a decrease in the level of carbamazepine when coadministered with carbamazepine. Erythromycin, allopurinol, cimetidine, fluoxetine, fluvoxamine, and lamotrigine lead to an increase in carbamazepine concentration when coadministered.

157. Answer: C. Nicotine leads to a decrease in the haloperidol concentration. Carbamazepine, phenobarbital, and rifampin lead to decreased concentration of haloperidol when coadministered.

158. Answer: D. Perphenazine (Trilafon) is a phenothiazine. In addition to the known antipsychotics, metoclopramide (Reglan) and prochlorperazine (Compazine) can lead to extrapyramidal side effects because of their D2-receptor-blocking properties.

159. Answer: E. According to the studies conducted by Farde et al., occupancy of more than 80% of the D2 receptors in the nigrostriatal tract leads to increased incidence of EPS. Occupancy of around 60–70% of the D2 receptors in the mesolimbic and mesocortical tract is necessary for therapeutic efficacy.

160. Answer: E. Patients who develop NMS can be rechallenged with the same antipsychotic medication or a different antipsychotic around 2 weeks after the resolution of NMS. The antipsychotic drug should be restarted at a low dosage and then slowly increased with monitoring.

161. Answer: D. It is not leucopenia but leukocytosis that is a feature of NMS. Atypical antipsychotics, including clozapine, can lead to the development of NMS. One of the first steps in the treatment of NMS is to stop the antipsychotics. Since this is not possible with depot preparations, they have a higher mortality rate.

162. Answer: E. Around 95% of the people who develop acute dystonia develop it within 3 days of being started on antipsychotics.

163. Answer: B. The main pathway involved in the metabolism of carbamazepine to its metabolite, carbamazepine 10,11-epoxide, is CYP 3A4 isoenzyme. So any substance that inhibits CYP 3A4 when coadministered with carbamazepine leads to an increase in carbamazepine levels. Oxcarbamazepine, a ketoderivative of carbamazepine, is minimally metabolized by CYP 3A4 isoenzyme.

164. Answer: B. Valproate can lead to hair loss not hirsutism. The other side effects associated with valproate are sedation, tremor, weight gain, dysarthria, elevation of hepatic transaminase levels, and fatal hepatotoxicity in pediatric patients, thrombocytopenia, agranulocytosis, hemorrhagic pancreatitis, and encephalopathy.

165. Answer: D. Low-potency antipsychotics lead to hypotension because of their alpha-blocking properties and can also lead to a worsening of cognitive functions because of their anticholinergic properties. Low-dosage, high-potency antipsychotics are preferred for elderly patients with dementia when they are agitated.

166. Answer: D. St. John's wort induces enzymes that increase the metabolism of oral contraceptive pills. Therefore, when treating sexually active women in the reproductive age group, it is necessary to discuss drug interaction with over-the-counter antidepressants like St. John's wort.

167. Answer: B. Tacrine is associated with liver toxicity. Therefore, a patient taking tacrine should be followed up with liver function tests. Serum glutamic pyruvic transaminase (SGPT), otherwise known as alanine amino transferase (ALT), is most specific for hepatic toxicity due to tacrine and its usage must be monitored for the first 16 weeks of treatment.

168. Answer: B. When the patient has been off clozapine for more than 36 hours, treatment needs to resume at the starting dosage and the dose slowly increased. Starting the patient on the same dosage as before the interruption can lead to development of orthostatic hypotension, which can result in a fall and injury to the patient.

169. Answer: D. Panic attacks can be provoked in patients with panic disorder by various methods like infusion of substances like lactate, flumazenil, and isoproterenol. Panic attacks can also be provoked by carbon dioxide inhalation. About 70% of the patients with panic disorder provoked by lactate develop panic attacks.

170. Answer: B. Amphetamines act by releasing dopamine from presynaptic terminals. Methyphenidate acts in the CNS mainly by inhibiting the reuptake of dopamine. Cocaine acts by leading to the release of dopamine in the CNS. Amphetamine intoxication leads to pupillary dilation.

171. Answer: B. Delta 9 tetrahydrocannabinol (THC) is the metabolite responsible for most of the psychoactive effects of cannabis. Less than 1% of the THC inhaled penetrates the blood–brain barrier.

172. Answer: C. Ingestion of lithium during the first trimester of pregnancy can lead to Ebstein's anomaly, which is characterized by a congenital anomaly of the tricuspid valve in which the septal and posterior leaflets are displaced into the right ventricle.

173. **Answer: B.** Cerletti and Bini were the two Italian physicians who did pioneering work with convulsive treatment. Delay and Deniker introduced chlorpromazine in the 1950s. Vaughn and Leff expounded the theory of "expressed emotions among highly critical relatives of schizophrenia with poor prognosis." Egaz Moniz, a Portuguese neurologist, along with his colleague Almeida Lima, introduced prefrontal leucotomy. Moniz was awarded the Nobel Prize in 1949.

174. **Answer: C.** Thioridazine when used in excess of 1,000 mg/day can lead to retinal pigmentation, known as retinitis pigmentosa, which can lead to visual impairment. Hence thioridazine should not be prescribed in dosages greater than 800 mg/day. The visual impairment associated with thioridazine is permanent and does not remit with stopping the medication.

175. **Answer: D.** Patients receiving chlorpromazine develop photosensitivity reactions leading to sunburns or rash when they are exposed to sunlight. This can be prevented by the use of sunscreen or by avoiding direct sunlight. People using chlorpromazine for a long time develop lenticular and corneal deposits leading to visual impairment. Some patients also develop slate gray discoloration of the skin when exposed to sunlight. Retinal pigmentation is a side effect of thioridazine.

Chapter 15

PSYCHOTHERAPY

QUESTIONS

1. Which of the following is essential for psychotherapy to proceed?
- A. Acting out
- B. Therapeutic alliance
- C. Splitting
- D. Idealization
- E. Repression

2. All of the following are examples of reconstructive psychotherapy *except*
- A. Freudian analysis
- B. Psychodrama
- C. Kleinian analysis
- D. Brief dynamic therapy
- E. Alderian therapy

3. Interpersonal psychotherapy differs from psychodynamic psychotherapy in that it does not use
- A. Empathy
- B. Transference analysis
- C. The "here and now" approach
- D. An attempt to improve social relationships
- E. Practical procedures

4. Interpersonal psychotherapy is very effective for the treatment of
- A. Depression
- B. Schizophrenia
- C. Anxiety disorders
- D. ADHD
- E. Borderline personality disorder

5. Who popularized Gestalt therapy?
  A. Freud
  B. Winnicott
  C. Jung
  D. Fritz Perls
  E. Eric Berne

6. Which of the following does Gestalt therapy involve?
  A. Gestalt psychology
  B. Psychodrama
  C. Existentialism
  D. Psychoanalysis
  E. All of the above

7. Which of the following includes the concept of auxiliary egos?
  A. Gestalt therapy
  B. Behavioral therapy
  C. Psychodrama
  D. Emotive relapse therapy
  E. Psychoanalysis

8. Which of the following is true for transactional analysis?
  A. It can be carried out only in individual therapy.
  B. Trust is established to facilitate the replacement of the child state by the adult state.
  C. People settle for no if they cannot obtain positive strokes rather than settle for negative strokes.
  D. It employs the gentle, understanding approach.
  E. It was founded by Moreno.

9. What do reconstructive psychotherapies aim to root out?
  A. Irrational impulses
  B. Transference
  C. Bio energy
  D. Ego
  E. Positive strokes

10. In which of the following is free association the key concept?
- A. Client-centered therapy
- B. Interpersonal therapy
- C. Psychodrama
- D. Transactional therapy
- E. Freudian psychoanalysis

11. Which of the following best describes the id?
- A. Self-critical
- B. Rational
- C. Unorganized
- D. Modified by external influences
- E. Self-loathing

12. Which of the following is true regarding interpretation in psychoanalysis?
- A. It should be done early in therapy.
- B. Its main function is to keep the patient happy.
- C. The analyst may interpret latent meanings.
- D. It should never be painful to the patient.
- E. The patient should agree with the analyst's interpretation.

13. Which of the following is a defense mechanism involved in the development of obsessive-compulsive disorder?
- A. Isolation
- B. Undoing
- C. Reaction formation
- D. Ambivalence
- E. All of the above

14. Which of the following is the means by which psychoanalysis achieves resolution of conflicts rooted in the past?
- A. Regression
- B. Denial
- C. Projection
- D. Projective identification
- E. Magical undoing

15. All of the following are seen in psychoanalysis *except*
   A. Remembering unconscious conflicts
   B. Developing transference to the analyst
   C. Developing countertransference to the analyst
   D. A single intense abreactive experience that results in cure
   E. Idealization of the analyst

16. All of the following are predictors of a poor response to psychotherapy *except*
   A. Poor impulse control
   B. Inability to tolerate frustration
   C. Patient on antidepressants
   D. Impaired social judgment
   E. Substance use

17. Behavior therapy has been shown to be useful in all of the following *except*
   A. Panic disorder
   B. Psychotic depression
   C. Specific phobia
   D. OCD
   E. Bulimia nervosa

18. For which of the following has biofeedback been used as treatment?
   A. Multiple sclerosis
   B. Hypertension
   C. Brain tumors
   D. Parkinsonism
   E. Diabetes insipidus

19. Systematic desensitization involves all of the following *except*
   A. Relaxation techniques
   B. Imagination of scenes
   C. Homework
   D. Hierarchical evaluation of a problem
   E. Resolution of childhood conflicts

20. How does the technique known as flooding expose patients to their phobic stimuli?
>   A. Gradually
>   B. In symbolic form
>   C. Along with benzodiazepines to allay anxiety
>   D. In massive amounts
>   E. Along with an interpretation of conflicts

21. All of the following are therapeutic factors in group therapy *except*
>   A. Altruism
>   B. Empathy
>   C. Acting out
>   D. Transference
>   E. Ventilation

22. Which of the following was pioneered by Maxwell Jones?
>   A. Couple therapy
>   B. Therapeutic community
>   C. Systemic approaches to couple therapy
>   D. Crisis intervention
>   E. None of the above

23. All of the following are examples of cognitive distortions *except*
>   A. Arbitrary inference
>   B. Depersonalization
>   C. Selective abstraction
>   D. Overgeneralization
>   E. Magnification

24. Which of the following is true regarding cognitive-behavioral therapy?
>   A. It is contraindicated in depressed in patients.
>   B. It can be effective in outpatients with depression.
>   C. It is more effective than antidepressants in severe depression.
>   D. It has faster onset of action than antidepressants in inpatients.
>   E. It should always be tried before medication.

25. Cognitive distortions are prominent in all of the following *except*

    A. Specific phobia

    B. OCD

    C. ADHD

    D. Eating disorders

    E. Depression

26. According to cognitive-behavioral therapy, which of the following is true regarding depression?

    A. Activity scheduling is discouraged.

    B. Thought diaries are not of much use.

    C. Cognitive content is a threat or danger.

    D. Depression can improve with correction of cognitive distortions.

    E. The therapy can be carried out by the passive therapist.

27. All of the following are true regarding cognitive-behavioral therapy (CBT) *except*

    A. It can be employed by a therapist without full CBT training.

    B. It is useful in depression secondary to life problems.

    C. It can be used in patients with dementia.

    D. It includes the three-column technique.

    E. It may need to be modified in the elderly.

28. Who originated dialectical behavior therapy (DBT)?

    A. Aaron Beck

    B. Sigmund Freud

    C. Isaac Marks

    D. Marsha Linehan

    E. Anthony Ryle

29. Which of the following is a component of dialectical behavior therapy?

    A. Admission to hospital

    B. Keeping a behavioral diary

    C. Daily skills training groups

    D. 24-hour telephone contact with the therapist

    E. Exploration of childhood traumas

30. Which of the following techniques is frequently used in DBT?
   A. Therapy sessions twice a week
   B. Total lack of communication with other professionals
   C. Transference interpretation
   D. Exploring alternative solutions to high risk suicidal behaviors
   E. Addressing life-threatening behaviors at the end of the session

31. Which of the following is true regarding systemic therapy?
   A. Systemic therapy often is used to refer to the Milan model of family therapy anxiety.
   B. It uses a cybernetic concept regarding family relationships.
   C. A special interview technique called circular questioning is used.
   D. Therapists maintain an attitude of neutrality.
   E. All of the above

32. All of the following are associated with structural family therapy *except*
   A. Challenging absent boundaries
   B. Challenging rigid boundaries
   C. Breaking down hierarchies
   D. Homework tasks
   E. Semipermeable boundaries

33. Which of the following effects has been found in family therapy for patients with schizophrenia?
   A. Reduced rates of relapse
   B. Decreased levels of expressed emotion
   C. Improved compliance
   D. Reduced overall cost of treatment
   E. All of the above

34. Which of the following is true regarding the technique called brief dynamic psychotherapy?
   A. It was pioneered by Sandor Ferenczi.
   B. It has time limits.
   C. Therapists maintain neutrality.
   D. It is based on principles of psychoanalytical therapy.
   E. All of the above

35. Which of the following is a function of ego?
   A. Primary desires
   B. Reality testing
   C. Object relationships
   D. Defense mechanisms
   E. All of the above

36. Which of the following is a defense mechanism associated with paranoia?
   A. Projection
   B. Magic undoing
   C. Turning against the self
   D. Denial
   E. Identification

37. Which of the following is a defense mechanism associated with depression?
   A. Isolation
   B. Regression
   C. Reaction formation
   D. Identification
   E. Turning against the self

38. Which of the following is a defense mechanism associated with obsessions?
   A. Reaction formation
   B. Splitting
   C. Denial
   D. Projective identification
   E. Projection

39. All of the following are true of institutional defense mechanisms *except*
   A. Splitting between staff
   B. Projection by staff onto patients
   C. Oedipal in nature
   D. Can decrease anxiety in staff
   E. Can cause anxiety in staff

40. All of the following are true regarding therapeutic milieu *except*
   A. Utilizes the total environment to promote change
   B. Is relevant only in therapeutic communities
   C. Is relevant in inpatient units
   D. Integrates physical, psychological, and social treatments
   E. Includes groups

41. The following are true about countertransference *except*
   A. Should be interpreted to the patient
   B. May be clarified with the supervisor
   C. Can be useful in understanding the patient
   D. May be stressful for the doctor
   E. Better understood by therapist having personal therapy

42. For which of the following is hypnosis a treatment?
   A. Smoking cessation
   B. Weight control
   C. Phobias
   D. Recall of memories
   E. All of the above

43. Which of the following is true regarding transference?
   A. It can assist treatment.
   B. It can impede treatment.
   C. It may lead to excessive dependency on the therapist.
   D. Transference becomes stronger as the treatment progresses.
   E. All of the above

44. Which of the following is an ego function according to Jung?
   A. Thinking
   B. Feeling
   C. Sensation
   D. Intuition
   E. All of the above

45. What was the real name of Freud's famous patient "Anna O."?

A. Martha Bernays

B. Bertha Pappenheim

C. Hippolyte Bernheim

D. Frau Emmy von N.

E. Fräulein Oesterlin

46. Which of the following was written by Sigmund Freud?

A. *Man and Woman*

B. *Studies in the Psychology of Sex*

C. *Sexual Inversion*

D. *Three Essays on the Theory of Sexuality*

E. *The Erotic Rights of Women*

47. Which of the following is not a mature defense mechanism?

A. Humor

B. Sublimation

C. Rationalization

D. Anticipation

E. Suppression

48. Which of the following is not a narcissistic defense mechanism?

A. Denial

B. Blocking

C. Distortion

D. Projection

E. None of the above

49. Which of the following terms was coined by Melanie Klein?

A. Paranoid-schizoid position

B. Good-enough mothering

C. Basic fault

D. Transitional object

E. True self and false self

50. Which of the following is not one of the eight stages of the life cycle described by Erikson?

    A. Identity vs. role confusion

    B. Generativity vs. despair

    C. Industry vs. inferiority

    D. Initiative vs. guilt

    E. Trust vs. mistrust

ANSWERS

1. **Answer: B.** Psychotherapy cannot proceed without a therapeutic alliance between patient and therapist.

   Acting out is the direct expression of an unconscious impulse in order to avoid the accompanying effect. Freud wrote about acting out in transference as the patient's acting toward the therapist as if the therapist were the patient's father, mother, or other significant figure from the patient's past life.

   Splitting is a primitive defense mechanism. The term refers to the division of an object into good and bad, "idealized" and "denigrated." The patient first idealizes the therapist, perhaps telling the therapist that he or she is perfect and is the only person who ever understood the patient. After the therapist disappoints the patient on one occasion, the patient denigrates him, describing him as being useless, incompetent, and irrelevant. The process of idealization followed by denigration is called splitting.

   Repression is the most basic defense mechanism. Thoughts or feelings that the conscious mind finds unacceptable are repressed from consciousness.

2. **Answer: B.** Reconstructive psychotherapy seeks not only to alleviate symptoms but also to produce alterations in maladaptive character structure and to expedite new adaptive potentials. This aim is achieved by bringing into consciousness an awareness of and insight into conflicts, fears, inhibitions, and their manifestations.

3. **Answer: B.** Interpersonal psychotherapy, a form of reeducative psychotherapy for treatment of depression, is not interpretive and does not involve transference analysis, which is one of the most important components of psychoanalytic psychotherapy. Based on the premise that depressed people have difficulties with relationships, it uses a practical "here and now" approach to improving interpersonal skills, rather than a more theoretical exploration of childhood experiences and unconscious motivation.

4. **Answer: A.** Interpersonal therapy is used in the treatment of depressed individuals. It is based on the premise that depressed patients have difficulties with social relationships.

5. **Answer: D.** Fritz Perls popularized Gestalt therapy, which emphasizes the patient's life experiences. Eric Berne developed transactional analysis.

6. **Answer: E.** Gestalt therapy draws on Gestalt psychology, existentialism, psychodrama, and psychoanalysis. Gestalt therapists observe an individual's gestures and bodily movements to discern aspects that reflect unconscious feelings.

7. **Answer: C.** Psychodrama is an approach to release emotion using verbal exploration, suggestion, interpretation, and experimental reliving of earlier traumatic experiences. The elements of psychodrama are the "director" (the therapist), the "protagonist" (the patient, who is the central figure or actor in the psychodrama), and other players, or "auxiliary egos." Auxiliary egos are other group members or trained assistants of the "director," who play roles in the protagonist's life.

8. **Answer: B.** The basic principle of transactional analysis is that ego manifests as an overbearing "parent," a rational "adult," or a helpless "child." Problems occur when there is incongruence and a clash between the egos of the participants in an interaction, for example between adult and child or between parent and child. In therapy, the ego states are explored and interpreted to the client in individual or group therapy. The adult state eventually is strengthened and the child and parent states are displaced. Stroke is the unit of social interaction of the positive (loving, supporting) and negative (hateful, critical); people seek positive strokes, and if they are unable to achieve them, they settle for negative strokes rather than have no strokes at all. Transactional therapy is sharp, gritty, abrasive, and blunt.

9. **Answer:** A. The ultimate goal of reconstructive psychotherapy (Kleinian, Freudian, Neo-Freudian, Alderian, ego analysis) is to root out irrational, immature impulses. Interpretation of transference is an important component of psychotherapy.

10. **Answer: E.** Free association, interpretation, and transference are considered among the key concepts in psychoanalysis. Free association is described as a "psychoanalytic procedure in which a person is encouraged to give free rein to his or her thoughts and feelings, verbalizing whatever comes to the mind without monitoring its content." Over time, this technique is supposed to help bring forth repressed thoughts and feelings that the person can then work through to gain a better sense of self.

11. **Answer: C.** The id is unorganized, unconscious, and instinctual. The ego is modified by direct external influences and is rational. The superego spawns self-hatred, self-criticism, self-control, and self-recrimination.

12. **Answer: C.** The analyst may interpret latent meanings. There is no specific time for interpretations. The function of the analyst is not to keep the patient happy but to help the patient understand the dynamics of the patient's present situation. Sometimes the interpretations might be painful to the patient, but that is necessary.

13. **Answer: E.** Isolation, undoing, reaction formation, and ambivalence are all defense mechanisms involved in the development of obsessive-compulsive disorder.

14. Answer: A. Regression to a childhood stage is necessary for resolution of conflicts from the past. Denial is a primitive defense mechanism whereby the patient refuses to accept the external reality. In projection, one attributes one's disowned or unacknowledged thoughts or feelings to others. Unlike simple projection, the individual does not fully disavow what is projected. Instead, the individual remains aware of his or her own affects or impulses but misattributes them as justifiable reactions to the other person.

15. Answer: D. A single intense abreactive experience does not by itself lead to cure. It does help on the path toward cure, however.

16. Answer: C. Being treated with antidepressants is neither a poor prognosticator for treatment with psychoanalysis nor a contraindication to it. Poor impulse control, inability to tolerate frustration, not being psychologically sophisticated, impaired social judgment, and substance use are all considered poor prognosticators for treatment with psychoanalysis.

17. Answer: B. Behavior therapy is useful in treating panic disorder, depression without psychotic features, specific phobias, OCD, and bulimia nervosa. However, psychotic depression needs treatment with antidepressants and antipsychotics or electroconvulsive therapy.

18. Answer: B. Biofeedback provides invaluable information about the impact of stress, cognitions, and emotional states on our bodies. In combination with stress management, biofeedback serves as a useful tool for people to learn to increase sympathetic nervous system activity and control the harmful effects of stress on their bodies. Hence biofeedback can be used in the treatment of hypertension.

19. Answer: E. Systematic desensitization was developed by Joseph Wolpe as a treatment for phobias. It involves exposing the patient to increasingly vivid cues of the phobic object and teaching the patient to relax during such exposure.

20. Answer: D. Flooding is a behavior-therapy technique for phobias and other problems involving maladaptive anxiety. In this technique, situations or objects producing anxiety are presented to the patient in intense forms either in imagination or in real life.

21. Answer: C. Acting out is considered a poor prognostic factor for group psychotherapy. Group therapy is especially useful to patients who have interpersonal problems. The results with group therapy are better in patients who are young, well motivated, able to express themselves fluently, and who do not have severe personality disorder.

22. Answer: B. Maxwell Jones pioneered the therapeutic community movement. In this approach, every shared activity is considered a potential source of change. Members learn about themselves through the responses and reaction of others in the group, and they learn to appreciate the point of view of others. The staff ensures the basic structure of the communities.

23. Answer: B. Examples of cognitive distortions include arbitrary inference, selective abstraction, overgeneralization, minimization, magnification, and personalization (not depersonalization). Cognitive distortions can lead to various types of psychopathology, like depression, anxiety, and false beliefs.

24. Answer: B. Cognitive therapy is especially useful in patients with depression without psychotic features. In severely depressed patients, however, treatment with antidepressants should be used before starting cognitive therapy.

25. Answer: C. Cognitive therapy has not proved to be effective in the treatment of ADHD. However, it has proven to be useful for correcting the cognitive distortions that are present in a number of disorders, including specific phobias, social phobia, OCD, eating disorders, and depression.

26. Answer: D. Cognitive therapy has proven useful in the treatment of depression by correcting the cognitive distortions that lead to the development of depression.

27. Answer: C. Cognitive-behavioral therapy cannot be used in patients with dementia. "Triple-column therapy" is a cognitive technique developed by David Burns in which a sheet of paper is divided into three columns and labeled from left to right: "Automatic Thoughts," "Cognitive Distortions," and "Rational Responses."

28. Answer: D. Dialectical behavioral therapy (DBT) was pioneered by Marsha Linehan, who maintained that some people overreact to emotional stimulation because of "invalidating environments" during upbringing and undetermined biological factors. DBT is a method for teaching skills for coping with the surges of emotion.

29. Answer: B. Dialectical behavioral therapy consists of individual psychotherapy once a week to review the patient's crises of the week and discuss ways to cope, as well as longer weekly group therapy sessions focusing on improving interpersonal interactions and finding ways to bear stress, accept reality, regulate emotion, and keep aware or "mindful."

30. Answer: D. Dialectical behavior therapy consists of once-weekly sessions in which a problematic behavior is explored, going through alternative solutions and determining what stopped the patient from using more adaptive solutions to the problem.

31. Answer: E. This term "systemic therapy" refers to the Milan model of family therapy but also is used with a wider meaning by family therapists who apply principles of systems theory in their work and use the term interchangeably with "systems therapy." The Milan model of family therapy consistently uses a cybernetic concept regarding family relationships. A special interview technique, circular questioning, allows the formation and verification or falsification of dynamic hypotheses about the interactional bases and functions of family problems. The therapist assumes a metaposition vis-à-vis the family system by maintaining an attitude of neutrality.

32. Answer: C. The term "family structure" refers to a set of unspoken rules governing how family members relate. Hypotheses about these rules are explained to the family members in structural therapy to bring about change.

33. Answer: E. Family therapy with families of patients with schizophrenia leads to reduced rates of relapse, improved compliance, reduced overall cost of treatment, and reduced levels of expressed emotion.

34. Answer: E. The origin of brief dynamic psychotherapy can be traced to the work of Sandor Ferenczi, who recognized a need for a treatment shorter than psychoanalysis. The basic principles are the same as in psychoanalysis, but this method is more focused and time limited.

35. Answer: E. The functions of ego include control and regulation of instinctual drives, judgment, reality testing, object relationships, synthetic function (ability to integrate different elements into an overall unitary structure), and defensive functions.

36. Answer: A. Projection involves the attribution of one's own unacknowledged or disowned feelings onto others. For example, a husband with powerful sexual fantasies may attribute his impulses and desires to his wife and become extremely jealous and possessive toward her. This defense is associated with hysteria as well.

Magic undoing is associated with obsessions. Turning against the self is a defense mechanism of depression in which unacceptable aggression to others is turned onto oneself. Denial, the refusal to recognize external reality, is the defense mechanism used in hysteria. An example would be a patient denying having been told he has cancer although his physician reports have given him a clear and concise explanation that he obviously understood and registered at the time.

In identification, a defense mechanism seen in hysteria, one may attempt to resolve an emotional conflict by attributing to oneself the attributes of another.

37. Answer: E. In "turning against the self," unacceptable aggression to others is turned onto oneself. In his classic paper "Mourning and Melancholia," Freud described this defense mechanism, which is used in depression and hypochondriasis.

A defense mechanism seen in obsessions is isolation, whereby a traumatic memory is denuded of any feelings. Regression is the abandonment of one's adult functioning and reverting to a more childlike mood of acting, feeling, and behaving. Reaction formation, a defense mechanism in obsessions, entails behaving or feeling in the way directly opposite to unacceptable or hostile instinctual impulses (for example someone who is fascinated by feces denies all interest in it and develops an obsessional need to wash his hands). In identification, one may attempt to resolve an emotional conflict by attributing to oneself the attributes of another.

38. Answer: A. Reaction formation is a defense mechanism in obsessions. It refers to behaving or feeling in the way directly opposite to unacceptable or hostile instinctual impulses (for example, showing excessive deference to a person in authority who one actually resents or despises).

Splitting, the defense mechanism frequently used by borderline personality disorders, is the division of an object or person into good and bad, idealized and denigrated. In simple projection, the defense mechanism of paranoia, the individual attributes his own disowned feelings to others. Projective identification, another defense mechanism used in paranoia, combines features of projection with that of identification, but unlike simple projection, the individual does not fully disavow what is projected. Instead, the individual remains aware of his or her own affects or impulses but misattributes them as justifiable reactions to the other person.

39. Answer: C. The various institutional defense mechanisms of a dynamic therapeutic institution include projection by patients onto staff, projection by staff onto patients, patients splitting the staff, and staff splitting the patients. They can lead to both increase and decrease in anxiety of the staff and patients and can have both beneficial and deleterious effects.

40. Answer: B. The concept of a therapeutic community (TC) is used mainly for the treatment of drug abuse and addiction but is also useful in the treatment of various other psychiatric disorders. In this method, treatment staff and patients interact to change attitudes, perceptions, and behaviors associated with drug use.

41. Answer: A. In countertransference, therapists displace onto their patients feelings and attitudes from their past personal relationships, which can lead to inappropriate involvement. Like transference, it is more likely to occur in long-term psychotherapeutic relationships and can either assist or impede the therapeutic effect.

42. Answer: E. Hypnosis can be used in the treatment of smoking cessation, weight control, phobias, to relieve symptoms of conversion disorder, and to aid recall of memories.

43. Answer: E. Transference is a phenomenon in psychotherapy whereby the patient transfers feelings and attitudes from past relationships with significant persons in his or her life onto the therapist with either positive or negative effects on the therapeutic process. Transference becomes increasingly strong as the treatment progresses and can lead to excessive dependency on the therapist, making it difficult to terminate the therapy.

44. Answer: E. According to Jung, the ego has four functions grouped in diametrically opposed pairs: thinking vs. feeling and sensation vs. intuition.

45. Answer: B. "Anna O." was Bertha Pappenheim. Martha Bernays was Freud's wife. Hippolyte Bernheim is famous for his work on hypnosis and his book *Suggestive Therapeutics*. Fräulein Oesterlin is one of Anton Mesmer's patients. Frau Emmy von N. is the patient with whom Freud used the technique of abreaction for the first time.

46. Answer: D. Havelock Ellis was the author of the seven-volume *Studies in the Psychology of Sex, Man and Woman, Sexual Inversion,* and *The Erotic Rights of Women* in the late nineteenth century. Greatly influenced by Ellis's work, Freud wrote *Three Essays on the Theory of Sexuality* (1905).

47. Answer: C. Rationalization is a neurotic defense mechanism. The mature defense mechanisms include altruism, anticipation, ascetism, humor, sublimation, and suppression.

48. Answer: B. The narcissistic defense mechanisms include denial, distortion, and projection. Blocking is an immature defense mechanism. The other immature defense mechanisms are acting out, hypochondriasis, introjection, passive-aggressive behavior, regression, schizoid fantasy, and somatization.

49. Answer: A. According to Melanie Klein there is a fear of annihilation in the first few months of an infant's life and the child suffers persecutory anxiety. The child uses projection and introjection as the primary defensive operations in that stage of life. This persecutory anxiety is a characteristic of the "paranoid-schizoid position" described by Klein, which she says is the infant's way of splitting all aspects of infant and mother into good and bad. "Good enough mothering," "transitional object," and "true self and false self" are terms coined by Donald Winnicott. Michael Balint described the "basic fault."

50. Answer: B. The eight stages of the life cycle described by Erikson are trust vs. mistrust, autonomy vs. shame and doubt, initiative vs. guilt, industry vs. inferiority, ego-identity vs. role-confusion, intimacy vs. isolation, generativity vs. self-absorption, and integrity vs. despair.

Chapter 16

PSYCHOLOGY

QUESTIONS

1. Which of the following is elicited by the conditioned stimulus in classic conditioning?
- A. Unconditioned response
- B. Shaping
- C. Conditioned response
- D. Operant conditioning
- E. Observational learning

2. Which of the following is necessary for classic conditioning to occur?
- A. The animal must be willing to learn.
- B. Compliance is essential.
- C. There should be resistance.
- D. The subject must be a dog.
- E. A temporal relationship between the conditioned and unconditioned stimuli must exist.

3. Which of the following is true regarding classic conditioning?
- A. The strength of conditioned stimulus is inversely proportional to the intensity of the unconditioned stimulus.
- B. Extinction is the same as forgetting.
- C. Spontaneous recovery occurs only after a short delay.
- D. Thorndike is a key figure.
- E. In forward conditioning, the conditioned stimulus always precedes the unconditioned stimulus.

4. Which of the following is true regarding operant conditioning?
- A. Positive reinforcers are inherently rewarding.
- B. Negative reinforcers weaken a particular response.
- C. It is associated with Skinner.
- D. It is not the same as instrumental conditioning.
- E. Extinction and spontaneous recovery do not occur.

5. What is the name of the process by which behavior leading to the removal of an aversive event strengthens the behavior?
    A. Negative reinforcement
    B. Punishment
    C. Penalty
    D. Habituation
    E. Positive reinforcement

6. Which of the following is true regarding operant conditioning?
    A. Punishment is the same as penalty.
    B. Punishment is the same as negative reinforcement.
    C. Toilet training is an example of backward chaining.
    D. Punishment strengthens positive response.
    E. Shaping is best used when the complete response desired is simple.

7. At what age do most infants learn to walk?
    A. 2–4 months
    B. 5–8 months
    C. 10–14 months
    D. 14–18 months
    E. 18–24 months

8. What form of learning did Pavlov study?
    A. Law of effect
    B. Observational learning
    C. Operant conditioning
    D. Classic conditioning
    E. Learned hopelessness

9. What is the result of imprinting?
    A. Children become the same as their parents.
    B. Offspring become independent of the mother.
    C. Proximity between mother and offspring is achieved.
    D. It supports Piaget's theory of development.
    E. Newborn animals follow their mothers.

10. Which of the following terms denotes an increase in undesired behavior before extinction of the behavior?

    A. Extinction burst

    B. Chaining

    C. Shaping

    D. Reciprocal inhibition

    E. Cueing

11. Who created the first modern intelligence test?

    A. Piaget

    B. Wechsler

    C. Skinner

    D. Seligman

    E. Binet

12. At what age does the sensorimotor stage occur in Piaget's theory of cognitive development?

    A. 0–2 years

    B. 0–3 years

    C. 2–7 years

    D. 7–11 years

    E. 6–9 years

13. What is the first sensory system to develop?

    A. Hearing

    B. Touch

    C. Taste

    D. Vision

    E. Vestibular

14. By what age do infants begin to search for hidden objects?

    A. 1 month

    B. 3 months

    C. 9 months

    D. 3 years

    E. 5 years

15. All of the following are stages of development postulated by Piaget *except*

    A. Sensorimotor

    B. Postconventional

    C. Preoperational

    D. Concrete operational

    E. Formal operational

16. According to Franz Alexander, what is the central curative factor in analytic psychotherapy?

    A. Intellectual insight

    B. Corrective emotional experience

    C. Abreaction

    D. None of the above

17. According to Piaget, by what age do children start to solve logic-related problems?

    A. 12 months

    B. 2 years

    C. 5 years

    D. 7 years

    E. 12 years

18. According to Piaget, in what stage is the concept of object permanence achieved?

    A. Sensorimotor stage

    B. Preoperational stage

    C. Concrete operational stage

    D. Formal operational stage

    E. Adolescence

19. According to Piaget, up to what age are children egocentric?

    A. 2 years

    B. 4 years

    C. 7 years

    D. 10 years

    E. 14 years

20. Which of the following is tested by the question, "Are there more dogs or more animals?" that is used in Piaget's logic tasks?

    A. Class inclusion

    B. Transitive inference

    C. Conservation

    D. Spatial cognition

    E. Separation

21. In infants, which of the following is the first to emerge?

    A. Repetitive babbling

    B. Reflexive babbling

    C. Vocal play

    D. "Mama"

22. About how large is the vocabulary of a preschool child?

    A. 1,000 words

    B. 2,000 words

    C. 4,000 words

    D. 8,000 words

    E. 14,000 words

23. Slow language development is associated with all of the following *except*

    A. Intrauterine growth retardation

    B. Large family size

    C. Twins

    D. Prolonged second-stage labor

    E. Childhood maternal loss

24. In which stage of Kohlberg's theory of moral development does authority orientation develop?

    A. Stage 1

    B. Stage 2

    C. Stage 4

    D. Stage 5

    E. Stage 6

25. In which stage of Kohlberg's theory of moral development are individuals most likely to focus on violation of laws and rules?

    A. Stage 1

    B. Stage 2

    C. Stage 3

    D. Stage 4

    E. Stage 5

26. According to Kohlberg's theory, which stage of morality may never be reached even in adulthood?

    A. Punishment orientation

    B. Authority orientation

    C. Reward orientation

    D. Social contract orientation

    E. Good boy/good girl orientation

27. Which of the following types of memory is impaired in amnesia?

    A. Nondeclarative memory

    B. Nonconscious memory

    C. Declarative memory

    D. Unconscious memory

    E. Potentiation memory

28. What is the final process in memory?

    A. Rehearsal

    B. Encoding

    C. Storage

    D. Retrieval

    E. Attention

29. Which of the following is the classification of items to be remembered into meaningful groups?

    A. Elaboration

    B. Selection

    C. Organization

    D. Rehearsal

    E. Priming

30. What kind of memory is commonly referred to in daily use?
   - A. Explicit memory
   - B. Implicit memory
   - C. Iconic memory
   - D. Nondeclarative memory
   - E. Long-term memory

31. According to Holmes and Rahe, what is the most stressful event?
   - A. Moving home
   - B. Divorce
   - C. Christmas
   - D. Death of spouse
   - E. Marriage

32. Which of the following activities do girls aged 2 to 4 years usually prefer?
   - A. Kicking a ball
   - B. Playing with blocks
   - C. Dressing up
   - D. Playing with trucks
   - E. Rough and tumble play

33. Which of the following is exemplified by an infant banging objects together to make noise?
   - A. Pretend play
   - B. Attention-seeking behavior
   - C. Disruptive behavior
   - D. Sensorimotor play
   - E. Early game

34. What is prosocial behavior?
   - A. Motivation to help others
   - B. Being concerned about others' distress
   - C. Actions that help society
   - D. Being very sociable

35. According to Piaget, what governs young children's moral judgments?
  - **A.** Concern for others' feelings
  - **B.** Concerns for their own feelings
  - **C.** Respect for adults and adult rules
  - **D.** Intentions of others
  - **E.** Desire to please others

36. What are digit-span tasks used to measure?
  - **A.** Speed of processing
  - **B.** Attention
  - **C.** Long-term memory
  - **D.** Short-term memory
  - **E.** Episodic memory

37. Which of the following develops the most during adolescence?
  - **A.** Vocabulary
  - **B.** Digit span
  - **C.** Arithmetic
  - **D.** Comprehension
  - **E.** Information

38. Which of the following changes the most during puberty?
  - **A.** Emotion
  - **B.** Behavior
  - **C.** Appetite
  - **D.** TV viewing
  - **E.** Interaction with parents

39. All of the following are true regarding the neurophysiology of memory *except*
  - **A.** Endorphins are involved in memory.
  - **B.** RNA is involved in memory transfer.
  - **C.** 5HT agonists impair cognition.
  - **D.** Bilateral damage to hippocampus can cause retrograde amnesia.
  - **E.** Basal forebrain lesions can result in memory deficit of the Korsakoff type.

40. Which of the following names is matched correctly with the theory the person proposed?
   A. Eysenck: striving for superiority
   B. Adler: dimensional approach to personality
   C. Freud: attachment theory
   D. Jung: introversion and extroversion
   E. Klein: grief

41. Which of the following is true?
   A. Cannon–Bard theory describes transferred excitation.
   B. Social referencing occurs only in brain-damaged patients.
   C. According to Schachter and Singer, facial feedback drives emotional experience.
   D. James–Lange theory emphasizes importance of physiologic responses.
   E. Facial movements are controlled by the pyramidal system.

42. All of the following are true regarding aggression *except*
   A. The amygdala and hippocampus are involved.
   B. Immediate rewards can alter the frequency of aggression.
   C. Aggressive behaviors are less likely in collective cultures.
   D. Aggression is more likely following an expected failure than an unexpected one.
   E. According to Freud, aggression is a biological urge.

43. The likelihood of an accident victim receiving help is greatest if the number of bystanders witnessing the accident is
   A. 1
   B. 5
   C. 15
   D. 50
   E. More than 100

44. Who proposed the concept of client-centered therapy?
   A. Sigmund Freud
   B. Carl Rogers
   C. Festinger
   D. Anna Freud
   E. Donald Winnicott

45. Which of the following tests is used to assess sustained attention?
- **A.** MMPI
- **B.** MMSE
- **C.** Rorschach test
- **D.** IQ test
- **E.** Continuous Performance Test

46. In which of the following are increased errors seen in the span of apprehension test?
- **A.** Schizophrenia
- **B.** Depression
- **C.** Anxiety
- **D.** Obsessive-compulsive disorder
- **E.** Panic disorder

47. In which of the following stages of sleep do newborns spend half of their time?
- **A.** Stage 1
- **B.** Stage 2
- **C.** Stage 3
- **D.** Stage 4
- **E.** REM sleep

48. What is the capacity of short-term memory?
- **A.** 12 items
- **B.** 4 items
- **C.** 7 ± 2 items
- **D.** 9 ± 2 items
- **E.** 15 items

49. A child has been negligent about doing his homework. His father tells him that, from then on, he will not be permitted to watch TV until he has finished his homework. What behavioral principle is being utilized by the parent?
- **A.** Premack principle
- **B.** Peter principle
- **C.** Dilbert principle
- **D.** None of the above

50. Which of the following is the dominant theme in adolescence according to Erikson?

    A. Initiative vs. guilt

    B. Identity vs. confusion

    C. Integrity vs. despair

    D. Autonomy vs. doubt

    E. Intimacy vs. isolation

ANSWERS

1. **Answer: C.** Classic conditioning is the pairing of two stimuli. In Pavlov's experiments, he initially used food as the unconditioned stimulus and rang a bell as the conditioned stimulus to elicit an unconditioned response of salivation from a dog. He then removed the unconditioned stimulus and presented the dog only with the conditioned stimulus (the bell). The dog continued to salivate. This is called the conditioned response.

2. **Answer: E.** Classic conditioning has been noted in many animals. Willingness to learn, compliance, resistance, etc. are not important factors.

3. **Answer: E.** Pavlov did pioneering work in classic conditioning. In forward conditioning, the conditioned stimulus is presented before the unconditioned stimulus and remains on while the unconditioned stimulus is presented until the unconditioned response appears. The longer the interval between the conditioned and unconditioned stimulus, the poorer the learning. The strongest learning occurs when the delay is no longer than 0.5 seconds.

   In backward conditioning, the conditioned stimulus is presented after the unconditioned stimulus.

   The conditioned response ceases to occur in both classic and operant conditioning when the reinforcement ceases. The conditioned response can reappear spontaneously over time.

   In forgetting, if the conditioned stimulus is repeatedly presented alone without the unconditioned stimulus, the conditioned response ceases to occur.

   Thorndike proposed the law of effect, which states that an organism learns from experiences that are reinforced by reward.

4. **Answer: C.** Operant conditioning is the method of behavior modification that B. F. Skinner developed by using rats as experimental subjects. Positive reinforcement causes a person or animal to repeat a behavior so that a pleasant stimulus will be repeated. Negative reinforcement causes a person or animal to behave so that an aversive stimulus is removed. Both positive and negative reinforcement strengthen behavior. Extinction and spontaneous recovery can occur in operant conditioning.

5. Answer: A. Punishment is the situation that occurs if an aversive stimulus is presented whenever the given behavior occurs, thereby reducing the probability of occurrence of this behavior. An example of negative reinforcement would be that in order to avoid an aversive stimulus such as an electric shock, the animal must press a lever. Habituation is the form of counterconditioning whereby successive presentations of the stimulus lead to a gradual reduction of the intensity of the response. An example would be a captive wild animal getting used to the presence of its captors.

6. Answer: C. In shaping, successively closer approximations to the desired behavior are reinforced in order to achieve the desired behavior. In chaining, the behavior is broken into a sequence of steps and each step is learned separately. The entire chain of steps is then brought together until the complex behavior is performed in its entirety. This can be done either forward or backward. Backward chaining may be more effective because the reward associated with the final links in the chain may be used to reinforce the learning of successively earlier links in the chain.

7. Answer: C.

8. Answer: D. Pavlov did the pioneering work in classic conditioning. Thorndike proposed the law of effect. Operant conditioning was demonstrated by Skinner. Bandura proposed the observational learning theory. Learned helplessness was proposed by Martin Seligman.

9. Answer: C. In imprinting, the animal forms strong and lasting attachments in the early stages of its life. This attachment may be toward the mother, food, and surroundings. Imprinting is very resistant to extinction. The theory of social development was proposed by Konrad Lorenz.

10. Answer: A. The frequency of desired behavior may be increased with reward, and the frequency of undesired behavior may be reduced by punishment. This is reciprocal inhibition. A cue is an object or stimulus that elicits the conditioned behavior in operant conditioning.

11. Answer: E. The first modern intelligence test, the Binet–Simon test, was developed in France in 1904 and published in 1905; its name was changed to Stanford–Binet after the test was revised at Stanford University. Piaget proposed a model of cognitive development that suggested that infantile and childhood intellectual development involves interactions with the outside world. Weschler responded to limitations in the Stanford–Binet test by devising his own test, called the Weschler Adult Intelligence Scales (WAIS). Skinner was a behaviorist who worked on operant conditioning. Seligman proposed the concept of learned helplessness.

12. Answer: A. The sensorimotor stage is the first stage of cognitive development, occurring in the first two years of life according to Piaget, who identified four stages of cognitive development:

Stage of Cognitive Development	*Description*
Sensorimotor stage (0–2 years)	The infant is egocentric and believes that everything happens in relation to him. Object permanence is fully developed around the age of 18 months.
Preoperational stage (2–7 years)	The child learns to use the symbols of language and exhibits thought processes like animism, artificialism, authoritarian morality, finalism, egocentrism, precausal reasoning, and creationism.
Concrete operational stage (7–14 years)	The child exhibits logical thought processes and more subjective moral judgments. The child also understands the law of conservation, initially of number and volume and then weight.
Formal operational stage: (>14 years)	The child has the ability to think in abstract terms and to systematically test hypotheses.

13. Answer: B. Touch is the first sense to develop. Embryos just 5–6 weeks sense touch on the nose and lips. Touch sensitivity continues to develop from head to toes as the spinal cord myelinates and continues to develop until the child is 6 years old.

14. Answer: C. Babies fail to search for hidden objects before 9 months. The baby has to possess a mental representation of the object to search for it.

15. Answer: B. Postconventional is a stage of moral development proposed by Lawrence Kohlberg. The other terms denote the four stages of cognitive development according to the theory of Piaget.

16. Answer: B. Franz Alexander considered "corrective emotional experience" to be the central agent of change in any psychotherapeutic relationship. This involves a disconfirmation of previously held wrong assumptions and projections.

17. Answer: D. Children start to solve logic-related problems at about 7 years of age. See Answer 12 for the list of stages of cognitive development according to Piaget.

18. Answer: A. Object permanence is achieved at around 18 months of age. See Answer 12.

19. Answer: C. Children are egocentric in the sensorimotor and preoperational stages. Egocentrism disappears in the concrete operational stage beginning at about age 7.

20. Answer: A. According to Piaget, class inclusion is not understood by children until the age of 10.

21. Answer: B. Reflexive babbling occurs by 3 to 4 months. This is followed by repetitive babbling by 8 months. Irrespective of the language the parents speak, by 1 year the baby is able to say "mama" and "dada," along with one additional word. By 18 months, infants have a vocabulary of 2 to 50 words, which they use in one-word utterances. By 2 years, two-word or three-word utterances can be strung together with some understanding of grammar. By 3 years, the child can usually understand a request containing three parts.

22. Answer: C. A preschool child has a vocabulary of about 4,000 words. A 1-year-old child learns approximately one new word a day, a 2-year-old child two words, and a 3-year-old child learns approximately three new words per day.

23. Answer: D. Language development can be influenced by a variety of factors. All the factors listed in the question, along with physical abuse, deafness, poor communication at home, and large family size can retard language development. Language development is slightly quicker in girls than in boys. Being middle class is also associated with relatively faster language development. Bilingual home has no negative effect on this.

24. Answer: C. Authority orientation develops in stage 4 of the six stages of development of moral judgment categorized into three levels proposed by Lawrence Kohlberg:

Level 1, preconventional morality	Stage 1, punishment orientation: The individual obeys rules in order to avoid punishment.
	Stage 2. Reward orientation: The individual conforms to rules in order to be rewarded.
Level 2, conventional morality	Stage 3, good boy/good girl orientation: The child conforms to rules in order to avoid the disapproval of others.
	Stage 4, authority orientation: The person upholds laws and social roles in order to avoid the censure

of authorities and the guilt about not doing one's duty.

Level 3, postconventional morality

Stage 5, social contract orientation: Movement actions are guided by principles of public welfare in order to maintain the respect of peers and self-respect.

Stage 6. Ethical principle orientation: Actions are guided by the principles of dignity, equality, and justice. These principles are upheld to avoid self-condemnation.

25. **Answer: D.** Individuals in stage 4 of moral development, authority orientation, focus on law and order. See Answer 24 for details of the other stages.

26. **Answer: D.** Some people never reach the level of postconventional morality (Level 3) even in adulthood. It requires individuals to have achieved the later stages of Piaget's formal operational stage.

27. **Answer: C.** Declarative memory is impaired by amnesia. It is the aspect of memory that stores facts and figures and that pairs a stimulus and the correct response. Unconscious memory is a subsystem within long-term memory. It is the basis for skills acquired through repetition and practice (e.g., dance, playing the piano, driving a car).

28. **Answer: D.** The three main processes of memory are encoding, storage, and retrieval. The first step, encoding, also called registration, is the process whereby information is received and assimilated. The information then goes to the next process, storage into long-term memory. Retrieval returns material from long-term memory to short-term memory and thereby reverses the process of encoding. Rehearsal is a strategy employed in order to increase the storage in the short-term memory systems. Attention is the process of selection of highly salient or relevant sensory input for action; it is divided into focused attention and divided attention.

29. **Answer: C.** Organization is the classification of items into groups to be remembered.

30. **Answer: A.** Explicit memory is retrieved with an awareness of remembering. The person is able to cite the memories that he or she is recalling as being a memory of a particular event. Implicit memory is used without conscious retrieval effort. Iconic memory is the temporary persistence of visual impressions after the stimulus has been removed. Declarative/nondeclarative is a distinction of long-term memory based on content; declarative memory stores information that can be proclaimed or described, whereas information in nondeclarative memory is not easily stated. Long-term memory (LTM) is a permanent store with practically unlimited capacity.

31. Answer: D. The Holmes-Rahe Social Readjustment Scale measures stress by according "life crisis units" to stressful life events: death of a spouse (100 units), divorce (73 units), marriage (50 units), moving home (20 units), Christmas (12 units).

32. Answer: C. At age 2 to 3, girls prefer dressing up and playing with dolls whereas boys prefer the other activities mentioned.

33. Answer: D. By 6 months of age, infants have developed simple but consistent action schemes through trial and error and much practice, which they use to make interesting things happen. For example, an infant will push a ball and make it roll in order to experience the sensation and pleasure of seeing the ball's movement.

Between 2 and 5 years, as children develop the ability to represent experience symbolically, pretend play becomes a prominent activity. In this complex type of play, children carry out action plans, take on roles, and transform objects as they express their ideas and feelings about the social world.

Children become interested in formal games with peers by age 5 or younger. The main organizing element in game play consists of explicit rules that guide children's group behavior.

34. Answer: C. Prosocial behaviors are voluntary actions that are intended to help or benefit another individual or group of individuals. Motivation to help others is altruism.

35. Answer: C. Young children's moral judgments are determined by respect for adults and adult rules.

36. Answer: D. Digit span is a common measure of short-term memory; it measures the number of digits a person can absorb and recall in correct serial order after hearing them or seeing them.

37. Answer: A. Vocabulary develops most during adolescence.

38. Answer: E. During adolescence, there is less interaction with parents and more with peers.

39. Answer: D. The hippocampus is responsible for the conversion of short-term memory to long-term memory. Individuals with damaged hippocampus (Korsakoff syndrome) have anterograde amnesia because they are unable to process and learn new information. They are able to learn new skills but are incapable of remembering how they learned them.

40. Answer: D. Carl Jung introduced the notions of introvert and extrovert. Jung's theory divides the psyche into three levels: the ego, the personal unconscious, and the collective unconscious. He founded the school of analytic psychology.

Eysenck developed the personality inventory, a self-reported questionnaire to assess the personality dimensions of extraversion, neuroticism, and psychoticism.

Adler emphasized the social factors in development of human personality. According to his theory, striving for power and superiority may reveal itself by its apparent opposite, a retreat into meditative weakness. He also played an important part in founding social and preventive psychiatry and in the development of day hospitals, therapeutic clubs, and group therapies.

Sigmund Freud did pioneering work on models of the mind, ego-defense mechanisms, and personality development.

Melanie Klein proposed two modes of functioning: the paranoid schizoid position and the depressive position.

41. **Answer: D.** The James–Lange theory views emotional response to a situation as the result of physiologic reactions. Cannon–Bard theory suggests that the autonomic nervous system responds in the same way to all emotional stimuli. The theory of emotion described by Schachter argues that emotional reaction is composed of initial peripheral physiologic changes and the interpretation of these changes. Social referencing is the means by which the normal child develops an understanding of both people and objects. It helps the child develop an understanding of emotional expressions.

42. **Answer: D.** Aggression is more likely in unexpected failure than in expected failure. The amygdala and hippocampus are important parts of the limbic system, which is concerned with memory, behavior, and emotional expression. Stimulation of the amygdala produces aggression, while ablation produces placidity. Various theories of aggression exist, and operant conditioning clearly suggests that positive reinforcement can occur with aggression. That is, if goals are achieved by aggression, the behavior is likely to be repeated. According to Freud, the two basic drives that motivate all thoughts are sex and aggression (Eros and Thanatos).

43. **Answer: A.** In bystander intervention, the presence of others is likely to deter an individual from intervening. When each individual knows that others are present, the burden of intervention does not fall solely on him or her and there is a diffusion of responsibility.

44. **Answer: B.** Client-centered therapy was proposed by Carl Rogers, who saw people as rational, whole beings who know their feelings and reactions; the Q Sort technique was developed from this theory. Freud's psychoanalytic approach divided personality into id, ego, and superego. Festinger proposed the concept of cognitive consistency and dissonance. Anna Freud continued to work on the principles of her father, Sigmund Freud, primarily with children. She published *The Ego and the Mechanisms of Defense.* Donald Winicott, a pediatrician, suggested the concepts of good-enough mother, false self, and transitional objects.

45. Answer: E. The Continuous Performance Test (CPT) measures sustained attention. It is used in the diagnosis and monitoring of children and adults with ADHD. The Minnesota Multiphasic Personality Inventory (MMPI) is a widely used test in the study of adult psychopathology. The Rorschach test is used to measure attitudes and personality.

46. Answer: A.

47. Answer: E. In neonates, the predominant sleep pattern is REM sleep, which occupies more than 50% of the sleep time. This gradually reduces until, by 5 to 6 years of age, the child is in REM sleep for about 25% of the sleep time. This proportion continues into adult life. In contrast, stages 3 and 4 of NREM sleep progressively shorten as the child grows older. They are gradually replaced by stages 1 and 2 of NREM sleep.

48. Answer: C. The capacity of short-term memory is 7 ± 2 items. This can be extended to some degree by chunking, which is a process where several items are grouped perceptually or cognitively into larger single units.

49. Answer: A. According to the Premack principle, a more probable behavior will reinforce less probable behaviors. This principle can be used for behavior modification. If a high-probability behavior (something the person desires or likes to do) is made contingent upon performance of a lower probability behavior (something the person finds less desirable), then the lower probability behavior will be more likely to occur.

50. Answer: B. Erikson's stages of psychosocial and personal development are as follows:

Stage	*Crisis*
First year	Trust vs. mistrust
Second year	Autonomy vs. self-doubt
Third to fifth years	Initiative vs. guilt
Sixth to thirteenth years	Competence vs. inferiority
Adolescence	Identity vs. confusion
Adulthood	Intimacy vs. isolation
Middle age	Generativity vs. stagnation
Later life	Integrity vs. despair

Chapter 17

EMERGENCY PSYCHIATRY

QUESTIONS

1. Which of the following is among the steps to be taken in the case of a very depressed patient with significant suicidal ideation?
   - A. Patient should be hospitalized, preferably in a locked unit.
   - B. The patient's clothes and baggage should be searched thoroughly for any items that the patient could potentially use for self-harm.
   - C. ECT therapy should be considered if the patient does not show rapid response to vigorous treatment with antidepressants.
   - D. The patient should be kept in a room near the nursing unit, so the patient can be easily monitored.
   - E. All of the above

2. Which of the following medical emergencies can present as a psychiatric emergency?
   - A. Hypocalcemia
   - B. Hyperthyroidism
   - C. Urinary tract infection (UTI)
   - D. Hepatic encephalopathy
   - E. All of the above

3. Which of the following is the first step to be taken in the treatment of neuroleptic malignant syndrome (NMS)?
   - A. Maintain electrolyte balance.
   - B. Start amantadine.
   - C. Cool the patient.
   - D. Start dantrolene.
   - E. None of the above

4. A 47-year-old man with a long history of alcohol dependence presents to the Emergency Room by himself in an inebriated state. He looks dehydrated and malnourished. Which of the following is the first step to be taken?

    A. Start the patient on benzodiazepines to prevent seizures.

    B. Start intravenous fluids since the patient is dehydrated, probably has electrolyte imbalance, and is malnourished.

    C. Put the patient in a bed with rails to prevent him from falling off the bed if he develops seizures.

    D. None of the above

5. Which medical emergency can be caused by magnesium deficiency in alcohol-dependent persons?

    A. Hepatic encephalopathy

    B. Cognitive deterioration

    C. Seizures

    D. None of the above

    E. All of the above

6. Which of the following side effects associated with antipsychotic medications can be lethal and requires the most emergent treatment?

    A. Oculogyric crises

    B. Torticollis

    C. Trismus

    D. Opisthotonus

    E. Laryngeal dystonia

7. A 42-year-old patient with schizophrenia who was being treated with risperidone and benztropine took an intentional overdose of benztropine and was found unconscious by his brother. When the patient was brought to the ER, he had increased heart rate, his mouth was dry, he appeared flushed, and his body temperature was elevated. Which of the following should be used to treat the patient's situation?

    A. Stop the antipsychotic

    B. Propranolol

    C. Physostigmine

    D. Trihexyphenidyl

    E. None of the above

8. Which of the following medications can be used in the treatment of acute dystonia?

    A. Benztropine

    B. Diphenhydramine

    C. Promethazine

    D. None of the above

    E. All of the above

9. Which of the following is not seen in barbiturate overdose?

    A. Respiratory depression

    B. Absent deep tendon reflexes

    C. Exaggerated deep tendon reflexes

    D. Hypothermia

    E. Coma

10. A 57-year-old woman with a history of recurrent depression is brought to the Emergency Room after an intentional overdose of benzodiazepines and tricyclic antidepressants. The patient has severe respiratory depression. A medical student assigned to the ER wants to know why she isn't given flumazenil. Why is flumazenil contraindicated in this patient?

    A. Flumazenil can lead to further respiratory depression.

    B. Flumazenil can lead to development of coma.

    C. Giving flumazenil can lead to seizures in this patient.

    D. All of the above

    E. None of the above

11. Which of the following cannot be used to treat orthostatic hypotension caused by typical antipsychotic medications?

    A. Compression stockings

    B. Advising the patient to get up slowly

    C. Epinephrine

    D. Metaraminol

    E. Norepinephrine

12. Which of the following is true regarding lithium toxicity?

    A. Dysarthria, ataxia, and tremor can be the primary manifestations.

    B. Gastric lavage using cation exchange resins like Kayexalate is helpful in treating toxicity.

    C. The treatment of choice for acute intoxication with very high blood levels is hemodialysis.

    D. It can lead to permanent cerebellar damage.

    E. All of the above

13. Which of the following medications can be used in the treatment of a patient taking MAOIs who presents to ER with hypertensive crisis?

    A. Epinephrine

    B. Phentolamine

    C. Metaraminol

    D. Norepinephrine

    E. None of the above

14. Which of the following medications should not be used for acute treatment of opioid withdrawal?

    A. Clonidine

    B. Buprenorphine

    C. Methadone

    D. Naltrexone

    E. None of the above

15. Which of the following benzodiazepines is considered as the treatment of choice in the treatment of catatonia?

    A. Diazepam

    B. Oxazepam

    C. Lorazepam

    D. Flurazepam

    E. None of the above

16. What percentage of patients suffering from schizophrenia commit suicide?

    A. Less than 1%

    B. Less than 5%

    C. More than 15%

    D. Around 10%

    E. Around 20%

17. When is the peak incidence of suicide among men?
   A. 15–25 years
   B. After age 55 years
   C. After age 45 years
   D. 25–35 years
   E. None of the above

18. Which of the following is true regarding suicide?
   A. The incidence is higher in men.
   B. Men use more violent methods.
   C. Suicide rates of single persons are double the rate for married persons.
   D. In the United States, Whites commit suicide twice more than non-Whites.
   E. All of the above

19. What percentage of persons attempting suicide have made a previous suicide attempt?
   A. Less than 10%
   B. Less than 5%
   C. 70%
   D. 40%
   E. None of the above

20. Which of the following findings is more common in people who commit suicide by violent means?
   A. Dopamine deficiency
   B. Serotonergic excess
   C. Increased levels of CSF 5-HIAA
   D. Low levels of CSF 5-HIAA
   E. None of the above

21. Which of the following is the strongest predictor of suicide?
   A. Ideas of worthlessness
   B. Ideas of hopelessness
   C. Inability to enjoy anything in life
   D. Early morning awakening
   E. None of the above

22. Which of the following measures can be used for the treatment of phency-
     clidine intoxication?
     A. Minimizing sensory stimulation
     B. Using physical restraints if necessary
     C. Treatment with benzodiazepines
     D. Treatment with antipsychotic medications
     E. All of the above

23. Which of the following psychiatric conditions increases the risk for suicide?
     A. Borderline personality disorder
     B. Alcohol dependence
     C. Antisocial personality disorder
     D. Panic disorder
     E. All of the above

24. A 35-year-old man presents to the ER, where he reports that he is in a
     methadone program but has missed that day's dosage of methadone. He
     states that he has been receiving 160 mg of methadone per day. Which of
     the following steps should *not* be taken in the treatment of this patient?
     A. Give the patient 160 mg of methadone.
     B. Evaluate the patient for any opioid withdrawal features.
     C. Check with the program from which the patient receives the
        methadone before giving methadone to the patient.
     D. None of the above
     E. All of the above

25. Which of the following sexual behaviors can lead to death?
     A. Hypoxyphilia
     B. Transvestic fetishism
     C. Fetishism
     D. Exhibitionism
     E. None of the above

ANSWERS

1. Answer: E. A highly depressed patient with suicidal ideation is best treated as an inpatient in a locked unit. Any potentially harmful objects should be searched for and removed. Patient should be vigorously treated with antidepressants, and ECT should be considered if the patient's condition does not show adequate response to the antidepressants.

2. Answer: E. Many medical emergencies can present as a psychiatric emergency to the Emergency Room. Calcium abnormalities can present with anxiety symptoms, especially panic symptoms. Hyperthyroidism can present with anxiety or manic symptoms. Urinary tract infection, especially in the elderly, can present with change in mental status also associated with perceptual abnormalities. Hepatic encephalopathy can present with change in mental status and at times with perceptual abnormalities.

3. Answer: E. The first step in the management of suspected NMS is to stop the antipsychotic medication immediately. Patient should be cooled and adequately hydrated, and electrolyte balance should be maintained. Electrolytes, liver function, creatinine phosphokinase (CK), renal function, and white blood cell count should be tested. Dopamine agonist and muscle relaxants can be used if the NMS does not start remitting with the primary measures taken.

4. Answer: D. The first step to take in treating a patient with a long history of alcohol dependence and malnourishment is to give thiamine supplements. The initial dose is best given parenterally. This should be done before giving the patient any intravenous fluids containing dextrose. The stores of thiamine in the patient's body might already be depleted, and giving intravenous fluids can exacerbate the condition and lead to the development of Korsakoff's psychosis with permanent sequelae.

5. Answer: C. Until the magnesium imbalance is corrected. Magnesium deficiency in alcohol-dependent persons can lead to persistent seizures. If the patient develops prolonged seizures associated with alcohol withdrawal, check for magnesium deficiency.

6. Answer: E. Laryngeal dystonia is a medical emergency and can lead to respiratory distress. It needs to be treated with intravenous antiparkinsonian agents like benztropine or diphenhydramine. If dystonia does not respond to the IV antiparkinsonian agents, an emergent tracheostomy may be necessary.

7. **Answer: C.** This patient has taken an overdose of benztropine, an anticholinergic agent, leading to anticholinergic toxicity. The symptoms of anticholinergic toxicity are tachycardia, autonomic instability, elevated body temperature, dry mucosa, dry skin, and delirium with hallucinations. This is best treated in an Emergency Room setting by administering physostigmine in a dosage of 0.5 to 2.0 mg IV. Because physostigmine is metabolized very fast when given parenterally, it needs to be given every 2 hours.

8. **Answer: E.** Acute dystonia is one of the first side effects usually seen with antipsychotic medications. More than 90% of the onset of dystonia occurs within the first 72 hours of starting the medications. Acute dystonia can be treated with benztropine, diphenhydramine, and promethazine. These medications can be given orally, intramuscularly, or intravenously.

9. **Answer: C.** Overdose with barbiturates can lead to respiratory depression, absent deep tendon reflexes, hypothermia, coma, and even death.

10. **Answer: C.** An overdose of tricyclic antidepressants can lead to seizures because tricyclics lower the seizure threshold. This patient has taken both benzodiazepines and tricyclics. If the amount of tricyclics taken was substantial, seizures may result. Seizures are probably being prevented by the benzodiazepines, which the patient has taken along with the tricyclics. Flumazenil is contraindicated for the overdose because flumazenil can negate this effect of benzodiazepines and thus induce seizures.

11. **Answer: C.** Epinephrine can lead to paradoxical worsening of orthostatic hypotension induced through beta-adrenergic stimulation. Pure alpha-adrenergic agents like metaraminol and norepinephrine can be used in the treatment of hypotension. Postural advice (telling the patient to get up slowly from a reclining position) and having the patient wear compression stockings also helps.

12. **Answer: E.** Lithium toxicity is manifested in the initial stages with tremor, dysarthria, and coarse tremor. It can also lead to vomiting and diarrhea resulting in further loss of fluids and thereby exacerbating the toxic effects. Lithium toxicity can also lead to permanent neurologic damage, especially to the cerebellum. Hemodialysis is the treatment of choice for acute toxicity.

13. **Answer: B.** Phentolamine either intramuscularly or intravenously can be used for acute treatment of hypertensive crisis that occurs with monoamine oxidase inhibitor antidepressants. If the patient takes any food substance containing tyramine when taking an MAOI, the patient can develop tyramine-induced hypertensive crisis. The food substances to be avoided are red wine, cheese, beer, yeast extracts, and pickled foods.

14. Answer: D. Clonidine, buprenorphine, and methadone can be used to mitigate the effects of acute opioid withdrawal. Naltrexone can be used in the maintenance treatment of persons addicted to opioids, but only after the patient has abstained from opioids for 7 to 10 days.

15. Answer: C. Lorazepam administered either intramuscularly or intravenously is the treatment of choice for catatonic states.

16. Answer: D. Around 10% of the patients suffering from schizophrenia ultimately commit suicide. Most of the patients who commit suicide are young. Schizophrenic patients with comorbid depression are at a higher risk for depression.

17. Answer: C. The peak incidence of suicide among men is after age 45 for men and after age 55 for women. The suicide rate in those above 75 is three times that in younger people.

18. Answer: E. In the United States, Whites commit suicide at twice the rate of non-White populations. Single persons commit suicide at twice the rate of married persons. Males are more likely to commit suicide than females and they use more violent methods than females.

19. Answer: D. Around 40% of the depressed persons who attempt suicide have attempted suicide before. Thus a suicide attempt is a good predictor of further suicide attempts.

20. Answer: D. It has been shown that serotonergic deficiency in the CNS plays a pivotal role in the incidence of suicide. People who commit suicide have low CSF 5-HIAA levels. A low level of CSF 5-HIAA is a strong predictor of future suicide.

21. Answer: B. Ideas of hopelessness are considered to be a strong predictor of suicidal behavior. Hopelessness further impedes the problem-solving abilities of the suicidal person, which increases despair and furthers suicidal thoughts.

22. Answer: E. Persons intoxicated with phencyclidine (PCP) can be very agitated, aggressive, and dangerous. They should be treated in a quiet room with minimal sensory stimulation. Precautionary physical restraints are not recommended because the intoxicated person may struggle against the restraints, sustaining injuries that can lead to rhabdomyolysis. The patient can be sedated using parenteral benzodiazepines or antipsychotics. Acidifying the urine also leads to increased elimination of phencyclidine.

23. **Answer: E.** Patients with antisocial personality disorder and borderline personality disorder are at higher risk of suicide. Alcohol-dependent persons have a higher rate of suicide. Studies have shown that 20% of patients suffering from panic disorder attempt suicide. Mood disorder is the psychiatric condition most frequently associated with suicide.

24. **Answer: A.** Some of the patients in opioid withdrawal programs are known to abuse or sell methadone. It is always prudent to check with the program from which the patient receives the methadone before giving methadone to the patient. If it is not possible to confirm the dosage the patient has been receiving, prescribe methadone according to the opioid withdrawal protocols. Giving a high dose of methadone to a patient who doesn't get such high doses can lead to respiratory depression.

25. **Answer: A.** Hypoxyphilia, also known as autoerotic asphyxia, is an extreme form of sexual masochism in which self-strangulation or other means of oxygen deprivation is used to achieve sexual gratification. Oxygen deprivation is achieved by means of ligature, noose, plastic bag, or nitrates. The asphyxiation is sometimes fatal.

Chapter 18

NEUROLOGY

QUESTIONS

1. Which of the following is most likely to be the cause of multiple ring enhancing lesions observed by means of computed tomography (CT scan)?
- A. Meningitis
- B. Neurosyphilis
- C. Cerebral embolism
- D. Brain abscess
- E. Dementia

2. An electroencephalogram (EEG) is most helpful to diagnose tumors in which of the following areas?
- A. Posterior fossa
- B. Deep in the cerebrum
- C. The base of the brain
- D. Near the surface of the cerebral hemispheres
- E. None of the above

3. Which of the following is associated with impaired consciousness?
- A. Alcoholic hallucinosis
- B. Wernicke's encephalopathy
- C. Korsakoff syndrome
- D. Dementia
- E. Schizophrenia

4. Which of the following diagnoses is strongly suggested by lower limb areflexia with Babinski sign?
- A. Infectious polymyalgia
- B. Motor neuron disease
- C. Tabes dorsalis
- D. Friedreich ataxia
- E. Cervical spine lesion

5. Which of the following terms describes the primary mechanism of neuro-transmission in the autonomic ganglia?
  A. Serotoninergic
  B. Noradrenergic
  C. Cholinergic
  D. GABAergic

6. All of the following can occur in seizures with a temporal lobe focus *except*
  A. Tinnitus
  B. Smell of burning rubber
  C. Rising epigastric sensation
  D. Aggression
  E. Micropsia

7. Which of the following is *not* true about magnetic resonance imaging (MRI)?
  A. It is the investigation of choice for multiple sclerosis.
  B. The presence of a pacemaker is an absolute contraindication.
  C. It demonstrates calcification better than does CT.
  D. Claustrophobia is a relative contraindication.
  E. MRI is not as good as CT to detect intracranial bleeding.

8. A 36-year-old man complains of double vision and difficulty walking down stairs. The physician examining him suspects a lesion in the brain. What is the most likely site of lesion?
  A. Venteromedial pons
  B. Medulla
  C. Midbrain
  D. Spinal cord
  E. None of the above

9. Which of the following psychological tests can detect organic brain damage?
  A. Thematic Apperception Test (TAT)
  B. Rorschach test
  C. Stanford-Binet test
  D. Wisconsin Card Sorting Test
  E. Minnesota Multiphasic Personality Inventory (MMPI)

10. What is the most common form of migraine?
   A. Classic migraine
   B. Migraine without aura
   C. Hemiplegic migraine
   D. Childhood migraine
   E. Basilar migraine

11. Which of the following is not a feature of migraine?
   A. Occurrence in the evening
   B. Aggravation by oral contraceptives
   C. Onset at menarche
   D. Higher incidence in women
   E. Relief during pregnancy

12. During which stage of sleep does nocturnal migraine tend to arise?
   A. Stage 1 sleep
   B. Stage 2 sleep
   C. Stage 3 sleep
   D. Stage 4 sleep
   E. REM sleep

13. A 38-year-old man presents with unilateral periorbital pain with ipsilateral tearing and nasal discharge. He also has ptosis and miosis. The pain is sharp and lasts for about 1 hour. What is the most likely diagnosis?
   A. Brain tumor
   B. Migraines
   C. Tension headache
   D. Cluster headache
   E. Retinal detachment

14. Which of the following is a common feature of cluster headache?
   A. Increased prevalence in women
   B. Familial predisposition
   C. Association with smoking
   D. Relieved by alcohol
   E. A preceding aura

15. A 60-year-old male presents with a continual headache on both sides of his head. He also complains of his jaws aching when he chews. What is the most important intervention for this patient?
- A. Reassurance
- B. CT scan
- C. Temporal artery biopsy
- D. NSAIDs
- E. High-dose steroids

16. A 55-year-old male being treated for hypertension has a headache of sudden onset that he describes as the worst ever in his life. What is the most likely cause of the headache?
- A. Subarachnoid hemorrhage
- B. Migraine
- C. Cluster headache
- D. Brain tumor
- E. Meningitis

17. All of the following awaken patients from sleep *except*
- A. Cluster headaches
- B. Brain tumors
- C. Tension headaches
- D. Subarachnoid hemorrhage
- E. Migraine

18. Which of the following does not cause chronic headaches?
- A. Depression
- B. Analgesic abuse
- C. Tension headaches
- D. Trigeminal neuralgia
- E. Regular use of benzodiazepines

19. For what percentage of persons with seizure disorder does an interictal EEG appear normal?
- A. 1%
- B. 5%
- C. 10%
- D. 20%
- E. 50%

20. Which of the following is not a feature of generalized seizures?
   A. Origin from a discrete region of the cerebral cortex
   B. Unconsciousness
   C. Generalized EEG abnormalities
   D. Bilateral occurrence
   E. Symmetric occurrence

21. Which of the following is the phenomenon in which a focal seizure undergoes secondary generalization and spreads along the entire cortex?
   A. Todd's palsy
   B. Generalized status epilepticus
   C. Jacksonian march
   D. Uncinate seizures
   E. Rolandic seizures

22. Post-traumatic seizures are associated with all of the following *except*
   A. Increased incidence as time passes after injury
   B. Increased incidence with alcohol abuse
   C. Depressed skull fracture
   D. Linear fracture
   E. Intracranial hematoma
   F. Penetrating wound

23. Which of the following is not a manifestation of partial complex seizures?
   A. They always have impaired consciousness.
   B. Patients may have amnesia for the event.
   C. They are usually accompanied by violent acts.
   D. Tonic-clonic activity is not usually present.
   E. They may consist only of simple purposeless repetitive movements.

24. Which of the following is a feature of frontal lobe seizures?
   A. Gradual onset
   B. Absence of aura
   C. Duration longer than 1 hour
   D. Detectable by EEG
   E. Postictal confusion lasting more than 1 hour

25. Which of the following is not associated with seizures?

    A. Random kicking

    B. Verbal abuse

    C. Screaming

    D. Murder

    E. Damage to property

26. Which of the following is true of psychosis related to epilepsy?

    A. Symptoms are usually depressive.

    B. Affect is normal.

    C. Deterioration of personality is seen.

    D. Increased family incidence of schizophrenia.

    E. Symptoms arise in late teens.

27. Which of the following may be the cause of confusion in a person with epilepsy?

    A. Postictal confusion

    B. Antiepileptic drug intoxication

    C. Status epilepticus

    D. Stopping drugs

    E. All of the above

28. What is the most common site of lesion in partial complex seizures?

    A. Parietal lobe

    B. Temporal lobe

    C. Occipital lobe

    D. Frontal lobe

    E. Cerebellum

29. When do absence seizures begin?

    A. Childhood

    B. Adolescence

    C. Early adulthood

    D. Middle age

    E. Old age

30. A 7-year-old boy suddenly starts staring while in the middle of a conversation. He is mute, rolls up his eyes, and blinks. After about 3 seconds, he resumes talking. What is the most likely diagnosis?

 A. Partial complex seizure

 B. Tonic-clonic seizures

 C. Rolandic seizures

 D. Absence seizure

 E. Focal seizure

31. Which of the following is characteristic of absence seizures?

 A. Presence of aura

 B. Simple repetitive movements

 C. Treatment with carbamazepine

 D. Duration of 1 to 10 seconds

 E. Autosomal recessive inheritance

32. Which of the following is more likely to occur in a pseudoseizure than in a true seizure?

 A. A tonic phase

 B. Incontinence

 C. Elevated prolactin level after the seizure

 D. Absence of postictal depression on the EEG

 E. Self-injury

33. Ipsilateral paralysis of the soft palate and pharynx, producing hoarseness and dysphagia is caused by paralysis of which of the following?

 A. Fifth cranial nerve

 B. Seventh cranial nerve

 C. Tenth cranial nerve

 D. Eleventh cranial nerve

 E. Twelfth cranial nerve

34. Which of the following is required for a definitive diagnosis of carotid artery stenosis?

 A. CT scan

 B. Arteriography

 C. Doppler ultrasound

 D. EEG

 E. SPECT

35. A 45-year-old man presents vertigo and tinnitus, the onset of which was sudden. He also reports vomiting. Upon examination, he is observed to have numbness around the mouth and nystagmus and to be ataxic. Which artery is most likely involved?

- A. Anterior cerebral
- B. Middle cerebral
- C. Vertebrobasilar
- D. Carotid
- E. Anterior common

36. Which of the following is seen in transient global amnesia?

- A. Impaired general knowledge
- B. Amnesia for personal information
- C. Inability to perform tasks learned before the event
- D. Confabulation
- E. Anterograde amnesia

37. Transient global amnesia is most commonly caused by a TIA in which of the following arteries?

- A. Anterior cerebral
- B. Posterior cerebral
- C. Anterior communicating
- D. Anterior common
- E. Carotid

38. Which of the following is not a risk factor for stroke?

- A. Atrial fibrillation
- B. Diabetes mellitus
- C. Migraine
- D. Cigarette smoking
- E. Type A personality

39. Which of the following is caused by a lesion in the pons?

- A. Oculomotor nerve paresis
- B. Limb ataxia
- C. Horner syndrome
- D. Palatal paresis
- E. Abducens nerve palsy

40. All of the following can occur in cerebellar hemorrhage *except*
   A. Contralateral lower limb hemiparesis
   B. Occipital headache
   C. Gait ataxia
   D. Dysarthria
   E. Lethargy

41. Poststroke depression is classically associated with lesion in which of the following?
   A. Right frontal lobe
   B. Right parietal lobe
   C. Left frontal lobe
   D. Left temporal lobe
   E. Occipital lobe

42. Poststroke depression is associated with all of the following *except*
   A. Older age of patient
   B. Greater functional disability
   C. Increased risk of subsequent stroke
   D. Increased risk of subsequent myocardial infarction
   E. Good response to MAOIs

43. Which of the following is not seen in locked-in syndrome?
   A. Quadriplegia
   B. Muteness
   C. Cognitive deficits
   D. Normal EEG

44. Which of the following is seen in persistent vegetative state?
   A. Absence of all reflexes
   B. Suspended animation
   C. Incontinence
   D. Lack of eye movements

45. Which of the following is a feature of carotid artery occlusion?

    A. Vertigo

    B. Nystagmus

    C. Diplopia

    D. Monocular amaurosis fugax

    E. Cortical blindness

46. A 58-year-old man presents with paralysis of the right side of the lower face, deviation of the tongue with no atrophy or loss of taste, and right spastic paralysis of the limbs. Where is the lesion most likely to be?

    A. Left internal capsule

    B. Right internal capsule

    C. Right base of medulla

    D. Left base of medulla

47. Which of the following most accurately describes the pathologic process in multiple sclerosis?

    A. Inflammatory

    B. Infectious

    C. Degenerative

    D. Demyelinating

    E. Metabolic

48. Which of the following is *not* true of multiple sclerosis?

    A. It is a multiphasic disease.

    B. It is asymmetric.

    C. It affects deep white matter.

    D. It is associated with perivascular infiltration of plasma cells.

    E. Spontaneous recovery never occurs.

49. Which of the following is true of multiple sclerosis?

    A. Seizures are common.

    B. Mean age of onset is 15 years.

    C. Incidence is equal worldwide.

    D. Onset is usually monosymptomatic.

    E. Progressive relapse is the most common variety.

50. Which of the following is not a feature of multiple sclerosis?
- A. Optic neuritis
- B. Involuntary movement disorders
- C. Incontinence
- D. Impaired gait
- E. Impotence

51. Which MRI finding is most closely correlated with cognitive impairment?
- A. Enlarged lateral ventricles
- B. Atrophy of the corpus callosum
- C. Total lesion load
- D. Periventricular lesions
- E. Cerebellar atrophy

52. What is the concordance rates of multiple sclerosis in monozygotic twins?
- A. 5%
- B. 10%
- C. 30%
- D. 50%
- E. 100%

53. All of the following are features of Guillain-Barre syndrome *except*
- A. Symmetric paresis
- B. Psychosis
- C. Flaccidity
- D. Areflexia
- E. Monophasic paresis

54. Which of the following may be the cause of central pontine myelinolysis?
- A. Hypokalemia
- B. Hyponatremia
- C. Rapid correction of hyponatremia
- D. Hypernatremia
- E. Hyperthyroidism

55. Postinfectious encephalomyelitis is commonly seen after which of the following?

    A. Chickenpox

    B. Rubella

    C. Measles

    D. Mumps

    E. Herpes simplex

56. Loss of which of the following occurs in Huntington disease?

    A. Serotonin

    B. Dopamine

    C. Substance P

    D. Acetylcholine and GABA

57. Which of the following is not a feature of Parkinson disease?

    A. Tremor

    B. Rigidity

    C. Bradykinesia

    D. Increased blinking

    E. Micrographia

58. Which of the following is seen in Parkinson disease?

    A. Bilateral onset

    B. Essential tremors

    C. Loss of postural reflexes

    D. Loud speech

    E. Lead-pipe rigidity

59. All of the following are common presentations of psychosis in patients with Parkinson disease *except*

    A. Auditory hallucinations

    B. Visual hallucinations

    C. Delusions

    D. Paranoid ideas

    E. Nighttime worsening of symptoms

60. Which of the following describes dementia associated with Parkinson disease?

    A. Aphasia

    B. Apraxia

    C. Agnosia

    D. Sudden onset

    E. Difficulty shifting mental sets

61. Which of the following symptoms does not respond to antiparkinsonian agents?

    A. Tremor

    B. Rigidity

    C. Hallucinations

    D. Bradykinesia

    E. Disturbances of gait

62. Antipsychotic-induced parkinsonism is related to blockade of which of the following receptors?

    A. D1

    B. D2

    C. D3

    D. D4

    E. D5

63. Which of the following antipsychotic medications has no effect on dopamine 2 (D2) receptors?

    A. Risperidone

    B. Quetiapine

    C. Haloperidol

    D. Olanzapine

    E. Chlorpromazine

64. Which of the following is the most disabling feature of Parkinson disease?

    A. Tremor

    B. Rigidity

    C. Masklike facies

    D. Bradykinesia

    E. Micrographia

65. Which of the following causes the abrupt onset and remission of parkinsonian symptoms after years of well-controlled antiparkinsonian treatment?
   A. Absence attacks
   B. Drug toxicity
   C. On–off phenomenon
   D. Treatment resistance
   E. Acute dystonia

66. Which of the following denotes slow, regular, twisting movements that are bilateral and affect distal parts of limbs?
   A. Tremors
   B. Athetosis
   C. Dystonia
   D. Chorea
   E. Tardive dyskinesia

67. What is the mode of transmission of Huntington disease?
   A. X-linked recessive
   B. Autosomal recessive
   C. Autosomal dominant
   D. Polygenic inheritance
   E. Sex-linked dominant

68. Which of the following is seen in Huntington disease?
   A. Depression
   B. Psychosis
   C. Euphoria
   D. Suicide
   E. All of the above

69. What is most common initial site of development of chorea in patients with Huntington disease?
   A. Face
   B. Upper limbs
   C. Trunk
   D. Lower limbs
   E. Muscles of deglutition

70. Which of the following pathologic changes is seen in Huntington disease?
  A. Cortical atrophy
  B. Atrophy of corpus striatum
  C. Dilatation of lateral ventricles
  D. Atrophy of thalamus
  E. All of the above

71. Where is the gene responsible for Huntington disease located?
  A. Chromosome 4
  B. Chromosome 5
  C. Chromosome 11
  D. Chromosome 13
  E. Chromosome 17

72. Which of the following is a feature of hemiballismus?
  A. Cognitive impairment
  B. Contralateral hemiparesis
  C. Unilateral flinging motion
  D. Spasticity
  E. Hyperreflexia

73. Which of the following is caused by lesion in the subthalamic nucleus?
  A. Tremors
  B. Tardive dyskinesia
  C. Hemiballismus
  D. Akathisia

74. Akinetic mutism is caused by lesions in which of the following areas?
  A. Right temporal lobe
  B. Left parietal lobe
  C. Right frontal lobe
  D. Pons and midbrain
  E. Right parietal lobe

75. Which of the following is produced by lesions of the lateral hypothalamus?
  A. Increased thirst
  B. Aphagia
  C. Hyperthermia
  D. Hyperphagia

76. All of the following are features of Lesch-Nyhan syndrome *except*
   A. Dystonia
   B. Self-mutilation
   C. Seizures
   D. Normal intelligence
   E. Hyperuricemia

77. What is the most common involuntary movement disorder?
   A. Parkinson disease
   B. Acute dystonia
   C. Essential tremor
   D. Focal dystonia
   E. Tardive dystonia

78. Which of the following is *not* true of essential tremor?
   A. It has a frequency of 6–9 Hz.
   B. It develops in young adults.
   C. Anxiety may increase the tremor.
   D. Alcohol worsens the tremor.
   E. Beta-blockers suppress the tremor.

79. Klüver-Bucy syndrome is caused by lesions in which of the following regions?
   A. Cingulate gyrus
   B. Medial hypothalamus
   C. Lateral hypothalamus
   D. Amygdala

80. Which of the following is true regarding chronic inflammatory demyelinating polyneuropathy?
   A. It is most common in the third and fourth decades of life.
   B. It typically shows predominantly motor involvement.
   C. Proximal and distal groups of muscles are equally involved.
   D. Muscle wasting is commonly seen.
   E. Pain is common.

81. What is the most common central nervous system infection in patients with AIDS?

    A. Tuberculosis

    B. Cytomegalovirus

    C. Toxoplasmosis

    D. Cryptococcus

    E. Herpes simplex

82. Which of the following characterizes astrocytomas in adults?

    A. The cure rate is 90%.

    B. Extensive infiltration to surrounding structures occurs.

    C. The cerebellum is the most common site.

    D. They do not evolve into more malignant forms.

    E. Total surgical removal is possible without sacrificing surrounding structures.

83. Which of the following is true about meningiomas?

    A. They arise from glial cells.

    B. They are associated with neurofibromatosis type 1.

    C. They are common in children.

    D. Radiotherapy is the treatment of choice.

    E. They are metastatic tumors.

84. Which of the following is the most common origin of metastatic tumor in the brain?

    A. Breast

    B. Bone

    C. Prostate

    D. Kidney

    E. Lung

85. Which of the following is not a typical feature of an intracranial neoplasm?

    A. Partial complex seizure

    B. Headache accompanied by vomiting

    C. Petit mal seizures

    D. Headache worse in the morning

    E. Headache is the presenting clinical feature in almost 35% of the patients.

86. Which of the following visual field effects is classically produced by pituitary adenomas?

A. Left central scotoma

B. Bilateral scotoma

C. Bitemporal hemianopia

D. Left homonymous hemianopia

E. Bitemporal inferior quadrant hemianopia

87. Which of the following is not a feature of acoustic neuroma?

A. Tinnitus

B. Vertigo

C. Loss of smell

D. Hearing impairment

E. Imbalance

88. Spinal-cord compression can cause all of the following *except*

A. Depression

B. Cognitive impairment

C. Paraplegia

D. Loss of sensation

E. Incontinence of urine

89. Alpha activity on an EEG is most prominent with which of the following?

A. Eyes open

B. Concentration

C. Anxiety

D. Eyes closed

90. A thin 68-year-old man presents with headaches that began 1 month earlier. Likely causes include all of the following *except*

A. Brain tumor

B. Subdural hematoma

C. Pseudotumor cerebri

D. Temporal arteritis

E. Nitroglycerin medication

91. A 50-year-old woman presents with a complaint of "the worst headache in my life." This was followed by a loss of consciousness, after which the patient recovers. What is the most likely cause?

    A. Middle meningeal artery occlusion

    B. Trauma of bridging meningeal veins

    C. Vertebrobasilar artery occlusion

    D. Rupture of a berry aneurysm

    E. Rupture of posterior cerebral artery

92. What is the most common cause of major head trauma in persons 15 to 24 years old?

    A. Physical assaults

    B. Sporting injuries

    C. Motor vehicle accidents

    D. Suicide attempts

    E. Domestic falls

93. In traumatic brain injury, lesion in which of the following regions is most closely correlated with the impairment it produces?

    A. Right parietal

    B. Left frontal

    C. Left temporal

    D. Occipital

    E. Right temporal

94. All of the following are features of postconcussional syndrome *except*

    A. Anxiety

    B. Depression

    C. Fatigue

    D. Poor concentration

    E. Schizophrenia

95. Personality change following head injury is most commonly seen after injury to which of the following?

    A. Caudate nuclei

    B. Frontal lobe

    C. Parietal lobe

    D. Occipital lobe

    E. Cerebellum

96. What is the most commonly seen psychiatric manifestation of neurosyphilis?

  A. Mania
  B. Schizophrenia
  C. Depression
  D. Anxiety
  E. Obsessive-compulsive disorder

97. In which of the following conditions is the cerebrospinal fluid clear on lumbar puncture?

  A. Bacterial meningitis
  B. Neurosyphilis
  C. Tuberculus meningitis
  D. Subarachnoid hemorrhage
  E. Fungal meningitis

98. Decreased glucose levels in the cerebrospinal fluid on lumbar puncture is seen in all of the following *except*

  A. Bacterial meningitis
  B. Viral meningitis
  C. Tuberculous meningitis
  D. Fungal meningitis

99. Which of the following is true regarding Creutzfeldt-Jakob disease?

  A. The age group most commonly affected is young adults.
  B. The disease is self-limiting.
  C. Presents with dementia and myoclonus.
  D. It is a viral infection.
  E. Patients have a lifespan of about a decade from diagnosis.

100. Which of the following is *not* true regarding HIV-associated dementia?

  A. It develops late in the course of disease.
  B. It is a cortical dementia.
  C. It causes decreased concentration and increased forgetfulness.
  D. Aphasia and apraxia are uncommon.
  E. Behavior problems may be present.

101. What is the most common neuropathy seen in HIV-positive patients?
- A. Distal symmetric polyneuropathy
- B. Autonomic neuropathy
- C. Toxic neuropathy
- D. Mononeuritis multiplex
- E. Myeloradiculopathy

102. Which of the following has been proven conclusively to be a risk factor for Alzheimer disease?
- A. NSAIDs
- B. Aluminum
- C. Maternal age
- D. Age
- E. Male sex

103. Gene mutation on all of the following chromosomes is associated with Alzheimer disease *except*
- A. Chromosome 1
- B. Chromosome 15
- C. Chromosome 14
- D. Chromosome 19
- E. Chromosome 21

104. The progression of Alzheimer disease may be delayed by the use of all of the following *except*
- A. Radical scavengers
- B. Antioxidants
- C. Cholinesterase inhibitors
- D. Anti-inflammatory drugs
- E. Antipsychotics

105. In Alzheimer disease, neuroimaging shows all of the following changes *except*
- A. Enlargement of ventricles
- B. Periventricular hyperintensities shown by MRI
- C. Extensive deep white-matter hyperintensities
- D. Medial temporal lobe atrophy
- E. Temporoparietal hypoperfusion shown by SPECT

106. What is the most frequently seen disturbance of behavior in patients with Alzheimer disease?

    A. Agitation

    B. Anxiety

    C. Irritability

    D. Apathy

    E. Dysphoria

107. All of the following are features of linguistic deficits in patients with early Alzheimer disease *except*

    A. Impaired word retrieval

    B. Meaningless speech and nonsense sounds

    C. Circumlocutionary language

    D. Impaired comprehension of verbal material

    E. Simplification of syntax

108. All of the following are seen in Alzheimer disease *except*

    A. Neuronal loss

    B. Cortical gliosis

    C. Extraneuronal neurofibrillary tangles

    D. Neuritic plaques

    E. Granulovacuolar degeneration

109. All of the following are suggestive of vascular dementia *except*

    A. Dementia within 3 months of a stroke

    B. Presence of delirium

    C. Abrupt deterioration in cognitive ability

    D. Stepwise progression of impairment

    E. Early gait disturbance

110. Which of the following is not a risk factor for vascular dementia?

    A. Hypertension

    B. Diabetes mellitus

    C. Elevated lipids

    D. Age

    E. Female sex

111. In vascular dementia, which of the following does imaging reveal?
- A. Reduced medial temporal lobe width
- B. Caudate atrophy
- C. Cortical atrophy
- D. Shrinkage of ventricles
- E. Hypoperfusion of frontal lobes

112. Which of the following dementias does not have a vascular etiology?
- A. Multi-infarct dementia
- B. Strategic single-vessel-infarct dementia
- C. Binswanger disease
- D. Progressive supranuclear palsy
- E. Lacunar dementia

113. Which of the following features is most likely to distinguish dementia with Lewy bodies from Alzheimer disease?
- A. Dementia
- B. Fluctuations in cognitive functions
- C. Auditory hallucinations
- D. Depression
- E. Falls

114. Which of the following is not seen by neuroimaging in dementia with Lewy bodies?
- A. Atrophy of medial temporal lobes
- B. Periventricular white-matter lesions shown by MRI
- C. Blood flow patterns similar to Alzheimer disease
- D. Decreased blood flow in basal ganglia

115. Which of the following does not suggest a diagnosis of dementia with Lewy bodies?
- A. Recurrent visual hallucinations
- B. Parkinsonian features
- C. History of strokes
- D. Neuroleptic sensitivity
- E. Syncope

116. All of the following are features of frontotemporal dementia *except*
- A. Disinhibition
- B. Delusions
- C. Preservation of affect
- D. Overeating
- E. Stereotyped behaviors

117. Which of the following is seen in frontotemporal dementia?
- A. Myoclonus
- B. Cerebellar ataxia
- C. Choreoathetosis
- D. Apraxia
- E. Hyperorality

118. In frontotemporal dementia, which of the following is revealed by neuroimaging?
- A. Generalized atrophy, more prominent in the parietal regions
- B. Frontal hypermetabolism, found by PET
- C. Parietal hypoperfusion, found by SPECT
- D. Parietal hypometabolism
- E. Frontal hypometabolism, found by PET

119. Which of the following is not a feature of dementia of normal pressure hydrocephalus?
- A. Impaired attention
- B. Poor learning
- C. Impaired judgment
- D. Apraxia
- E. Gait disturbance

120. All of the following are clinical features of Alzheimer dementia *except*
- A. Disorder of language and praxis
- B. Depression
- C. Loss of primitive reflexes
- D. Persecutory delusions
- E. Long-term memory loss

121. Which of the following is true about vascular dementia?

    A. Slow, gradual deterioration occurs.

    B. MRI shows areas of multiple infarction.

    C. Depression is rare.

    D. PET shows symmetric changes in the cortex.

    E. SPECT shows global hyperperfusion.

122. Which of the following is seen in Pick disease?

    A. Senile plaques

    B. Neurofibrillary tangles

    C. Atrophy of frontal and parietal lobes

    D. Knife-blade atrophy

123. All of the following are features of dementia of Lewy bodies *except*

    A. Extrapyramidal symptoms

    B. Clouding of consciousness

    C. Longer clinical course than Alzheimer disease

    D. Sensitivity to antipsychotic drugs

124. Which of the following is true regarding HIV encephalopathy associated with AIDS?

    A. Insight is preserved until late in the course of the disease.

    B. EEG is abnormal in the early stages.

    C. Frank dysphoria is common.

    D. Memory is usually preserved.

    E. Treatment has no influence on course of the disease.

125. Which of the following is true regarding Lewy bodies?

    A. They do not occur in normal brains.

    B. Their presence confirms Parkinson disease.

    C. They are extracellular bodies.

    D. They occur in Alzheimer disease.

126. Which of the following is commonly seen following frontal lobe injury?

    A. Contralateral optic atrophy

    B. Dyspraxia

    C. Ipsilateral spastic paresis

    D. Disinhibition

    E. Anosognosia

127. Which of the following is seen in nondominant parietal lobe lesions?
- A. Prosopagnosia
- B. Dyspraxia
- C. Alexia
- D. Body image disorders
- E. Hyperorality

128. Which of the following is seen in lesions of the dominant temporal lobe?
- A. Impaired visual memory
- B. Dysprosody
- C. Deep prosopagnosia
- D. Retained verbal memory
- E. Visual object agnosia

129. Which of the following is not caused by bilateral temporal lobe lesion?
- A. Hyperorality
- B. Hypersexuality
- C. Cortical blindness
- D. Amnestic syndrome
- E. Visual agnosia

130. Occipital lobe lesions can cause all of the following *except*
- A. Visual field defects
- B. Anton syndrome
- C. Visual hallucinations
- D. Sensory neglect
- E. Prosopagnosia

131. Parietal lobe lesions can cause all of the following *except*
- A. Dressing apraxia
- B. Gerstmann syndrome
- C. Pure agraphia without aphasia
- D. Personality changes
- E. Visual field defects

132. Which of the following can be caused by frontal lobe lesion?
   A. Hypersexuality
   B. Indifference to feelings of others
   C. Dyscalculia
   D. Pure alexia
   E. Ocular apraxia

133. Which of the following is the most commonly affected muscle in myasthenia gravis?
   A. Upper limb
   B. Lower limb
   C. Oropharyngeal
   D. Respiratory
   E. Ocular

134. All of the following are true about Gilles de la Tourette syndrome *except*
   A. Echolalia
   B. Improves with haloperidol
   C. High incidence of complex partial seizures
   D. Autosomal dominant with low penetrance
   E. Associated with obsessive-compulsive disorder

135. Which of the following is true about severe closed head injury?
   A. Headaches are inevitable.
   B. Recovery is completed within a year.
   C. Dementia is never seen.
   D. About 20% suffer from post-traumatic seizures.
   E. Post-traumatic amnesia is the best prognostic indicator.

136. Which of the following suggests that seizures may be pseudoseizures?
   A. Presence of interictal EEG abnormalities
   B. Incontinence
   C. Seizures occurring at night
   D. Seizures lasting longer than 30 minutes
   E. Seizures always occurring when patient is alone

137. A 70-year-old presents for evaluation of forgetfulness. Early dementia is suspected. Alzheimer dementia is most likely with which of the following symptoms?

    A. Sudden onset of forgetfulness

    B. Seizures

    C. Gait disturbance

    D. Progressive agnosia

    E. Incontinence

138. Which of the following is not seen in Gerstmann syndrome?

    A. Finger agnosia

    B. Alexia

    C. Acalculia

    D. Agraphia

    E. Right–left disorientation

139. Which of the following is caused by lesion at the level of C5?

    A. Sensory loss over little finger

    B. Motor loss of triceps function

    C. Loss of triceps tendon jerk

    D. Sensory loss over biceps

    E. Loss of flexion in interphalangeal joints

140. Which of the following is seen in Tourette syndrome?

    A. Coprophagia

    B. Paralysis of limbs

    C. Choreiform movements

    D. Subjective sudden release of tension

    E. Violent automatisms

141. Which of the following is a feature of transient global amnesia?

    A. Loss of identity

    B. Confabulation

    C. Decreased attention span

    D. Dissociative phenomena

    E. Global memory deficits

142. Which of the following is not seen in damage to the frontal lobes?
  A. Emotional changes
  B. Visual distortion
  C. Difficulty planning tasks
  D. Grasp reflex
  E. Incontinence

143. Which of the following is not seen with parietal lesions?
  A. Left–right disorientation
  B. Alexia with agraphia
  C. Topopagnosia
  D. Perseveration

144. What is the most sensitive test for detection of multiple sclerosis?
  A. CT
  B. MRI
  C. Evoked potentials
  D. SPECT
  E. EEG

145. In which stage of sleep is vivid dreaming most common?
  A. Stage 1
  B. Stage 2
  C. Stage 3
  D. Stage 4
  E. REM sleep

146. In which region of the spine are spinal epidural abscesses most commonly found?
  A. Cervical
  B. Thoracic
  C. Lumbar
  D. Sacral
  E. Coccygeal

147. What is the treatment of choice for subacute combined degeneration?
   A. Oral folic acid
   B. Parenteral folic acid
   C. Oral vitamin B12
   D. Parenteral vitamin B12
   E. Parenteral iron

148. Which of the following can result from brainstem ischemia?
   A. Jacksonian seizures
   B. Complex partial seizures
   C. Drop attacks
   D. Todd's palsy
   E. Grand mal epilepsy

149. Which of the following is not a feature of pseudobulbar palsy?
   A. Brisk jaw jerk
   B. Emotional lability
   C. Fasciculating tongue
   D. Presence of gag reflex
   E. Dysphagia

150. Which of the following is true of acute porphyria?
   A. Presence of abdominal pain
   B. Cloudy urine
   C. Widespread necrosis in the central nervous system
   D. Convulsions
   E. Weakness

151. Memory deficits can occur with lesion in which of the following areas?
   A. Wernicke's area
   B. Wall of the third ventricle
   C. Broaca's area
   D. Parietal cortex
   E. Lateral nucleus

152. Which of the following is not a part of the limbic system?
- A. Corpus callosum
- B. Parahippocampal gyrus
- C. Anterior nucleus of thalamus
- D. Subcallosal gyrus
- E. Hypothalamus

153. In which of the following does diplopia occur?
- A. Huntington disease
- B. Diabetes insipidus
- C. Facial nerve neuropathy
- D. Oculomotor nerve neuropathy
- E. Parkinson disease

154. Which of the following is not associated with benign intracranial hypertension?
- A. Polycythemia
- B. Oral contraceptives
- C. Myxedema
- D. Hypoparathyroidism
- E. Tetracyclines

155. A 55-year-old presents with a cerebrovascular accident. Which of the following suggests occlusion of a posterior inferior cerebellar artery?
- A. Ipsilateral Horner syndrome
- B. Dissociated analgesia
- C. Contralateral facial analgesia
- D. Ipsilateral limb analgesia
- E. Contralateral ataxia

156. Nystagmus can occur in
- A. Brainstem legions
- B. Cerebellar lesions
- C. Healthy subjects
- D. Rotational stimulation
- E. All of the above

157. Which of the following features would arouse a suspicion of basilar artery occlusion?

   A. Monoplegia
   B. Contralateral cerebellar signs
   C. Hypopyrexia
   D. Contralateral cranial nerve palsies

158. A 40-year-old man presents with sudden onset of blindness. Possible causes include all of the following *except*

   A. Vitreous hemorrhage
   B. Acute glaucoma
   C. Methanol ingestion
   D. Prolapsed intervertebral disc
   E. Retinal detachment

159. Which of the following is a function of the limbic system?

   A. Emotional behavior
   B. Motivation
   C. Sexual activity
   D. Conditioned reflexes
   E. All of the above

160. Which of the following is a feature of Brown-Séquard syndrome?

   A. Contralateral loss of kinesthesia
   B. Ipsilateral loss of crude touch
   C. Contralateral loss of temperature
   D. Contralateral loss of two-point discrimination

161. Which of the following is a feature of complete spinal-cord transection?

   A. Retention of voluntary movements below the lesion
   B. Hyperactive reflexes
   C. Loss of all sensation below the lesion
   D. Loss of all reflexes after 3 weeks
   E. Development of automatic bladder within first 3 days

162. Dopaminergic cells are found in all of the following *except*

   A. Median raphe nucleus
   B. Ventral tegmental area
   C. Substantia nigra
   D. Arcuate nucleus of hypothalamus

163. Which of the following occurs on carotid sinus stimulation?
- **A.** Hypertension
- **B.** Tachycardia
- **C.** Peripheral vasodilatation
- **D.** Raised intracranial pressure
- **E.** Hyperventilation

164. Components of the pyramidal system include all of the following *except*
- **A.** Anterior horn cells
- **B.** Vestibular nuclei
- **C.** Pyramidal tract
- **D.** Corticospinal tract

165. Which of the following is a component of the circle of Willis?
- **A.** Anterior inferior cerebellar artery
- **B.** Posterior spinal artery
- **C.** Superior cerebellar artery
- **D.** Posterior communicating artery

166. Which of the following is not a feature of cerebellar disease?
- **A.** Dysdiadochokinesis
- **B.** Past pointing
- **C.** Scanning dysarthria
- **D.** Resting tremor

167. Which of the following is not a sign of posterior column damage?
- **A.** Impaired two-point discrimination
- **B.** Loss of perception of pain
- **C.** Inability to detect direction and speed of a moving stimulus on the skin
- **D.** Loss of proprioception
- **E.** Loss of vibration sense

168. Which of the following is a feature of upper motor neuron disease?
- **A.** Clonus
- **B.** Flexor plantar response
- **C.** Wasting of muscles
- **D.** Decreased tendon reflexes
- **E.** Cogwheel rigidity

169. Which of the following is a feature of lower motor neuron lesion?
- **A.** Hypertonicity
- **B.** Clasp-knife rigidity
- **C.** Parkinsonism
- **D.** Absent reflexes
- **E.** Tardive dyskinesia

170. Which of the following can be caused by posterior cerebral artery occlusion?
- **A.** Ipsilateral hemianesthesia
- **B.** Ipsilateral hemianalgesia
- **C.** Ipsilateral hemiplegia
- **D.** Ipsilateral hemianopia
- **E.** Spontaneous pain

171. Which of the following can result in papilledema?
- **A.** Hypoparathyroidism
- **B.** Hypercapnia
- **C.** Cranial arteritis
- **D.** Cavernous sinus thrombosis
- **E.** All of the above

172. All of the following are due to disorders of the extrapyramidal system *except*
- **A.** Tremor
- **B.** Spasmodic torticollis
- **C.** Clasp-knife rigidity
- **D.** Akathisia
- **E.** Festinant gait

173. Which of the following is true about essential tremor?
- **A.** It has a frequency of 2–4 Hz.
- **B.** It is abolished on action.
- **C.** Alcohol may reduce essential tremor.
- **D.** It most commonly affects the head.

174. All of the following can occur with lesions of the parietal lobe *except*
- **A.** Astereognosis
- **B.** Gerstmann syndrome
- **C.** Dressing apraxia
- **D.** Tactile inattention
- **E.** Expressive dysphagia

175. Which of the following is a feature of Horner syndrome?
- A. Paralysis of lower part of face
- B. Ptosis of the eyelid
- C. Pupillary dilatation
- D. Sweating on the affected side
- E. Ataxia

176. A 62-year-old man with diabetes and hypertension is admitted to the emergency department because he has a severe headache and acute onset of double vision. Examination reveals that the man has ptosis on the right side and an inability to elevate or adduct the right eye, although lateral eye movements are spared. The man's right pupil is dilated and unreactive. What is the most likely diagnosis?
- A. Myasthenia gravis
- B. Pontine hemorrhage
- C. Extradural hemorrhage
- D. Diabetic palsy of cranial nerve III
- E. Berry aneurysm of the right posterior communicating artery

177. For which of the following is a CT scan superior to an MRI scan?
- A. Detecting lesions in the spinal cord
- B. Detecting demyelination secondary to multiple sclerosis
- C. Differentiating hemorrhage from edema
- D. Showing early ischemic changes
- E. Detecting small tumor

178. A 42-year-old man is referred for a psychiatric evaluation 4 years after sustaining a head injury in a car accident. Prior to the accident, he was a stable, happily married man. Since the accident, he has been described as very talkative and irresponsible. His marriage has ended in a divorce and he lost his job. Neuropsychiatic testing reveals that the man has average intelligence and no detectable memory deficits. The patient's clinical presentation is most consistent with damage to which of the following brain areas?
- A. Thalamus
- B. Temporal lobe
- C. Corpus striatum
- D. Amygdaloid body
- E. Frontal lobe

179. When examined, a 65-year-old man is found to be apathetic, forgetful, and confused, with psychomotor retardation. When he is admitted to the hospital for a routine transurethral retrograde prostatectomy, a psychiatric consultation is requested. The only medication the man has been taking is over-the-counter (OTC) cold remedies. Which of the following is included in the differential diagnoses for this patient?

  A. Parkinson disease
  B. Dementia
  C. Depression
  D. Anticholinergic side effects
  E. All of the above

180. Episodes of staring, lip smacking, and amnesia preceded by fear and a smell of burning rubber are most commonly associated with an electrical abnormality in which of the following?

  A. Cerebellum
  B. Occipital lobe
  C. Temporal lobe
  D. Frontal lobe
  E. Parietal lobe

181. A 50-year-old man is assessed for headaches and memory problems. CT and MRI scans reveal ventriculomegaly that is out of proportion to sulcal atrophy. Which diagnosis does this finding support?

  A. Pick disease
  B. Normal pressure hydrocephalus
  C. Alzheimer disease
  D. Huntington disease
  E. Parkinson disease

182. Which of the following statements is true about early-onset Alzheimer disease?

  A. Occurs sporadically
  B. Autosomal dominant inheritance
  C. No response to cholinesterase inhibitors
  D. More common in Black population
  E. More agitation and aggression

183. Prosopagnosia means the inability to do which of the following?

    A. Recognize faces

    B. Understand written text

    C. Follow directions

    D. Remember names

    E. Read fluently

184. A 56-year-old patient who is an alcoholic experiences unsteadiness of gait. He has a history of drinking alcohol every day for the past 30 years. Examination reveals minimal appendicular ataxia in the patient's lower extremities only and normal eye movements. The patient walks with a lurching, broad-based gait. What is the most appropriate diagnosis?

    A. Hysterical gait disorder

    B. Alcoholic cerebellar degeneration

    C. Chronic subdural hematoma

    D. Spinocerebellar degeneration

    E. Multiple sclerosis

185. A 65-year-old patient is diagnosed with severe Alzheimer disease. Where would you expect to see the maximum density of senile plaques and neurofibrillary tangles?

    A. Substantia nigra

    B. Subthalamic nucleus of Luys

    C. Hippocampus

    D. Dentate nucleus

    E. Parietal lobe

186. With which of the following is internuclear ophthalmoplegia most commonly seen?

    A. Optic neuritis

    B. Multiple sclerosis

    C. Amyotrophic lateral sclerosis

    D. Cerebellar dysfunction

    E. Pituitary tumor

187. Which of the following does MRI of the brain show in Huntington disease?

    A. Bilateral caudate atrophy

    B. Enlargement of ventricles

    C. Narrowing of pars compacta of substantia nigra

    D. Basal ganglia atrophy

    E. Frontotemporal atrophy

188. A 45-year-old man experiences a sudden onset of back pain while playing tennis. Examination reveals some spasms in the paraspinal muscles in the right lumbar region. He is able to perform a straight leg raise to 90 degrees with some increase in pain. Knee jerks and ankle jerks are normal and symmetric with no weakness in the muscles of the hip, leg, or foot. Sensory examination is within normal limits. What is the most appropriate next step in management?

    A. MRI of the lumbar spine

    B. Refer to physical therapy

    C. X-ray of the lumbar spine

    D. Psychiatric consultation for somatization disorder

    E. Bed rest and administration of analgesics

189. A 64-year-old woman is examined because she has been getting lost on her way home in her neighborhood during the past several weeks. A Mini-Mental Status examination is administered to screen for cognitive deficits. She answers all of the questions correctly, but she has difficulty copying intersecting pentagons. In which of the following regions of the brain has this woman most likely experienced a stroke?

    A. Left occipital lobe

    B. Left frontal lobe

    C. Left parietal lobe

    D. Right parietal lobe

    E. Right temporal lobe

190. A 58-year-old man suffers a stroke and is admitted to a rehabilitation unit for physical therapy. He is unable to wash the left side of his body and denies that his left arm belongs to him even though he clearly visualizes it. Examination reveals that the patient's somatosensory system is intact. These findings indicate that the patient may have a lesion. In which area of the brain is the lesion?

    A. Substantia nigra

    B. Caudate nucleus

    C. Right parietal cortex

    D. Left parietal cortex

    E. Right frontal cortex

191. A 36-year-old woman has experienced anxiety with intrusive mental images involving sex with animals. These experiences are accompanied by intense distress and unsuccessful attempts at resisting the thoughts. She relieves this anxiety by counting up to 100. In the last few weeks, she has been having severe problems with these episodes and they have caused significant distress. What is a PET scan in this patient likely to reveal?

A. Increased metabolic rates in the temporoparietal cortex

B. Increased metabolic rates in the temporofrontal cortex

C. Increased metabolic rates in the caudate nucleus and the prefrontal cortex

D. Decreased metabolic rates in the caudate nucleus and the prefrontal cortex

E. Decreased metabolic rates in the temporal and frontal cortex

192. A 34-year-male is assessed for speech problems following a "small stroke." Examination reveals no obvious language problems except for severe difficulty with fluency. The man has no problems with comprehension. His articulation is good, and nothing abnormal is detected on examination of the articulation muscles. What is the most likely site of the lesion?

A. Right parietal lobe

B. Right temporal lobe

C. Right caudate nucleus

D. Left parietal lobe

E. Left frontal lobe

193. A 20-year-old man is assessed for new onset psychosis. He is observed to have paranoid delusions and occasional auditory hallucinations. On physical examination, the psychiatrist also notices some abnormal movements of the arms and legs. Examination of the eyes reveals some abnormality with the cornea, but the physician is not sure what exactly the problem is. What is the most important next step in the management of this patient?

A. Start treatment with antipsychotic medications

B. Order a blood test to measure the level of ceruloplasmin

C. Order an MRI of the brain

D. Order a CT scan of the brain

E. Refer the patient to a neurologist

194. Characteristics of Huntington disease include all of the following *except*
- **A.** Progressive dementia
- **B.** Autosomal dominant transmission
- **C.** Caudate nucleus atrophy
- **D.** Transient neurologic abnormalities
- **E.** Personality changes

195. On an EEG, which of the following characterizes the second stage of NREM sleep?
- **A.** Predominant (more than 50%) delta waves
- **B.** Predominant alpha waves
- **C.** Sleep spindles and K complexes
- **D.** Rapid eye movements
- **E.** Less than 50% of delta waves

196. A 54-year-old woman with a history of depression is currently in remission after 6 months of treatment. However, she had sleep problems preceding the depression, and she continues to complain of daytime fatigue and nonrefreshing sleep. A detailed history reveals that she has a history of snoring and currently is borderline overweight. She had rhinoplasty a few years ago. Which of the following conditions does this patient probably have?
- **A.** Sleep problems secondary to depression
- **B.** Obstructive sleep apnea
- **C.** Somatization disorder
- **D.** Narcolepsy
- **E.** Psychophysiologic insomnia

197. A 54-year-old woman presents for assessment because of headaches and vision problems. Examination reveals that the patient has bitemporal hemianopia. What is the most likely cause of the patient's problems?
- **A.** Meningioma
- **B.** Lesion of optic nerve
- **C.** Multiple sclerosis
- **D.** Pituitary tumor
- **E.** Migraine

198. All of the following are true about Pick disease *except*
- A. Age of onset is 40–60 years.
- B. Memory loss occurs early in the course of the disease.
- C. Autosomal dominant inheritance is present in 20% of cases.
- D. Psychiatric symptoms are often the first manifestations.
- E. Linkage to chromosome 17 is established in some cases.

199. All of the following are features of Gerstmann syndrome *except*
- A. Lesion in the nondominant parietal lobe
- B. Right–left disorientation
- C. Acalculia
- D. Finger agnosia
- E. Agraphia

200. Which of the following do patients with Anton syndrome have?
- A. Language problems
- B. Articulation problems
- C. Denial of blindness
- D. Auditory problems
- E. Olfactory problems

ANSWERS

1. **Answer: D.** Ring-enhancing lesions seen on CT scan are indicative of brain abscess. Abscesses follow intravenous drug use, dental procedures, sinusitis, bacterial endocarditis, and immunodeficiency. Bacterial infections are the most common cause, but in AIDS, toxoplasmosis is the most common cause.

2. **Answer: D.** Electroencephalography (EEG), which traces brain waves, is the most helpful investigative method for determining pathology near the surface of the cerebral hemispheres. (Note that the abbreviation EEG also is used to refer to the tracing itself, the electroencephalogram.) Magnetic resonance imaging (MRI) is the best method for visualizing the posterior fossa, pituitary gland, and optic nerves. It is also the best for visualizing the white-matter changes of multiple sclerosis. Computed tomography (CT scan) can rapidly detect acute hemorrhage from acute intracranial hematomas, subdural hematomas, and subarachnoid hemorrhages.

3. **Answer: C.** Wernicke's encephalopathy is characterized by impairment of consciousness, ataxia, and ophthalmoplegia, typically palsy of the sixth cranial nerve. These symptoms reverse rapidly with administration of vitamin B1 (thiamine). Alcohol hallucinosis, schizophrenia, and dementia by definition occur without impairment of consciousness. Korsakoff syndrome is characterized by anterograde and retrograde amnesia and impairment in learning.

4. **Answer: D.** Friedreich ataxia is an autosomal recessive spinocerebellar degeneration. Eighty percent of persons diagnosed with Friedreich ataxia developed the disease before the age of 20 years. The most frequent presenting symptom is gait ataxia, followed by lower limb weakness and clumsiness. Lower limb reflexes are usually absent. Muscle tone is usually reduced. The coexistence of lower limb areflexia and Babinski sign strongly suggests Friedreich ataxia.

5. **Answer: C.** The transmitter that is mainly released from the preganglionic endings of sympathetic and parasympathetic fibers is acetylcholine.

6. **Answer: D.** Planned, goal-directed aggression is virtually never seen in seizure disorder. Ictal violence associated with seizures may injure people and damage property, but it is not directed or purposefully destructive and not based on aggression. Tinnitus, smell of burning rubber, rising epigastric sensation, and micropsia (seeing things as smaller than they actually are) are all part of aura in seizures with a temporal lobe focus.

7. **Answer: C.** CT scan is better than MRI to demonstrate calcification and bleeding in the brain. MRI is more useful to differentiate between white and gray matter. The presence of devices made of ferromagnetic (iron) metals such as older model pacemakers, intracranial aneurysm clip, or cochlear implants is a contraindication to performing an MRI.

8. **Answer: C.** Double vision is associated with damage to the fourth cranial nerve (trochlear), which originates in the midbrain. Walking down stairs requires that the eyes be able to move down, an ability that is governed by trochlear nerve. Because the trochlear nucleus is in the midbrain and the trochlear fibers cross the midbrain, the lesion is most likely to be in the midbrain.

9. **Answer: D.** The Wisconsin Card Sorting Test detects frontal lobe damage. The Thematic Apperception Test, Rorschach test, and MMPI are used for personality evaluation. Stanford-Binet is an intelligence test.

10. **Answer: B.** Common migraine, which is migraine without aura, affects about 75% of patients who have migraine headaches. The headaches last for 4 to 24 hours and are throbbing or pulsating, hemicranial, and temporal, retro-orbital, or periorbital; they may be accompanied by nausea and vomiting. Classic migraine, which is migraine with aura, affects only about 15% of patients and is preceded by an aura, although the subsequent headache is similar to migraine without aura. Hemiplegic migraine is characterized by a combination of hemiparesis or aphasia preceding or accompanying typical migraine symptoms. In childhood migraine, the headache is more likely to be bilateral, briefer, and more severe; other symptoms, like nausea, may be prominent. In basilar migraine, headache is accompanied by symptoms suggestive of basilar artery dysfunction such as ataxia, vertigo, dysarthria, and diplopia.

11. **Answer: A.** In contrast to tension headaches, which tend to occur in the evening, migraine headaches begin in the early morning. They are more common in women and start at menarche, occur premenstrually, and are aggravated by oral contraceptives. The majority of women experience relief from the symptoms during pregnancy.

12. **Answer: E.** Nocturnal migraine headaches tend to occur during REM sleep. Some people have migraine headaches only during sleep.

13. **Answer: D.** Cluster headache is a condition in which severe headaches occur daily for a period of 4 to 8 weeks, usually in the spring. The headaches are sharp, nonthrobbing, and bore into one eye and around the eye. The pain is excruciating and is associated with tearing, conjunctival injection, nasal congestion, and Horner-like syndrome. Cluster headache condition is more common in men aged 20–40 years than in others. Brain tumors and tension headaches are unlikely to present in such a dramatic manner. Retinal detachment does not typically cause pain.

14. Answer: C. Among persons diagnosed with cluster headache, more than 80% smoke and 50% drink alcohol excessively (although, unlike tension headache, the condition is not relieved by alcohol). The condition has no familial tendency. In the vast majority of cases, the symptoms are not preceded by an aura. The headaches may be treated with sumatriptan and oxygen inhalation.

15. Answer: E. The symptoms with which this patient presents are typical of temporal arteritis, a condition in which the temporal and other cranial arteries become inflamed. Patients present with dull, continual headache in one or both temples. There is also pain on chewing. Systemic signs such as malaise, fever, and weight loss may be present. Serious complications may occur, such as ophthalmic artery occlusion, causing blindness, or cerebral artery occlusion, causing cerebral infarcts. A blood test showing estimated sedimentation rate (ESR) greater than 40 mm per hour supports the diagnosis, and temporal artery biopsy is a definitive test. The most important intervention is the administration of high-dose steroids, which will relieve the headaches and prevent complications. CT and MRI are not indicated.

16. Answer: A. Subarachnoid hemorrhage is most commonly caused by rupture of a berry aneurysm. It can cause severe headaches and nuchal rigidity and can occur during exertion, including exercise or sexual intercourse. Blood can be seen on CT or MRI and on lumbar puncture. Headaches of such sudden onset are not characteristic of the other conditions listed in the question.

17. Answer: C. Tension headaches and trigeminal neuralgia do not awaken people from sleep. Subarachnoid hemorrhage and brain tumors can wake people up from sleep. Migraine can occur during sleep, as can cluster headaches.

18. Answer: D. In trigeminal neuralgia, patients suffer from dozens of brief jabs of sharp excruciating facial pain lasting 20 to 30 seconds, which can be provoked by touching the affected area and which recur for days, weeks, or months. On touching the trigger area, usually around the mouth, patients may experience a shocklike sensation. Depression, chronic analgesic abuse, tension headaches, use of drugs like benzodiazepines, ergotamines, and narcotics can cause chronic daily headaches. NSAIDs are least likely to cause chronic daily headaches; however, other antimigraine medications, aspirin, and caffeine compounds can cause them.

19. Answer: D. Interictal EEG is normal for about 20% of patients with a seizure disorder. Therefore, normal interictal EEGs do not rule out a diagnosis of seizure disorder.

20. Answer: A. There are two major seizure categories: partial seizures and primary generalized seizures. In primary generalized seizures, the thalamus or subcortical structures generate discharges, which spread upward to excite the entire cerebral cortex; these seizures are bilateral, symmetric, and without focal clinical or EEG findings.

21. Answer: C. A partial seizure with elementary motor symptoms may begin in a limited body region and undergo secondary generalization. This progression is called Jacksonian march. A postictal monoparesis or hemiparesis is called Todd's palsy and may persist for up to 24 hours. Partial seizures with olfactory symptoms are called uncinate seizures because olfactory hallucinations result from discharges in the amygdala or uncus. Rolandic epilepsy is the most common cause of childhood epilepsy; it begins between the ages of 5 and 9 and occurs in boys.

22. Answer: D. Post-traumatic seizure disorder is one of the most common complications of major traumatic brain injury, occurring in up to 50% of patients following major injury. Incidence increases in association with penetrating injuries, the presence of intracranial bleeding, and depressed fractures of the skull. The disorder is not particularly associated with linear fractures of the skull. The incidence is higher in patients using alcohol. The incidence increases, rather than decreases, as time passes after injury.

23. Answer: C. Violent acts may accompany the seizure but are not common. Partial complex seizures begin in late childhood through the early 30s. This is the most common seizure variety, affecting about 65% of patients. Most patients only display a blank stare during which they are inattentive or uncommunicative. They always have impaired consciousness and may have memory loss. Physical manifestations usually only consist of automatisms like lip smacking, fumbling, scratching, and rubbing. About 40% of patients have elevated prolactin level after the seizure.

24. Answer: B. Frontal lobe seizures often arise abruptly without an aura and are of relatively short duration (<1 minute). They cause minimal postictal confusion. They tend to begin in adult years, occur frequently, are more common during sleep, and may not be detected by EEG. Their manifestations are bizarre and may mimic pseudoseizures.

25. Answer: D. Planned aggressive acts do not happen during a seizure episode. Random violent acts like kicking, verbal abuse, screaming, and damage to property can occur.

26. Answer: B. Schizophrenia-like symptoms are seen in up to 10% of patients with partial complex seizures. Symptoms such as hallucinations and paranoia are seen. However, their affect is relatively normal, they do not deteriorate, and the incidence of schizophrenia in the family is not increased. There is no deterioration of personality and symptoms arise on an average when patients are about 30 years old.

27. **Answer: E.** Confusion can be caused by postictal confusion, antiepileptic drug intoxication, status epilepticus, or stopping antiepileptic drugs.

28. **Answer: B.** Partial complex seizures have a temporal lobe focus in about 90% of patients.

29. **Answer: A.** Absence seizures begin between the ages of 4 and 10 years and disappear in early adulthood. They consist of lapses of attention lasting 2 to 10 seconds, which are accompanied by automatisms, clonic limb movements, or blinking. These seizures are not associated with amnesia, confusion, or agitation. EEG shows generalized 3-Hz spike and wave complexes.

30. **Answer: D.** These symptoms are typical of absence seizures.

31. **Answer: D.** Absence seizures do not have auras or postictal confusion. Valproate and ethosuximide are the preferred treatments.

32. **Answer: D.** Pseudoseizures or psychogenic nonepileptic seizures are psychogenic seizure-like episodes. They can be present in patients with true seizures. They develop slowly and are accompanied by prominent flailing, struggling, agitation, and alternating limb movements. The duration of 2 to 5 minutes is longer than the average epileptic seizure. They usually have no tonic phase or incontinence. Consciousness is preserved and patients have no postictal symptoms like confusion, headache, or retrograde amnesia. The EEG obtained during a pseudoseizure is normal, and a postictal EEG does not show postictal depression. The serum prolactin concentration is not elevated. EEG video monitoring can help differentiate pseudoseizures from an epileptic seizure. Self-injury is rare, although patients may bite the lip or tip of the tongue rather than the side of the tongue as in epilepsy.

33. **Answer: C.** Axons of the tenth cranial nerve innervate the soft palate and pharynx. Damage to these axons causes dysphagia, hoarseness, and paralysis of the soft palate. These symptoms can be caused by damage to the ninth cranial nerve as well.

34. **Answer: B.** A definitive diagnosis of carotid artery stenosis is made by arteriography. However, because arteriography acquires catheterization, magnetic resonance angiography is preferred. Doppler ultrasonography (ultrasound) is also reliable for revealing carotid artery stenosis.

35. **Answer: C.** The symptoms are most suggestive of involvement of the vertebrobasilar system, which supplies the brainstem, cerebellum, and posterior inferior cerebrum. The symptoms result from brainstem ischemia and include circumoral paresthesias, dysarthria, nystagmus, ataxia, and vertigo. Patients may have drop attacks when generalized brainstem ischemia impairs consciousness and body tone and causes them to collapse.

36. Answer: E. Basilar artery transient ischemic attacks (TIAs) are the most likely cause of transient global amnesia. TIAs impair circulation in the artery's terminal branches, the posterior cerebral arteries, which supply the temporal lobe, thus causing temporary amnesia. Patients cannot learn new information; that is, they have anterograde amnesia. They also have retrograde amnesia. General knowledge and personal information is retained. There is no confabulation, and the motor system is completely spared. The TIAs happen in middle-aged and older individuals. They have a sudden onset and the recurrence rate is about 10%.

37. Answer: B. See the preceding answer.

38. Answer: E. The greatest risk factor for strokes is age. Hypertension, valvular disease, acute MI, and atrial fibrillation are other cardiovascular risk factors. Diabetes mellitus, cigarette smoking, migraines, and drug abuse are also risk factors. Type A personality and stress have not been shown to be risk factors.

39. Answer: E. Lesions of the pons cause abducent nerve and contralateral palsy. Oculomotor nerve palsy is caused by lesions of the midbrain. Lateral medullary infarctions cause ipsilateral ataxia, Horner syndrome, contralateral hypalgesia, and palatal paresis.

40. Answer: A. Cerebral hemorrhages are characterized by occipital headaches, gait ataxia, dysarthria, and lethargy. They should be evacuated immediately as a life-saving step. Contralateral lower limb paresis is caused by occlusion of the anterior cerebral artery.

41. Answer: C. Poststroke depression may affect 30–50% of patients following a stroke. The classic association of depression following stroke is with lesion in the left frontal region of the brain. However, this has not been supported by recent studies. (It is still reasonable to answer "left frontal" to exam questions about lesion associated with depression nonetheless.) It has been suggested that depression immediately following stroke could be due to lesion in the left frontal region, whereas in the long term it is more likely to be associated with right occipital lesions.

42. Answer: E. A number of factors are associated with poststroke depression; among them are the age of the patient and the degree of functional disability. Being depressed also places patients at greater risk of a further stroke, myocardial infarction, and death. Only nortriptyline, citalopram, and fluoxetine have been studied in the treatment of poststroke depression.

43. Answer: C. The locked-in syndrome results from an infarction of the base or ventral surface of the pons due to occlusion of the basilar artery. Patients are mute because of bulbar palsy and quadriplegic because of interruption of the corticospinal tract. The upper brainstem and connections with the cerebral cortex are intact, and hence patients are alert and retain normal cognition.

44. Answer: C. Massive cerebral injury can result in a persistent vegetative state. Patients are unaware of themselves or their surroundings, devoid of cognitive capacity, and unable to interact or communicate in any manner. They are bedridden with quadriparesis and incontinence. Patients are neither in suspended animation nor prolonged sleep. Eye movements are present.

45. Answer: D. Carotid artery occlusion causes monocular amaurosis fugax. The other symptoms are caused by basilar artery occlusion.

46. Answer: A. All of these deficits are caused by lesion in the left internal capsule. Since the motor fibers from the cortex that supply all three of these regions are crossed, a lesion in the internal capsule will produce these deficits.

47. Answer: D. Multiple sclerosis is a demyelinating disease. Demyelinated plaques are scattered throughout the optic nerve, brain, and spinal cord. Demyelinated patches cause neurologic deficits because axons deprived of their myelin sheath cannot properly transmit nerve impulses. The deficits resolve as the inflammation spontaneously subsides. The most common course is relapsing-remitting, and it is also the most amenable to treatment.

48. Answer: E. See the preceding answer.

49. Answer: D. The most frequent symptoms of multiple sclerosis are caused by plaques on the white-matter tracts of the spinal cord, brainstem, and optic nerves. Symptoms may begin between 15 and 50 years of age; the mean age of onset is 33 years. The incidence is greatest in patients who have lived in cool northern latitudes of the United States and Europe. There are three variants of disease progression: the disease most commonly begins with a relapsing-remitting (RR) course; primary-progressive (PP) MS is a gradual decline; secondary-progressive (SS) is RR followed by PP. Progressive-relapsing (PR) MS is rare.

50. Answer: B. Multiple sclerosis does not cause involuntary movement disorders. Symptoms include ataxia, tremors, trigeminal neuralgia, optic neuritis, nystagmus, internuclear ophthalmoplegia, diplopia, paresis with hyperactive deep tendon reflexes and Babinski sign, sexual impairment, generalized fatigue, and depression.

51. Answer: C. Cognitive impairment and dementia induced by multiple sclerosis correlate with physical disability, duration of illness, enlarged cerebral ventricles, atrophy of the corpus callosum, periventricular white-matter demyelination, total lesion load as shown by MRI, and cerebral hypometabolism as shown by PET. Of these, the closest correlation is with "lesion load" (number of lesions) detected by MRI.

52. Answer: C. The concordance rate among monozygotic twins is 30%; among dizygotic twins it is 5%.

53. Answer: B. Guillain-Barre syndrome is a demyelinating disease of the peripheral nervous system. It affects young and middle-aged adults and causes paraparesis or quadriparesis. It is characterized by a single monophasic attack, lasting weeks to months, of symmetric, flaccid, areflexic paresis. It does not cause cognitive impairment or psychosis.

54. Answer: C. Central pontine myelinolysis is caused by rapid correction of hyponatremia. It is associated with severe debilitating illnesses. Delayed appearance of an acute spastic quadriparesis with pseudobulbar palsy is the classic manifestation. Behavioral changes and decreased consciousness are also seen.

55. Answer: C. Measles does not usually acutely affect the central nervous system, but in 1 in 1,000 patients with measles, on average at 5 days after the onset of the rash, it produces a postinfectious, immune-mediated encephalomyelitis. This results in death in 10% of patients and severe sequelae, with seizures, mental regression, and focal deficits in others.

56. Answer: D. In Huntington disease, there is a reduction in acetylcholine and GABA in the basal ganglia.

57. Answer: D. Parkinson disease is characterized by tremor, rigidity, bradykinesia, masked facies, paucity of movement, micrographia, and decreased blinking and facial expression.

58. Answer: C. Symptoms in Parkinson disease develop in an asymmetric or unilateral pattern. The tremor is most evident at rest. As the disease progresses, patients lose their postural reflexes. This, in combination with akinesia and rigidity results in a festinating gait, is characterized by a tendency to lean forward and accelerate the gait. The voice becomes low in volume and monotonous. Rigidity is classically of the cogwheel variety.

59. Answer: A. Psychosis is seen in about 10% of patients with Parkinson disease. It is associated with dementia, older age, long-standing illness, and excessive levels of antiparkinsonian medication. The most common manifestations are visual hallucinations, delusions, paranoia, and chronic confusion with a nighttime worsening of symptoms. Auditory hallucinations are rarely seen. Typical antipsychotics should be avoided. Clozapine and quetiapine are considered the best medications to use because they do not exacerbate parkinsonism.

60. Answer: E. Dementia affects about 20% of patients with Parkinson disease and is more common with increased duration of the illness. It increases in proportion to physical impairments, especially bradykinesia. The dementia associated with Parkinson disease is a subcortical dementia characterized by inattention, poor motivation, difficulty shifting mental sets, slowed thinking, and gait impairment. Aphasia, apraxia, and agnosia are symptoms of cortical dementia. A sudden onset usually excludes a diagnosis of dementia and warrants a search for other causes.

61. Answer: C. Hallucinations do not respond to antiparkinsonian drugs and may in fact be worsened by them because of increased dopamine.

62. Answer: B. The tendency of typical antipsychotics to produce parkinsonism is related to their ability to block D2 receptors. Risperidone in doses more than 6 mg also can cause parkinsonism. Other medications, like metoclopramide, cisapride, trimethobenzamide, and prochlorperazine, also block D2 receptors and cause parkinsonism.

63. Answer: B. Quetiapine and clozapine have very little affinity for D2 receptors and hence do not cause parkinsonism.

64. Answer: D. Bradykinesia is reported by patients to be the most disabling symptom of parkinsonism. Tremor and rigidity are also distressing. Masklike facies and micrographia do not cause disability.

65. Answer: C. Patients with Parkinson disease who have been well controlled on medication for years may suddenly develop symptoms of parkinsonism, which may remit abruptly. The mechanism for this is not well understood and is called on–off phenomenon.

66. Answer: B. Athetosis is the slow, regular, continual twisting movements that are typically bilateral and symmetric and affect distal parts of the limbs. Chorea consists of random, discrete, brisk movements that jerk the pelvis, trunk, and limbs. The walking gait has an irregular, jerky pattern. Dystonia consists of involuntary movements caused by muscle contraction.

67. Answer: C. Huntington disease is autosomal dominant and is characterized by chorea and dementia. Occasionally sporadic cases may be seen.

68. Answer: E. A variety of psychiatric sequelae are seen with Huntington disease. Depressive symptoms are the most common. A high rate of affective disorders, including bipolar disorder, has been reported. Paranoid symptoms and schizophrenia are more common than in the general population, although the incidence of schizophrenia among relatives is not increased. Dementia is usual in the later stages and insight is preserved until late. Patients are also prone to commit suicide.

69. Answer: A. The most common initial site of development of chorea is the face. The chorea may consist of only excessive facial gestures (grimaces) or hand gestures and twitchiness. It interferes with normal eye movements, and patients have difficulty making sudden and smooth shifts of gaze. It also affects movements of the upper limbs, trunk, lower limbs, and the swallowing muscles.

70. Answer: E. The characteristic gross pathologic finding in Huntington disease is atrophy of the caudate nuclei. The corpus striatum consists of the caudate, putamen, and globus pallidus. The loss of caudate nuclei permits the lateral ventricles to balloon outward and become voluminous. The cerebral cortex also undergoes atrophy as the illness progresses. There is atrophy of the thalamus as well. PET studies demonstrate caudate hypometabolism early in the illness.

71. Answer: A. The Huntington gene responsible for Huntington disease lies on the short arm of chromosome 4. The Huntington gene is unstable and tends to expand further in successive generations. The progressive expansion and amplification explains why carriers in successive generations show signs at younger ages.

72. Answer: C. Hemiballismus consists of intermittent gross movements on one side of the body. The movements are usually unilateral and consist of a flinging motion. The lesion is usually in the caudate nucleus or other basal ganglia structures. No cognitive impairment, paresis, or corticospinal tract signs accompany hemiballismus.

73. Answer: C. Lesions in the subthalamic nucleus result in hemiballismus.

74. Answer: D. Strokes in the pons and midbrain, which often result from occlusion of the basilar artery, can produce coma or a variant called akinetic mutism. The EEG shows a pattern associated with slow wave sleep, but eye movements are preserved.

75. Answer: B. Aphagia is produced by a lesion of the lateral hypothalamus. The lateral hypothalamus is the "hunger center" and the ventromedial hypothalamus is the "satiety center." The preoptic region regulates temperature and thirst.

76. **Answer: D.** Lesch-Nyhan syndrome is a sex-linked recessive condition. Affected children, aged between 2 and 6 develop dystonia, self-mutilation, mental retardation, corticospinal tract signs, seizures, and hyperuricemia. The basic abnormality is a deficiency of hypoxanthine guanine phosphoribosyl transferase (HGPRT), which is an enzyme required for urea metabolism.

77. **Answer: C.** The most common involuntary movement disorder is essential tremor. Parkinson disease is the second most common, but it causes the most disability.

78. **Answer: D.** Patients with essential tremor have fine tremors (measured as oscillation between 6 and 9 Hz) of the wrist, hands, or fingers. Essential tremor usually develops in young and middle-aged adults. It follows a pattern of autosomal dominant inheritance with variable penetrance. Family history is present in about 30%. Anxiety can intensify tremor. Almost 50% of patients have a resolution of the tremors with alcohol. Beta-blockers can suppress tremors.

79. **Answer: D.** Klüver-Bucy syndrome is manifested by hyperorality and hypersexuality. It results from lesions in the temporal lobe in which parts of the amygdala are involved.

80. **Answer: C.** CIDP is most commonly seen in the fifth and sixth decades of life. It typically shows symmetric motor and sensory involvement. Wasting is rarely seen, and pain is uncommon. Proximal and distal muscles are equally involved, and lower limbs are more severely involved.

81. **Answer: C.** The most common infection of the central nervous system in patients with AIDS is toxoplasmosis. Tuberculosis, cytomegalovirus, cryptococcus, and herpes simplex also have an increased prevalence in patients with AIDS.

82. **Answer: B.** Astrocytomas arise from the astrocytes, which are glial cells. They affect children and adults. In children, they tend to be cystic and are located in the cerebellum and brainstem. They may be totally removed and have a cure rate of about 90%. In adulthood, they occur predominantly in the cerebrum, infiltrate extensively, and may evolve into more malignant forms like glioblastomas. Total surgical removal requires sacrificing surrounding structures. Cure rates are low.

83. **Answer: B.** Meningiomas arise from cells of the meninges. They are often associated with neurofibromatosis type 1. They grow slowly and develop almost exclusively in adults. They cause symptoms by compressing the underlying brain and spinal cord. Most meningiomas can be totally removed by surgery.

84. Answer: E. Metastatic tumors spread through the blood into the brain and spinal cord. They tend to be multiple, surrounded by edema, and grow rapidly. The most common site of origin is the lung. Other sites include breast, kidney, skin, bone, and prostate. Gastrointestinal and pelvic cancers rarely spread to the brain.

85. Answer: C. Petit mal or absence seizures are not seen with intracranial neoplasms. Seizures are usually either partial elementary or partial complex. Tumors can cause headaches, accompanied by nausea and vomiting, which are worse early in the morning, predominantly unilateral, and may wake patients up from sleep. Increased intracranial pressure can develop and can cause generalized, nonspecific cognitive changes and papilledema. Tumors can also cause hemiparesis and cranial nerve palsies. Headache is the presenting clinical feature in almost 35% of patients.

86. Answer: C. Pituitary adenomas, by pressure on the optic chiasma, can cause bitemporal hemianopia. They also cause headaches, hormonal irregularities including infertility, amenorrhea, decreased libido, anergia, apathy, and listlessness. The investigation of choice is an MRI.

87. Answer: C. Acoustic neuroma is caused by the proliferation of the Schwann cells of the eighth cranial nerve. It develops in the internal auditory canal and cerebellopontine angle and may compress adjacent structures. Symptoms include hearing impairment, tinnitus, imbalance, and vertigo. If it compresses the fifth cranial nerve, patients develop facial sensory loss. With compression of the seventh cranial nerve, facial muscle weakness develops.

88. Answer: B. Spinal cord compression causes pain, quadriplegia, paraplegia, loss of sensation, and incontinence of urine and feces. Cognitive capacity is preserved though depression may ensue.

89. Answer: D. Alpha activity is EEG activity with a frequency of 8–13 Hz. It is most prominent on the occipital leads with eyes closed.

90. Answer: C. Pseudotumor cerebri is characterized by excessive fluid accumulation in the brain parenchyma. It may cause headache, papilledema, and visual field defects. It affects obese young women.

91. Answer: D. This is a typical presentation of subarachnoid hemorrhage, the most common cause of which is rupture of a berry aneurysm. Symptoms include sudden onset of headaches and nuchal rigidity. This is usually preceded by physical exertion. CT or MRI reveals blood in the subarachnoid space at the base of the brain, and lumbar puncture reveals bloody cerebrospinal fluid (CSF).

92. Answer: C. Motor vehicle accidents are the most common cause of head trauma in adolescence and early adulthood.

93. Answer: C. Lesion to the left temporal region has the closest correlation with the impairment produced. Frontal lobe trauma is the most common.

94. Answer: E. Schizophrenia, by definition, exists in the absence of any brain injury or substance use. Psychotic symptoms are not part of a postconcussional syndrome. Postconcussional syndrome is the most important long-term consequence of minor head trauma. The core symptoms are headaches, memory impairment, and insomnia lasting 2 to 3 months after a concussion. Other symptoms include anxiety, depression, fatigue, and poor concentration.

95. Answer: B. Personality change following head injury is most common after injury to the frontal or temporal lobe. Damage to the frontal lobe impairs the brain's inhibitory centers, which can lead to aggressiveness and emotional lability.

96. Answer: C. The most common psychiatric manifestation of neurosyphilis is depression. Dementia is common as well. Although euphoria and mania are also seen, they are not as common as depression.

97. Answer: B. When tested by means of lumbar puncture, cerebrospinal fluid is clear in neurosyphilis and also in Guillain-Barre (GB) syndrome. It is turbid with bacterial, tuberculous, and fungal meningitis. It may be either clear or turbid with viral meningitis. Bloody CSF is found in subarachnoid hemorrhage.

98. Answer: B. Normal CSF glucose of 50 to 80 mg per dl is seen in viral meningitis and Guillain-Barre syndrome. It is decreased in all the other conditions mentioned.

99. Answer: C. CJD is an infection with a prion, which is a subviral replicative protein. It causes a rapidly progressive cortical pattern dementia. The age of onset is in the sixth or seventh decade. Clinical symptoms initially may be nonspecific, but later, symptoms like dementia, myoclonus, and pyramidal and extrapyramidal signs develop. EEG shows diffuse symmetric slow waves. Definitive diagnosis is made on postmortem exam. Death usually ensues within 6 months to 2 years following onset of the illness.

100. Answer: B. AIDS dementia affects about 20% of all AIDS patients and about 30% to 60% of those in the late stages of their illness. It is a subcortical type of dementia with decreased concentration, forgetfulness, slowed mentation, apathy, and social withdrawal. Aphasia and apraxia, which are cortical signs, are uncommon, at least in the early stages. Motor symptoms like slow limb movements, clumsy and slow gait, frontal signs, ataxia, increased tone, and hyperactive reflexes may present. Behavior problems are common as well.

101. Answer: A. Distal symmetric polyneuropathy is the most frequent neuropathy seen in HIV disease. It is usually a painful sensorimotor polyneuropathy. The major symptoms are paresthesias and dysesthesias in the lower extremities, with the upper extremities affected later. Diminution or abolition of tendon reflexes is an invariable sign. Sensation is affected more than motor function in the distal segments, more in the legs than arms. Vibratory sense is involved more than position and tactile senses. Weakness is generally limited to the foot muscles. Toxic neuropathy is associated with antiretroviral treatment, and autonomic neuropathy is infrequently seen.

102. Answer: D. Age is the only proven risk factor for dementia, the incidence of which increases with increasing age. Women have a slightly greater risk of developing dementia. NSAIDs may confer a protective effect. Maternal age per se is not a risk factor for the development of Alzheimer disease. Exposure to aluminum has been postulated to be a risk factor but has not been proven.

103. Answer: B. Chromosome 15 is not associated with Alzheimer disease. Mutation in three genes (the APP gene on chromosome 21, presenilin-1 (PS1) on chromosome 14, and presenilin-2 (PS2) on chromosome 1) produce the autosomal dominant form of Alzheimer disease, which can manifest as early as the third decade of life. The mutations are rare, highly penetrant, and all carriers develop Alzheimer disease. A polymorphism of the APOE gene on chromosome 19 is also a susceptibility marker for Alzheimer disease. Not all patients with APOE4 develop Alzheimer disease.

104. Answer: E. Antipsychotic drugs may worsen the cognitive deficits. Agents shown to be helpful in delaying the progression of Alzheimer disease include radical scavengers, antioxidants like vitamin D and selegiline, cholinesterase inhibitors like donepezil, galantamine, and rivastigmine, and anti-inflammatory drugs.

105. Answer: C. Deep white-matter hyperintensities are seen in vascular dementia not Alzheimer's. Imaging studies in Alzheimer disease show generalized atrophy and ventricular enlargement with reduced medial temporal lobe width and periventricular white-matter lesions. Single photon emission computed tomography (SPECT) reveals temporoparietal hypoperfusion.

106. Answer: D. All of the symptoms mentioned are seen in patients with dementia. However, apathy has been reported most frequently in more than two-thirds of patients. This is followed by agitation, anxiety, irritability, and dysphoria. Disinhibition, delusions, and hallucinations are also common. The frequency and severity of apathy, agitation, dysphoria, and aberrant motor behavior correlate with the degree of cognitive impairment.

107. Answer: B. A number of abnormalities of speech are seen in Alzheimer disease. These include impaired word retrieval, circumloculatory language, impaired comprehension of verbal material, and simplification of syntax. In more advanced stages of the disease, speech deteriorates to meaningless speech and nonsense words.

108. Answer: C. The major pathologic changes in Alzheimer disease include neuronal loss, cortical gliosis, neuritic plaques, granulovacuolar degeneration, and amyloid angiopathy of cerebral vessels. Neurofibrillary tangles are composed of altered microtubule protein "tau." They are intraneuronal not extraneuronal.

109. Answer: B. The absence of delirium and psychosis are necessary criteria to diagnose vascular dementia. Vascular dementia is a dementing condition produced by ischemia or hemorrhage with brain injury. Classically it is characterized by an abrupt onset, stepwise deterioration, patchy pattern of intellectual deficits, focal neurologic symptoms and signs, history of hypertension, and associated cardiovascular disease. Vascular dementia is most common after the age of 50. Early gait disturbance with falls, urinary symptoms, pseudobulbar palsy, and personality changes also support a diagnosis of vascular dementia.

110. Answer: E. Vascular dementia is more common in men than in women. The other risk factors of stroke are also risk factors for vascular dementia.

111. Answer: C. Vascular dementia is associated with cortical and central atrophy. It is also associated with increased prevalence of infarcts and extensive white-matter change. In particular, bilateral left-sided lesions, diffuse white-matter change, and small infarcts in strategic regions are all important in causing cognitive impairment. SPECT shows patchy multifocal perfusion deficits.

112. Answer: D. Binswanger disease, one of the causes of multi-infarct dementia, is characterized by extensive ischemic injury of the white matter. Multi-infarct dementia results from the cumulative effect of multiple small-vessel and large-vessel occlusions. Strategic single-vessel infarct dementia is caused by strategically located solitary infarcts. Progressive supranuclear palsy is a chronic progressive disorder associated with eye movement abnormalities, parkinsonism, and dementia; mutations on chromosome 17 account for the majority of cases. Lacunar dementia is caused by multiple small lacunar infarctions of the basal ganglia and thalamus.

113.   Answer: B. Dementia with Lewy bodies (DLB) should be suspected in the presence of a dementia syndrome with the triad of fluctuating cognitive impairment, extrapyramidal symptoms, and visual hallucinations. Falls are also more likely in DLB although not they are not a feature that distinguishes DLB from Alzheimer disease. Auditory hallucinations, depression, and dementia are seen in both.

114.   Answer: A. In dementia with Lewy bodies, there is generalized ventricular enlargement with relative preservation of medial temporal lobe structures. White-matter changes are similar to Alzheimer disease but less extensive than vascular disease. SPECT shows posterior deficits and reduced D2 receptor density and dopamine transporters.

115.   Answer: C. A history of strokes is more suggestive of vascular dementia. Visual hallucinations and parkinsonian symptoms are features of DLB. More than one-third of patients are sensitive to antipsychotic drugs. They are also prone to falls and syncopal attacks.

116.   Answer: C. Frontotemporal dementia (FTD) is a group of disorders with atrophy of frontal and temporal lobes. The main features are personality alteration with disinhibition, emotional coarsening, loss of the ability to empathize, apathy, inability to interpret social cues, and poor judgment, planning, and insight. It begins between the ages of 40 and 65 years. Memory and visuospatial skills are relatively preserved, although language may be affected. FTD is sometimes associated with lability of affect.

117.   Answer: E. Hyperorality with oral exploration of objects is a prominent behavioral disturbance in frontotemporal dementia, or FTD. Abrupt onset with seizures, head trauma, early amnesia, apraxia, spatial disorientation, myoclonus, cerebellar ataxia, and choreoathetosis are not prominent features, and their presence goes against a diagnosis of FTD.

118.   Answer: B. Positron emission tomography (PET) reveals frontal hypermetabolism in frontotemporal dementia.

119.   Answer: D. Normal pressure hydrocephalus (NPH) is characterized by dementia, gait disturbance, and urinary incontinence. The dementia consists of impaired attention, poor learning, visuospatial disturbance, impaired attention and impaired judgment. Aphasia, apraxia, and agnosia are usually absent. Personality alterations, anxiety, mood changes, and rarely psychosis may also be present.

120.   Answer: C. Disorder of language, apraxia, and impaired naming; impaired auditory comprehension; poor calculation, abstraction, and judgment; depression; delusions; and both short-term and long-term memory loss are seen in Alzheimer disease. As the disease progresses, there is emergence of primitive reflexes.

121. **Answer: B.** In vascular dementia, MRI shows areas of multiple infarcts. About one-quarter to one-third of patients with vascular dementia also develop depression. Vascular dementia is characterized by a stepwise deterioration in cognitive abilities. SPECT shows global hypoperfusion.

122. **Answer: D.** Pick disease is a degenerative dementia seen in about 5% of demented patients. It is diagnosed by the autopsy finding of focal degeneration of the frontal or temporal lobes. "Knife-blade" atrophy of the frontal and temporal lobes is found. Personality changes and behavioral disturbance, along with apathy or impulsivity, sexual disinhibition, roaming, and hyperorality may be seen. Patients also demonstrate signs of frontal lobe impairment with loss of executive functions. The dementia syndrome is characterized by early disruption of expressive speech, with reduced verbal output and echolalia, and impairment of judgment.

123. **Answer: C.** Dementia with Lewy bodies (DLB) tends to be more rapidly progressive than Alzheimer disease. It is characterized by Lewy bodies found in the neurons in the neocortical (frontal, temporal, parietal lobe), allocortical (hippocampal complex, entorhinal cortex), and subcortical (substantia nigra and locus caeruleus) regions of the brain. The clinical characteristics include progressive dementia with relatively little memory impairment at first but with poor attention and executive function, fluctuating cognitions, visual hallucinations, extrapyramidal features, tremor, and sensitivity to neuroleptics in one-third of patients.

124. **Answer: A.** Insight is usually preserved until late in HIV encephalopathy (AIDS dementia complex). The EEG is normal early, with diffuse slowing as the illness progresses. Adjustment reactions are common; however, frank dysphoria is not. Impairment of memory is an early symptom. Treatment with antiviral drugs does influence the course of the disease.

125. **Answer: D.** Lewy bodies are intracellular inclusion bodies that are present in the normal brain and a wide variety of dementias, including Alzheimer disease. Their presence does not indicate Parkinson disease.

126. **Answer: D.** Frontal lobe injury causes a number of sequelae. Among them are disinhibition, Broaca's aphasia, anterograde and retrograde amnesia with confabulation, and, with left-sided lesions, impaired working memory for verbal material. Right-sided lesions cause expressive aprosody, akinetic mutism, amnesia, and impaired working memory for nonverbal spatial material and impaired nonverbal intellect.

127. **Answer: A.** In prosopagnosia, patients are unable to recognize familiar faces. This is caused by lesions in the nondominant parietal and temporal lobes. The other symptoms are neglect, anosognosia, tactile object agnosia, and defective music recognition.

128. Answer: C. Left temporal lobe lesion causes deep prosopagnosia (partial recognition defect). It also causes impaired verbal memory. Visual object agnosia is caused by a bilateral temporal lobe lesions.

129. Answer: C. Hyperorality, hypersexuality, amnestic syndrome, and visual agnosia are caused by bilateral temporal lobe lesions.

130. Answer: D. Sensory neglect is caused by parietal lobe lesions not by lesions of the occipital lobe. Parietal lobe lesions can cause visual field effects, visual hallucinations, and prosopagnosia, especially in lesions of occipitotemporal junction. Anton syndrome is denial of blindness, seen in patients with acquired cortical blindness, arising from bilateral occipital cortex damage.

131. Answer: D. Personality changes are associated with lesions of the frontal and temporal lobes. Parietal lobe lesions cause dressing apraxia, pure agraphia without aphasia, and visual field defects. Gerstmann syndrome consists of agraphia, acalculia, right–left disorientation, and finger agnosia.

132. Answer: B. Frontal lobe lesions cause indifference to the feelings of others, defective social conduct, and acquired sociopathy. Hypersexuality is caused by a temporal lobe lesion. Dyscalculia is caused by parietal lobe dysfunction. Pure alexia resulting in a complete or partial impairment in reading is caused by occipital lobe lesions. Ocular apraxia is an inability to voluntarily direct the gaze toward a stimulus located in the peripheral vision to bring it to a central focus. It is also due to occipital lobe dysfunction.

133. Answer: E. Ocular muscles are involved first in 40% of cases of myasthenia gravis and ultimately in 80%. Patients with oropharyngeal or respiratory muscle involvement may develop myasthenic crisis.

134. Answer: C. Tourette syndrome is a familial disorder with incomplete autosomal dominant transmission characterized by the association of tics and obsessive-compulsive features. It is not associated with a high incidence of seizures. Children with Tourette syndrome may have ADHD. The syndrome is believed to be due to an abnormality in the dopaminergic transmission. It is treated symptomatically with neuroleptics like haloperidol. Clonidine may also help.

135. Answer: E. The presence and duration of post-traumatic amnesia is the best prognostic indicator for the outcome of head injury. Headaches may or may not be present. Recovery may take longer than a year. Dementia is a known sequela. Only about 1–2% of persons affected with post-traumatic amnesia develop seizures.

136. **Answer: D.** Seizures lasting as long as 30 minutes are very strongly suggestive of pseudoseizure as absence of tonic phase and incontinence, lack of increased prolactin following a seizure, and absence of postictal confusion. If the seizures always occur in the presence of others, they are likely to be manifestations of pseudoseizure.

137. **Answer: D.** Progressive agnosia, apraxia, and aphasia are suggestive of Alzheimer disease. A sudden onset is highly unlikely in any dementing process. Seizures and incontinence are classically seen in more advanced stages.

138. **Answer: B.** Alexia and ataxia are absent in Gerstmann syndrome.

139. **Answer: D.** Lesions of the C5 can cause sensory loss over the lateral aspects of the biceps. Sensory loss over the little finger is seen in C8 injury, and loss of triceps tendon jerk is seen in lesions of C6, C7, and C8.

140. **Answer: D.** Subjective sudden release of tension is seen in Tourette syndrome.

141. **Answer: E.** Global memory deficits are seen in transient global amnesia. There is no loss of identity or confabulation. The attention span is normal. It is not a dissociative phenomenon.

142. **Answer: B.** Visual distortions are not seen in frontal lobe damage. Incontinence, difficulty planning tasks, emotional changes, and reemergence of grasp reflex are all seen in frontal lobe dementia.

143. **Answer: C.** Neglect of the left side of the body is seen with lesions of the right parietal lobe. It also causes impaired object recognition. The three other symptoms listed as answer choices are caused by lesions of the left parietal lobe.

144. **Answer: B.** MRI is the most sensitive test to differentiate between white and gray matter and hence is the most useful investigation in multiple sclerosis.

145. **Answer: E.** REM sleep is strongly associated with dreaming; in sleep lab studies, 80% of awakenings during REM sleep produce a dream report. Dreams occurring in REM sleep are more vivid and intense than in non-REM sleep.

146. **Answer: B.** Epidural abscess is most frequently seen in the thoracic spine. The clinical features are pain in a root distribution and transverse spinal cord syndrome with paraparesis, sensory impairment, and sphincter dysfunction.

147. Answer: D. Subacute combined degeneration of the cord is characterized by myelopathy with predominant pyramidal and posterior column deficits in association with polyneuropathy, mental changes, and optical neuropathy. It is caused by vitamin B12 deficiency and is treated with parenteral B12.

148. Answer: C. Brainstem ischemia results in drop attacks.

149. Answer: C. Pseudobulbar palsy arises from an upper motor neuron lesion of the bulbar muscles. The tongue is small and bunched and moves slowly. The jaw jerk is brisk and patients have emotional lability. Dysphagia may also be present.

150. Answer: A. Porphyria is an inherited disorder of enzymes in the hemibiosynthetic pathway. It is characterized by many features including abdominal pains and seizures. However, seizures are not common, and it is not a common cause of weakness.

151. Answer: B. Memory deficits occur with lesion of the wall of the third ventricle.

152. Answer: A. Parahippocampal gyrus, anterior nucleus of thalamus, subcallosal gyrus, and hypothalamus constitute the limbic system.

153. Answer: D. Oculomotor neuropathy can cause diplopia. Diabetes insipidus does not cause diplopia. Facial nerve neuropathy causes paralysis of the muscles of the face depending on the site of the lesion.

154. Answer: C. Benign intracranial hypertension is the term used to describe a persistent rise in CSF pressure in the absence of a space-occupying lesion and with ventricles of normal or reduced size. It usually occurs in women and has peak incidence in the third and fourth decades. The women are often obese, and there is an association with oral contraceptive use, pregnancy, and miscarriage. Headache is the most common complaint.

155. Answer: A. Posterior inferior cerebellar artery occlusion, also known as Wallenberg syndrome, is characterized by loss of ipsilateral pain and temperature sensation in the face with loss of pain and temperature sensation in the contralateral limbs, ipsilateral Horner syndrome, and ipsilateral weakness of the palate, pharynx, and larynx.

156. Answer: E. Nystagmus is an oscillation that is initiated by a slow eye movement. The direction of the nystagmus is determined by the direction of the quick phase.

157. Answer: A. Basilar artery occlusion can produce paralysis or weakness of extremities, diplopia, blindness, and visual field effects, bilateral cerebellar ataxia, and coma.

158. Answer: D. Prolapsed intervertebral disk does not cause blindness.

159. Answer: E. Limbic system mediates all of the functions mentioned.

160. Answer: C. Lesion on one side of the spinal cord causes Brown-Séquard syndrome, an ipsilateral paralysis with loss of vibratory and position sense on the same side and a contralateral loss of pain and temperature.

161. Answer: C. Complete spinal cord transection causes loss of all sensations and voluntary movements below the level of lesion. Pain may occur at the level of the lesion. Damage to the lateral and anterior columns will result in upper motor neuron signs below the level of lesion, with a pyramidal pattern of weakness, spasticity, and deep tendon hyperreflexia, with absent abdominal reflexes and extensor plantar responses. Acute severe cord lesions produce a flaccid paraplegia with a temporary phase of hypotonia and areflexia before appearance of upper motor neuron signs.

162. Answer: A. 5-HT neurons are found in the median raphe nucleus.

163. Answer: C. Stimulation of the carotid sinus in the young rarely causes any symptoms. In the elderly, it can cause bradykinesia and syncope. Most commonly, this is due to reflex vagal inhibition of the heart.

164. Answer: B. Vestibular nuclei is not part of the pyramidal system.

165. Answer: D. The circle of Willis is formed by the proximal part of the two anterior cerebral arteries connected by the anterior communicating artery and the proximal part of the two posterior cerebral arteries, which are connected to the distal internal carotid arteries by the posterior communicating artery.

166. Answer: D. Cerebellar hemisphere damage causes ipsilateral dysmetria or ataxia and hypotonicity. Midline damage to the cerebellar vermis causes gait ataxia, truncal ataxia, and dysarthria. Lesions of the flocculonodular lobe produce eye-movement abnormalities.

167. Answer: B. Posterior column syndrome causes loss of vibration and position sense below the lesion, but the perception of pain and temperature is affected very little. Loss of sensory functions that follow a posterior column lesion include impaired two-point discrimination, detection of size, shape, weight, and texture of objects and ability to detect the direction and speed of a moving stimulus on the skin.

168. Answer: A. Clonus, extensor plantar response, hypertonicity, and increased tendon reflexes are seen with upper motor neuron disease.

169. Answer: D. Lower motor neuron lesion causes absent reflexes and hypotonia.

170. Answer: E. Spontaneous pain can occur in association with paresthesias in peripheral nerve disorders. Spontaneous pain can also arise from thalamic and spinothalamic tract lesions.

171. Answer: E. The presence of papilledema signifies the presence of raised intracranial pressure.

172. Answer: C. Clasp-knife rigidity results from an exaggeration of the stretch reflex.

173. Answer: C. Essential tremor is characterized by action-induced and posture-induced rhythmic shaking with a frequency range of 4 to 12 Hz. The hands are most commonly affected. In about half of patients with essential tremor, small amounts of alcohol reduce the symptoms.

174. Answer: E. Expressive dysphasia is also called Broaca's aphasia. It is caused by a lesion in the Broaca's area, around the posterior part of the inferior frontal convolution.

175. Answer: B. Horner syndrome consists of miosis and ptosis. There may also be depigmentation of the affected iris. It may also be associated with vasomotor and sudomotor changes on the affected side of the face, such as loss of sweating and facial flushing.

176. Answer: E. In this patient, both the motor and the parasympathetic components of the oculomotor nerve are affected, which can result from a berry aneurysm of the posterior communicating artery. In diabetic palsy of the third cranial nerve, only the motor component is affected. Myasthenia gravis causes weakness of muscles.

177. Answer: C. CT scan is particularly useful in detecting hemorrhage. Ischemic changes are better seen in MRI. MRI is the investigation of choice in multiple sclerosis to detect demyelination. Small tumors and lesions in the spinal cord are, again, better seen by MRI.

178. Answer: E. This patient has signs and symptoms suggestive of frontal lobe injury. Disinhibition and irresponsible behavior (i.e., poor judgment) suggest frontal dysfunction. Injury to the amygdala is more likely to cause emotional problems than injury to the temporal lobe, which usually leads to seizures, memory problems, and other symptoms.

179. Answer: E. This elderly patient could be suffering from any of the conditions listed in the question. Parkinsonism, depression, and dementia can cause apathy and psychomotor retardation. Memory problems and confusion can be caused by depression, dementia, and anticholinergic side effects.

180. **Answer: C.** This is typical petit mal, or absence seizure, the focus of which is in the temporal lobe. An aura followed by a staring spell, automatic movements, and amnesia for the episode is characteristic of temporal lobe seizures.

181. **Answer: B.** Ventriculomegaly that is out of proportion to the sulcal atrophy in a middle-aged male is suggestive of normal pressure hydrocephalus. In Pick disease, there is frontotemporal atrophy. In Alzheimer disease, apart from ventriculomegaly, widening of sulci and narrowing of gyri are noticed. In Huntington disease, atrophy of the caudate nucleus is prominent. Progressive supranuclear palsy, results from lesions in the subcortical structures and ventricular volumes are relatively normal.

182. **Answer: B.** Early-onset Alzheimer disease is thought to have autosomal dominant inheritance and typically affects individuals as young as 45 to 50 years old. Cholinesterase inhibitors are found to be useful in controlling the cognitive decline in the early stages. It is no more prevalent in Blacks than in people of other races.

183. **Answer: A.** Prosopognosia is the inability to recognize faces. It is caused by a lesion in the nondominant parieto-occipital lobe.

184. **Answer: B.** A patient with chronic alcohol problems with the presentation described in the question is most likely to have alcoholic cerebellar degeneration. Frontal lobe dysfunction is more likely to cause behavioral disturbances. The patient does not have the transient neurologic deficits that are associated with multiple sclerosis.

185. **Answer: C.** Hippocampus, responsible for memory function, has the highest concentration of neurofibrillary tangles and senile plaques.

186. **Answer: B.** Internuclear ophthalmoplegia, a condition that affects the medial longitudinal fasciculus, is most commonly seen in patients with multiple sclerosis. It is a disturbance of the horizontal gaze leading to displacement of objects and nystagmus. In the elderly, stroke is a common cause of this condition.

187. **Answer: A.** In Huntington disease, bilateral caudate atrophy is noticed. On MRI, it gives a "box car" appearance. Frontotemporal atrophy is noticed in Pick disease. Enlargement of the ventricles associated with widening of the sulci and narrowing of the gyri is a feature of Alzheimer disease.

188. **Answer: E.** With the history of pain and absence of any signs or symptoms to suggest spinal cord compression, bed rest, and analgesics will be the most appropriate therapy.

189.   Answer: D. This patient has problems with topographic disorientation and visuospatial dysfunction, which are associated with lesions of the right (nondominant) parietal lobe.

190.   Answer: C. This patient has hemisensory neglect, which is typically seen in patients who have a lesion of the right parietal cortex.

191.   Answer: C. This patient has obsessive-compulsive disorder. PET scans have revealed increased glucose metabolism in the caudate nucleus and prefrontal cortex. Treatment with SSRIs or CBT results in normalization of the increased metabolism.

192.   Answer: E. This patient has expressive aphasia, which is caused by a lesion in the left frontal lobe secondary to a stroke. If the lesion were in the left temporal region, it would cause receptive aphasia and lead to problems with comprehension.

193.   Answer: B. Although all the options listed in the question are appropriate to a certain extent, a blood test to determine the ceruloplasmin level is the most important step in management of this patient. History of new onset psychosis, movement disorder, and abnormality in the eyes (maybe Kayser-Fleischer rings) are all suggestive of Wilson disease. This condition has a definitive treatment and should not be missed.

194.   Answer: D. Huntington disease is an abnormality of triplet gene repetition (CAG, CAG, . . .) and is inherited by autosomal dominant transmission. It is characterized by chorea, progressive dementia, personality changes, paranoia, and depression. Transient neurologic signs and symptoms are a feature of multiple sclerosis.

195.   Answer: C. Stage 2 of NREM (non–rapid eye movement) sleep is characterized by sleep spindles and K complexes. Alpha waves are seen predominantly in the arousal state. Delta waves are seen in deep sleep. Stage 3 has less than 50% of delta waves, and stage 4 has more than 50% of delta waves.

196.   Answer: B. From the history, this patient appears to be in remission from depression, and she does not have the sleep problem of early morning awakening typically associated with depression. She probably has obstructive sleep apnea. A polysomnogram or referral to a physician specializing in sleep disorders will be helpful for making the diagnosis.

197.   Answer: D. Pituitary tumor can cause these symptoms. Because of the crossing over of nerve fibers in optic chiasma, compression in the medial region typically causes bitemporal hemianopia.

198. **Answer: B.** In Pick disease, memory loss occurs relatively late. This lateness is one of the features that helps to distinguish Pick disease from Alzheimer disease. Psychiatric symptoms like personality changes, agitation, and lack of judgment are often seen before memory problems.

199. **Answer: A.** Gerstmann syndrome results from a lesion in the dominant parietal lobe and is characterized by right–left disorientation, finger agnosia, acalculia, and agraphia.

200. **Answer: C.** Patients with Anton syndrome have denial of blindness. They frequently bump into objects but, when confronted, they vehemently deny any visual problems. The condition is thought to be a form of anosognosia. The lesion is thought to be in both occipital cortex and higher order association cortex.

Chapter 19

MISCELLANEOUS QUESTIONS

QUESTIONS

1. Which of the following is a feature of phencyclidine intoxication?
- A. Vertical or horizontal nystagmus
- B. Belligerent and assaultive behavior
- C. Psychomotor agitation
- D. Hypertension
- E. All of the above

2. Who among the following was murdered by Daniel M'Naghten?
- A. Sir Robert Peel
- B. Edward Drummond
- C. John Hinckley
- D. Mark Chapman

3. How long after their psychological effects have worn off can cannabis and its metabolites be detected in urine?
- A. <12 hours
- B. <24 hours
- C. >1 week
- D. 42–72 hours

4. Who coined the term "psychobiology"?
- A. Adolph Meyer
- B. Sigmund Freud
- C. Karl Menninger
- D. Benjamin Rush

5. Which of the following is not one of the signs of cannabis intoxication according to DSM-IV-TR diagnostic criteria?

    A. Bradycardia

    B. Increased appetite

    C. Dry mouth

    D. Conjunctival injection

6. A 35-year-old woman is seen in the outpatient clinic, referred by her plastic surgeon. According to the referral letter, this person has consulted three cosmetic surgeons in the last 6 months about a perceived deformity of her upper lip. All the physicians have told her that there is no deformity and that there is no need for any surgery. But the woman firmly believes there is a deformity and this belief has hampered her socially and occupationally. What is the diagnosis?

    A. Hypochondriasis

    B. Somatization

    C. Body dysmorphic disorder

    D. Delusional disorder: somatic type

7. A 24-year-old woman has been referred to a psychiatrist by her primary care physician. The patient has been complaining of pain all over the body, frequent episodes of abdominal discomfort, decreased sexual desire, and occasional weakness of her right arm. According to the patient, all these symptoms have been present for less than a year. What is the most appropriate diagnosis?

    A. Somatization

    B. Undifferentiated somatoform disorder

    C. Conversion disorder

    D. Pain disorder

8. Which physician was awarded the Nobel Prize for medicine for work in psychosurgery?

    A. Cerletti

    B. Moniz

    C. Vaughn

    D. Delay

9. What percentage of American psychiatrists use electroconvulsive therapy?

    A. Less than 40%

    B. Less than 30%

    C. Less than 20%

    D. Less than 10%

10. A 42-year-old man presents to the Emergency Room accompanied by his wife, who reports that her husband has been behaving oddly over the last few months, has been very irritable and critical, and has become very suspicious of her. She also reports that he has been making "snakelike movements" with his upper arms. She says that her husband's father developed a similar illness in his early 40s and died of it. What is the location of the gene responsible for the condition described?

    A. Short arm of chromosome 4

    B. Long arm of chromosome 4

    C. Long arm of chromosome 7

    D. Short arm of chromosome 7

11. A dog trainer trying to housebreak a new puppy keeps rewarding the dog at a random rate for correct responses. The rate has no relation to time or sequence of responses. What reinforcement schedule of the operant conditioning is the trainer using?

    A. Fixed-ratio schedule

    B. Variable-ratio schedule

    C. Fixed-interval ratio

    D. Variable-interval ratio

12. A horse trainer rewards a horse only when the horse obeys him and never when the horse obeys it owners. The horse begins to obey only the trainer and never the owners. This is an example of what type of learning?

    A. Discriminative learning

    B. Partial reinforcement

    C. Partial learning

    D. None of the above

13. The phenomenon of long-term potentiation involved in the memory involves which of the following receptors?

    A. Glutamate

    B. NMDA

    C. GABA

    D. Aspartate

14. Which of the following abilities is not considered a component of emotional intelligence?
   A. Recognizing emotions in others
   B. Managing emotions
   C. Self-awareness
   D. An IQ of at least 105

15. A large percentage of Asians exhibit flushing in response to alcohol. To what is this response attributed?
   A. Atypical aldehyde dehydrogenase (ALDH2) genes
   B. Atypical alcohol dehydrogenase
   C. Poor metabolism of CYP2D6
   D. None of the above

16. According to a Epidemiological Catchment Area (ECA) survey, which of the following has the highest prevalence rate?
   A. Substance use disorder
   B. Schizophrenia and schizophreniform disorder
   C. Mood disorders
   D. Anxiety disorders

17. Which of the following is the system used for scoring responses to Rorschach test?
   A. John Exner's scoring system
   B. Murray's system
   C. Millon's scoring system
   D. None of the above

18. An applicant to the business school of a prestigious university scores 132 on an IQ test. How many standard deviations above the mean is his score?
   A. 3
   B. 4
   C. 2
   D. 1

19. A 17-year-old presents to the ER with her parents. Her parents report that she has been behaving very unusually in the last 6 months. She has developed what they term "strange beliefs," has become very suspicious of family members and friends, and claims that her high school teachers are actually members of a radical group who are enemies of the country. Physical examination of the young woman shows a minimal resting tremor and a grayish green ring around the edges of the cornea which is most marked at the superior and inferior pole. What is the location of the genetic abnormality that is responsible for the patient's disease condition?

    A. Chromosome 6

    B. Chromosome 13

    C. Chromosome 12

    D. Chromosome 9

20. A 32-year-old patient reports that when he was watching a movie he got the sense that he had heard the dialogues in the movie before although he had never seen that movie. What is this phenomenon called?

    A. Déjà vu

    B. Déjà pensé

    C. Déjà entendu

    D. Jamais entendu

21. Who introduced the term "neurosis"?

    A. James Braid

    B. William Cullen

    C. Eugen Kahn

    D. Ernst Feuchtersleben

22. The 1976 Nobel Prize for medicine was awarded to Carleton Gajdusek for describing which disease?

    A. Viral encephalitis

    B. Kuru

    C. Creutzfeldt-Jakob disease

    D. AIDS

23. A person with a long history of alcohol dependence has been abstinent for 2 months following attendance at a rehabilitation program for substance abuse. The patient has not met any criteria for dependence in the last 2 months. According to the DSM-IV-TR criteria, the person is in which stage of remission?

    A. Early full remission

    B. Early partial remission

    C. Sustained full remission

    D. Sustained partial remission

24. According to an NIMH Epidemiological Catchment Area (ECA) study conducted an 1980–1984, what percentage of the U.S. population aged 18 and older qualifies for a diagnosis of either abuse of or dependence on some substance?

    A. 25%

    B. 32%

    C. 12%

    D. 17%

25. Which of the following is not an indication for expressive psychoanalytic psychotherapy?

    A. Strong ego strength

    B. Good impulse control

    C. Cognitive deficits

    D. Ability to verbalize deficits

26. Who is considered the founder of modern group psychotherapy?

    A. Jacob Moreno

    B. Joseph Pratt

    C. Kurt Lewin

    D. Alexander Low

27. A driver who is stopped by the police for driving erratically has a blood alcohol level of 300 mg/dl. He does not show any sign of being under the influence of alcohol. He acts very sober and is able to answer all questions appropriately and perform all the tasks asked of him. This is an example of what kind of tolerance?

    A. Pharmacodynamic tolerance

    B. Pharmacokinetic tolerance

    C. Behavioral tolerance

    D. Cross-tolerance

28. Which of the following lab findings shows a distinct abnormality with long history of alcohol abuse?

  A. RDW

  B. MCV

  C. Hemoglobin

  D. Neutrophil count

29. A 35-year-old man miraculously survived a fall from the second floor with only a right clavicle bone fracture and a bruise on his face. He was discharged from the hospital 2 days after his fall. One month later, the man's girlfriend calls the hospital to report that the man is behaving abnormally. According to her, he has become very irritable and has started having explosive fits of anger. She also reports that he has become a philanderer and that he has been found to be making obscene jokes and acting disinhibited with some of her girlfriends. What could be the sequela of his injury that is leading to such behavior?

  A. Frontopolar syndrome

  B. Orbitofrontal syndrome

  C. Temporal lobe syndrome

  D. Postconcussional disorder

30. Which of the following is considered a characteristic of interictal behavioral syndrome?

  A. Decreased interest in sexual activities

  B. Hyperreligiosity

  C. Hypergraphia

  D. Viscosity or stickiness

  E. All of the above

31. The intoxicating effects of alcohol are more pronounced when the blood alcohol levels are increasing. What is this phenomenon called?

  A. Mallenby effect

  B. Pharmacodynamic tolerance

  C. Pharmacokinetic tolerance

  D. Reverse tolerance

32. Which French psychiatrist first described the concept of circular insanity, or "folie circulaire"?

    A. Jean-Pierre Falret

    B. Jules Baillarger

    C. Benjamin Rush

    D. Gabriel Langfeldt

33. Who coined the term "neurasthenia"?

    A. James Braid

    B. William Cullen

    C. George Beard

    D. Robert Post

34. A 35-year-old man tells his therapist that he has difficulty describing his emotions accurately. He says that he can't find the words to describe how he is feeling. What is the phenomenon that is causing this inability?

    A. Neurasthenia

    B. Alexithymia

    C. Mental fatigue

    D. Dysphoria

35. According to epidemiologic studies, in which of the following communities is suicide most common?

    A. Muslims

    B. Catholics

    C. Protestants

    D. Jews

36. Which of the following has been described by Emile Durkheim as a type of suicide?

    A. Anomic

    B. Egoistic

    C. Altruistic

    D. All of the above

37. After around 2.5 weeks of being treated with tricyclic antidepressants, a patient diagnosed with extreme depression with severe psychomotor retardation shows signs of improvement. There is marked improvement in his psychomotor retardation, although he continues to report severe ideas of worthlessness and hopelessness. One week later, he commits suicide by hanging himself. What description fits this suicide?

    A. Anomic

    B. Egoistic

    C. Paradoxical

    D. None of the above

38. What percentage of homeless people are estimated to be suffering from chronic mental illness?

    A. Less than 10%

    B. 10–15%

    C. 25–35%

    D. More than 50%

39. What is otherwise known as Ekbom syndrome?

    A. Restless leg syndrome

    B. Periodic limb movement disorder

    C. Nocturnal eating syndrome

    D. None of the above

40. A 19-year-old first-year college student reports that she feels very sleepy by 6 or 7 in the evening and has to go to bed. She says that she wakes up very early in the morning and finds herself to be more alert then. What best describes this sleep pattern?

    A. Delayed sleep phase syndrome

    B. Advanced sleep phase syndrome

    C. Hypersomnia

    D. None of the above

41. Which of the following is a feature of periodic limb movement disorder?

    A. It was formerly called nocturnal myoclonus.

    B. It involves brief, repetitive, stereotypic movements of the legs.

    C. It occurs during NREM sleep.

    D. All of the above

42. Which of the following is a feature of nightmare disorder?

A. The person awakens with detailed recall of frightening dreams.

B. After awakening, the person rapidly becomes oriented and alert.

C. The nightmares occur during REM.

D. All of the above

43. Which of the following is a feature of sleep terror disorder?

A. It occurs primarily in NREM sleep.

B. It is characterized by recurrent episodes of abrupt wakening from sleep during the first third of the sleep cycle.

C. The person is disoriented and unresponsive to the calming efforts of others during the episode.

D. The details of the dream cannot be recalled by the person.

E. All of the above

44. Which of the following is *not* true regarding kleptomania?

A. The person with kleptomania is not able to resist recurrent impulses to steal objects that are not needed.

B. The person describes feeling an intense sense of tension before committing the theft, which is relieved by committing the act.

C. There is always a comorbid diagnosis of antisocial personality disorder with kleptomania.

D. None of the above

45. Which of the following is considered a treatment for pathologic gambling?

A. Psychodynamic psychotherapy

B. Treating comorbid conditions like depression

C. Attending Gamblers Anonymous

D. Imaginal desensitization

E. All of the above

46. Which of the following is considered a feature of trichotillomania?

A. Patients display recurrent episodes of pulling out their hair.

B. Patients experience an intense sense of tension before pulling out their hair.

C. Patients report intense pleasure, relief, and sense of gratification after pulling out their hair.

D. Hair ingestion can lead to development of trichobezoars and bowel obstruction and resultant peritonitis.

E. All of the above

47. Which of the following is considered the treatment of choice for trichottilo-mania?

    A. Risperidone

    B. Imipramine

    C. Zoloft

    D. None of the above

48. Chronic use of which of the following can lead to delusions of parasitosis?

    A. Amphetamine

    B. Ritalin

    C. Cocaine

    D. All of the above

49. Which of the following did Franz Alexander consider to be a psychosomatic disease?

    A. Peptic ulcer disease

    B. Ulcerative colitis

    C. Essential hypertension

    D. Graves' disease

    E. All of the above

50. Which of the following is true regarding the dexamethasone suppression test (DST)?

    A. The test is considered positive if it shows that the level of serum cortisol is 5 micrograms or more after the patient has been given 1 mg of dexamethasone at 11 PM the previous day.

    B. Around 40% of the depressed patients have a positive DST result.

    C. Anorexia nervosa leads to positive DST results.

    D. All of the above

51. Which of the following terms was coined by Friedman and Rosenmann in 1959 in connection with stress and heart disease?

    A. Type A personality disorder

    B. Panic disorder

    C. Generalized anxiety

    D. None of the above

ANSWERS

1. **Answer: E.** The following signs are seen in people intoxicated with phencyclidine: vertical or horizontal nystagmus, hypertension or tachycardia, numbness, diminished responsiveness to pain, ataxia, dysarthria, muscle rigidity, seizures, coma, and hyperacusis.

2. **Answer: B.** M'Naghten is mentioned in connection with the insanity defense; he was a person suffering from paranoid delusions who, in 1843, killed John Drummond, secretary to British Prime Minister Sir Robert Peel, his intended target. John Hinckley, who suffered from paranoid schizophrenia, made an unsuccessful attempt to assassinate President Ronald Reagan. Mark David Chapman shot Beatles legend John Lennon because his hallucinatory voices told him to.

3. **Answer: D.** How long cannabis and its metabolites can be detected in the urine depends on the cutoff level used by the laboratory. Most labs use a cutoff level of 100 ng/ml, which can be detected in the urine up to 42 to 72 hours after the psychological effects of cannabis have worn off. Passive inhalation of cannabis smoke can also lead to the detection of cannabis and its metabolites in urine if the cutoff used is 25 ng/ml. Cocaine metabolites can be found for varying periods depending on the duration or dosage of cocaine use.

4. **Answer: A.** Adolph Meyer coined the term "psychobiology."

5. **Answer: A.** According to DSM-IV-TR, two of the following signs should develop within 2 hours of cannabis use: conjunctival injection, increased appetite, dry mouth, and tachycardia.

6. **Answer: D.** This patient firmly believes that there is a deformity in her upper lip even when presented evidence to the contrary. The belief is delusional. In body dysmorphic disorder, a belief such as this does not have the same intensity as in delusions.

7. **Answer: B.** Although the patient has multiple pain symptoms, gastrointestinal symptoms, sexual symptoms, and a pseudoneurologic symptom, the duration of these symptoms does not meet the duration criteria for somatization disorder. In somatization disorder, the symptoms must have been present for many years. In undifferentiated somatoform disorder, symptoms need to be present for at least 6 months.

8. **Answer: B.** Cerletti and Bini were two Italian physicians who did pioneering work with convulsive treatment. Vaughn and Leff expounded the theory of "expressed emotions among highly critical relatives of schizophrenia with poor prognosis." Delay and Deniker introduced chlorpromazine in 1950s.

9. Answer: D. It is only less than 8% of the psychiatrists in the United States that use ECT.

10. Answer: A. The patient most likely has Huntington disease, which is of autosomal dominant inheritance; the gene for this disease is located on the short arm of chromosome 4.

11. Answer: B. Among the different schedules that can be used for reinforcement in operant conditioning, the variable-ratio schedule has been proven to be the most effective and long lasting.

12. Answer: A. In discriminative learning, stimulus generalization is avoided and the person makes responses only to specific stimuli. In this example the horse learns to obey only the trainer and not the owner.

13. Answer: B. Cells possessing NMDA type of glutamate receptor develop increased responsivity to high-frequency stimulation. This phenomenon is called long-term potentiation. It is an example of synaptic plasticity, which plays a role in the process of memory and learning.

14. Answer: D. Emotional intelligence is a concept popularized by Daniel Goleman. According to Goleman the following are components of emotional intelligence: self-awareness, self-motivation, managing one's own emotions, recognizing emotions in others, and being able to handle relationships.

15. Answer: A. The presence of atypical aldehyde dehydrogenase leads to a decreased ability by the carriers to metabolize the aldehyde formed in the metabolism of alcohol by the enzyme alcohol dehydrogenase. In some Asians, this results in a flushing reaction following ingestion of alcohol.

16. Answer: D. Anxiety disorders were found to have the highest prevalence in the National Institute of Mental Health (NIMH) Epidemiological Catchment Area (ECA) Survey of the prevalence of mental disorders, conducted in the late 1970s. The 1-year prevalence rate of mental disorders and substance abuse disorders was 28.1%. This study was conducted in five areas: New Haven, Baltimore, Durham, St. Louis, and Los Angeles. Trained interviewers used the Diagnostic Interview Schedule (DIS) to assess symptoms in 18,571 household residents and 2,290 institutional residents.

17. Answer: A. John Exner's scoring system is the most widely used scoring system to score the responses to the Rorschach test. That test, developed in 1917 by Swiss psychiatrist Herman Rorschach, is a projective test consisting of 10 symmetric and ambiguous inkblots. Henry Murray developed another projective personality test, the Thematic Apperception Test.

18. Answer: C. The average IQ is around 90 to 109. A score of 115 is considered 1 standard deviation (SD) above mean, 130 is considered 2 SD above mean, and a score of 145 is considered 3 SD above mean. Two percent of the population scores above 130.

19. Answer: B. The patient has Wilson disease, an autosomal recessive disorder of copper metabolism that can present with movement disorder, personality changes, and psychosis. It usually presents in the first through third decade. The genetic defect, which is localized to chromosome 13, leads to a defect in copper-transporting adenosine triphosphatase in the liver, which in turn leads to accumulation of copper in the liver, kidney, brain, and cornea.

20. Answer: C. Déjà entendu is the sense that one has previously heard what is actually being heard for the first time.

21. Answer: B. William Cullen coined the term "neurosis." James Braid coined the term "hypnosis." Eugen Kahn coined the term "psychopathy" to describe conditions that lay between mental health and illness. Ernst Feuchtersleben introduced the term "psychosis" in 1945.

22. Answer: B. The 1976 Nobel Prize for Medicine was given to Carleton Gajdusek for his work on kuru, a fatal dementia similar to Creutzfeldt-Jakob disease. Twenty years later, Stanley Prusiner was awarded the 1997 Nobel Prize for Medicine for discovering the small infectious proteins, prions, which likely cause mad cow disease, kuru and Creutzfeldt-Jakob disease.

23. Answer: A. "Early full remission" is the term used if a person has been abstinent for at least 1 month but for less than 12 months and has not met any of the criteria for dependence or abuse during that period. "Sustained full remission" is used if the person has not met any criteria for dependence or abuse in the past 12 months. "Early partial remission" is used if the person has been abstinent for 1 month but less than 12 months but has met one or more criteria for substance dependence or abuse during that period. "Sustained partial remission" is used if the person has been abstinent for at least 12 months but has met one or more criteria for substance dependence or abuse during that time period.

24. Answer: D. According to an NIMH Epidemiological Catchment Area study conducted in 1980–1984, 16.7% of U.S. population aged 18 and older qualified for a diagnosis of either substance abuse or substance dependence for some substance.

25. Answer: C. Cognitive deficits are a contraindication for expressive psychoanalytic psychotherapy. Other contraindications are poor motivation, poor psychological mindedness, poor impulse control, poor social network, poor frustration tolerance, and inability to form therapeutic alliance.

26. Answer: B. Joseph Pratt, who treated tuberculosis patients in organized classes, is known as the father of modern group psychotherapy.

27. Answer: C. Behavioral tolerance is the ability of a person to perform tasks effectively despite the effects of the substance. Pharmacokinetic tolerance is the adaptation of the metabolic system to rid the body of alcohol rapidly by producing more enzymes. Pharmacodynamic tolerance is an adaptation of the nervous system so that it can function despite high blood alcohol concentrations. This is also known as cellular tolerance. Cross-tolerance occurs when a person shows a similar reaction to another drug of the same class.

28. Answer: B. Chronic use of alcohol can lead to increase in mean corpuscular volume (MCV).

29. Answer: B. Orbitofrontal syndrome is characterized by disinhibition, explosiveness, and inappropriate jocularity. Frontopolar syndrome is characterized by apathy, behavioral inertia, and indifference.

30. Answer: E. Some patients with epilepsy develop the following: schizophreniform psychosis; heightened significance of events and things; humorlessness. They may become overly religious, philosophical, or moral; become overly inclusive; write voluminously (hypergraphia); and talk repetitively and circumstantially about restricted topics (viscosity). Most of these features are associated with left-sided or bilateral or temporal foci.

31. Answer: A. The intoxicating effect of alcohol is highest when the blood alcohol levels are increasing. This is called Mallenby effect.

32. Answer: A. Jean-Pierre Falret described "folie circulaire." Jules Baillarger described "folie à double forme." Gabriel Langfeldt described schizophreniform psychosis. Benjamin Rush, a signer of the American Declaration of Independence, is considered the father of American psychiatry.

33. Answer: C. "Neurasthenia" is a term coined by George Beard in 1869 to describe a chronic condition characterized by anxious-depressive symptomatology. In this condition people are overly anxious and have a chronic predisposition to mental fatigue, lethargy, exhaustion, and irritability. This diagnosis is widely used in China.

34. Answer: B. "Alexithymia" is the inability to describe emotions in words. Individuals with this condition are unaware of their feelings. This is common in psychosomatic disorders and post-traumatic stress disorder.

35. Answer: C. Suicide rates differ among different communities. Suicide is much less among Catholic, Muslim, and Jewish communities than among Protestant Christians. Religious beliefs and cohesiveness of the communities is hypothesized to play a role in the differential rates of suicide in different communities.

36. Answer: D. Emile Durkheim described three social types of suicide: altruistic, anomic, and egoistic.

37. Answer: C. When patients are severely depressed, they sometimes have such severe psychomotor retardation that they are not even able to contemplate suicide, much less act upon their suicidal impulses. But when the intensity of depression begins to decrease as a result of treatment or as a natural course, there is an improvement in psychomotor retardation and patients are able to act upon their suicidal impulses. Suicide committed under these circumstances is called paradoxical suicide.

38. Answer: C. Between 25% and 35% of homeless people are estimated to have a mental illness. Cause and effect are unclear—it is not clear whether homelessness causes the mental illness or is the result of the downward drift of the people with mental illness.

39. Answer: A. Restless leg syndrome, otherwise known as Ekbom syndrome, is characterized by an irresistible urge to move the legs while trying to fall asleep. Persons with this syndrome also report a crawling feeling in their legs.

40. Answer: B. In advanced sleep phase syndrome, the person feels sleepy very early in the evening and goes to sleep early and wakes up very early in the morning. In delayed sleep phase syndrome the person does not fall asleep until very late and sleeps late into the morning or afternoon.

41. Answer: D. Periodic limb movement disorder consists of short, repetitive, stereotypic movements of limbs. The movement usually involves the legs, and extension of the toes is sometimes seen. The movement occurs in NREM sleep and leads to brief arousals from sleep. Benzodiazepines are the most commonly used treatment.

42. Answer: D. People with nightmare disorder report repeated awakenings with vivid recall of the frightening dreams. The awakenings usually occur in the second half of the sleep cycle, during REM sleep. These symptoms are sometimes seen with febrile illness. On awakening, the person does not have any prolonged disorientation like that seen in sleep terror.

43. Answer: E. Sleep terror usually occurs in the first half of the sleep cycle, during NREM sleep. It involves abrupt awakening from sleep, and the person is usually disoriented, terrified, and inconsolable and can't remember the content of the terrifying dream.

44. Answer: C. To meet the DSM-IV-TR diagnostic criteria for kleptomania, the stealing should not be better accounted for by antisocial personality disorder or manic-depressive illness.

45. Answer: E. All of the following are considered treatment modalities for pathologic gambling: treating comorbid depression, psychodynamic psychotherapy, Gamblers Anonymous, and imaginal desensitization.

46. Answer: E. Trichotillomania is characterized by recurrent pulling out of one's hair. Patients experience an increasing sense of tension before pulling the hair, which is followed by pleasure and relief. From 70% to 80% of hair pullers are female. Some of them also ingest the hair they pulled out, and this can lead to medical complications, such as intestinal obstruction.

47. Answer: C. SSRIs are now considered as the treatment of choice for trichottilomania. Tricyclic antidepressants also can be used. Cognitive-behavioral therapy and hypnosis have also been proved beneficial.

48. Answer: D. Delusional parasitosis is the belief that one is infested with worms, insects, lice, or vermin. It can develop as a side effect of substances like cocaine, amphetamine, and Ritalin.

49. Answer: E. The seven diseases studied by Franz Alexander are peptic ulcer disease, ulcerative colitis, essential hypertension, Graves' disease, neurodermatitis, rheumatoid arthritis, and bronchial asthma.

50. Answer: D. The dexamethasone suppression test cannot be used in diagnosing illness. At best it can be used to follow the response to treatment. The patient is given 1 mg of oral dexamethasone at 11 PM. The plasma cortisol levels are measured next morning at 8 AM and also at 4 PM. In ordinary circumstances the dexamethasone suppresses the cortisol response. If the level is above 5 mg/dl, it is considered abnormal. Dexamethasone test is positive in more than 50% of patients with depression. It also gives false positive results in the following conditions: dehydration, alcohol abuse, hypertension, weight loss, and diabetes.

51. Answer: A. Friedman and Rosenmann were two cardiologists from San Francisco who studied the relationship between behavior and heart disease and published the book *Type A Behavior and Your Heart in 1974.*

abdominal pain, 395
abducens nerve palsy, 381
abnormal affect, 41
abnormal association, 40–41
abscesses, spinal epidural, 363
absence seizures (petit mal seizures), 340–341, 380, 387
absent reflexes, 396
abstinence, 194
acetaminophen, 272
acetazolamide, 282
acetylcholine and GABA, 383
acoustic neuroma, 352
acquired immunodeficiency syndrome. see AIDS
acute stress disorder, 92
ADHD (attention-deficit hyperactivity disorder), 126, 133, 139, 140
adjustment disorder, 83
Adler, Alfred, 322
adolescence, 138, 227, 321, 323
adrenergic innervation, 90
advance directives, 148, 158
advanced sleep phase syndrome, 416
aesthetic agents, 24
affect, abnormal, 41
affective disorder, 79, 145, 155, 279
affective symptoms, 50
aggression, 211, 216, 266, 268, 313, 322
agranulocytosis, 256, 280, 283
AIDS, 150, 159, 351
  dementia in, 150, 159
  encephalitis in, 147, 157
akinetic mutism, 349
alcohol
  and benzodiazepines, 268
  and bulimia nervosa patients, 203
  and essential tremor, 386, 397
  REM sleep affected by, 189
  and sexual dysfunction, 205
alcohol abuse, 176, 186
alcohol dependence, 175–177, 188, 189, 334
alcohol detoxification, 172
alcohol infusion, 284
alcohol intoxication, 167
alcohol poisoning, methyl, 176
alcohol withdrawal, 172, 174–176, 187–189
alcohol withdrawal delirium, 184, 193
alcohol withdrawal tremors, 178, 190
alcoholic blackouts, 183
alcoholic cerebellar degeneration, 398
alcoholic hallucinations, 6
alcoholic hallucinosis, 178, 190
alcohol-induced mood disorder, 190
alcoholism, 172
  assessment of patients with, 187
  chronic, 177, 189
  Cloninger's type 1, 173
  and depression, 158
  family history of, 189
  personality types associated with, 186
  physical features seen in, 183, 193
  risk factors for, 171, 186
  and suicide, 173, 187
  treatment of, 190
Alderian therapy, 298

ALDH2 (atypical aldehyde dehydrogenase) genes, 413
Alexander, Franz, 318
alexithymia, 7, 15, 415
alkalosis, hypokalemic, 202
alpha activity, on EEG, 387
alpha-1 receptor, 275
alpha-2 receptors, 271
alpha-adrenergic blocking effect, 266
alpha-adrenergic receptors, 273
ALT liver enzyme, 284
altruism, 300
Alzheimer dementia, 358, 391
Alzheimer disease, 113, 116–117, 355–356
  delaying progression of, 389
  distinguished from dementia, 391
  early-onset, 370
  and gene mutation, 389
  linguistic deficits in, 390
  and neuroimaging, 121, 389
  prevalence of delusions in, 119
  risk factors for, 121, 389
  severe, 371
amaxophobia, 100, 110, 270
ambivalence, 40, 41, 299
amine, secondary, 238
amitriptyline, 269, 270
amnesia, 310
  anterograde, 193, 381
  discontinuous, 110
  dissociative, 96, 99, 108–109
  transient global, 342, 362
Amok, 110
amphetamines, 49, 191, 192, 205
  psychotic disorder induced by, 177, 190
  use of, 179, 417
amygdala, 48, 386
analyst, idealization of, 300
analytic psychotherapy, 308
anemia, hemolytic, 278
aneurysm, berry, 387, 397
anger, and suicide, 157
Angst, Jules, 76
anhedonia, 76
anorexia nervosa, 196–198, 202–203, 215
anorgasmia, 272
anosmia, 387
anosognosia, 16
anterior lens, granular deposits in, 285
anterograde amnesia, 193, 381
anticholinergics
  effects of, 238, 397
  properties of, 257, 281
anticipation, 136, 304
antidepressant discontinuation syndromes, 59, 79
antidepressant-induced hypomania, 76
antidepressants, 69, 70, 82. see also tricyclic antidepressants
  atypical, 277
antiemetics, 231
antiepileptics, 55
antipsychotic-induced parkinsonism, 347
antipsychotics, 21, 252, 256
  with antidepressant effect, 58, 78
  associations with classes, 277

  atypical, 28
  lethal side effects of, 326
  low-potency, 262, 284
  parenteral, 258, 281
  and seizures, 280
  and sexual dysfunction, 259, 282
  side effects of, 278
  treatment duration, 79
  weight gain with, 78
antisocial personality disorder, 132, 139, 186, 334
Anton syndrome, 375, 400
anxiety, 1, 11, 106, 187, 268
  pathological, 90, 106
anxiety disorders, 87–112, 88
  cardiac abnormalities in people with, 105
  features observed in, 105
  neurotransmitter abnormalities in, 88, 105
  prevalence rate of, 413
  treatment of, 298
anxiety-depressive disorder, mixed, 102
apathy, 389
aphagia, 385
appetite, lack of, 76
arbitrary inference, 301
areflexia, 383
areflexia, lower limb, 335
aripiprazole, 257, 281
arteriography, 380
Asperger syndrome, 135, 209, 211, 215, 216
asphyxia, autoerotic, 334
aspirin, 275
assaultive behavior, 412
association, loosening of, 7, 15
asthenic body types, 46
astrocytomas, 351, 386
asyndetic thinking, 47
ataxia, 193, 235, 250
  and benzodiazepine, 268
  and carbamazepine, 268, 275, 277
  Friedreich, 376
  and valproate, 276
athetosis, 384
atomoxetine (Strattera), 133
atrial fibrillation, 381
attention
  disturbance of, 156
  sustained, 314
attention-deficit hyperactivity disorder, 126, 133, 139, 140
atypical aldehyde dehydrogenase genes, 413
auditory hallucinations, 14, 16, 47, 49
augmenting agents, 80
authority orientation, 319
autism, 128
autistic behavior, 40, 41
autoerotic asphyxia, 334
autonomic ganglia, 336
autoscopy, 16
autosomal dominant, 384
autosomal dominant inheritance, 398
auxiliary egos, 288
avoidant personality disorder, 226
axis I psychiatric disorder, 150, 159

Babinski sign, 335
backward chaining, 317
Baillarger, Jules, 415
Balint, Michael, 137, 304
barbiturates
    intoxication with, 256, 280
    overdose of, 327, 332
    withdrawal from, 180, 191
basilar artery occlusion, 366, 381
BDI (Beck Depression Inventory), 17
BDZ receptors, 79
Beard, George, 85, 415
Beck, Aaron, 77, 85
Beck Depression Inventory, 17
behavior therapy, 290
behavioral diary, 301
behavioral tolerance, 415
bell and pad method of conditioning, 134
belligerent behavior, 412
benign intracranial hypertension, 365, 395
benzodiazepine withdrawal, 182, 191,
        234–235, 267, 268
benzodiazepines, 232–236, 269
    and alcohol, 268
    children born to mothers taking, 267
    and liver disease, 266
    side effects of, 267, 268
    tolerance to, 268
    use, 267
Bernays, Martha, 304
Berne, Eric, 298
Bernheim, Hippolyte, 304
berry aneurysm, 387, 397
Binet, Alfred, 317
binge eating disorders, 202
Bini, Lucio, 285, 412
Binswanger disease, 390
biofeedback, 290
bipolar disorder, 47, 54, 72, 246, 248
    and carbamazepine, 76
    epidemiology of, 71, 84
    and genetics, 73, 76
    medications for, 54
    prevalence of, 53, 76
    rapid-cycling, 54, 76
    relapse of, 55, 77
    and suicide, 74, 85
    type I, 71, 84, 86, 274
    type II, 274
    untreated depressive episodes in, 84
bitemporal hemianopia, 374, 387
bizarre delusions, 49
black eyes, bilateral, 138
blindness, sudden onset of, 396
blood/injection/injury phobia, 99, 110
blurred vision, 269, 271, 277
body dysmorphic disorder, 45, 103, 112
borderline personality disorder, 80, 223,
        226, 334
Bowlby, John, 85
bradycardia, 110
bradykinesia, 383, 384
Braid, James, 414
brain abscess, 376
brain damage, 10, 79, 336
brain injury, 279, 353
brain tumors, 378, 387
brainstem ischemia, 364
brainwashing, 103, 112
brief dynamic psychotherapy, 293, 298,
        302
Brown, George W., 77
Brown-Séquard syndrome, 366, 396
bucket-handle fractures, 138
bulimia nervosa, 195–198, 202, 203, 300
bupropion, 78, 277
buspirone, 87, 105, 282
butyrophenone, 277
bystander intervention, 322

C5, lesion at level of, 394
caffeine withdrawal, 184, 193, 194
caffeinism, 185

cancer patients, 149, 158
cannabis, 284, 401, 402, 412
Cannon-Bard theory, 322
Capgras syndrome, 3, 12, 16, 45
carbamazepine, 57, 248–249, 261
    and ataxia, 268, 277
    and bipolar affective disorder, 76
    and CYP 2D6 enzyme, 282
    levels of, 260
    and libido, 281
    metabolism of, 283
    side effects of, 275, 276
    when contraindicated, 276
cardiac abnormalities, 105
cardiac arrhythmias, 278
carotid artery occlusion, 344
carotid artery stenosis, 341
carotid sinus stimulation, 367
cataplexy, 15
catatonia, 6, 25, 328, 333
catatonic states, 43
catlike cry, 214
caudate nuclei, 47
    bilateral atrophy of, 398
cavernous sinus thrombosis, 397
CBT (cognitive-behavioral therapy), 83,
        203, 205, 291–292, 301
central pontine myelinolysis, 345
cerebellar disease, 367, 396
cerebral palsy, 213
cerebrospinal fluid, 5-HIAA in, 333
Cerletti, Ugo, 285, 412
ceruloplasmin, 399
change, theory of, 173, 188
Chapman, Mark David, 412
Charles Bonnet syndrome, 40
Chess, Stella, 137
child abuse, 129, 138
child psychiatry, 123–140
children
    and absence seizures, 380
    ADHD in, 140
    concept of death in, 136
    depression in, 124, 130
    and logic-related problems, 318
    with mental retardation, 210, 215
    moral judgments of, 321
    OCD in, 130, 138
    reactive attachment disorder in, 139
    schizophrenia in, 32, 134
    sexual abuse of, 138
    suicide in, 131, 138, 139
    and toxic levels of lead, 136
    vocabulary of, 319
chlordiazepoxide, 187, 266, 267
chlorpromazine, 203, 231, 252–254,
        264, 266
    as antiemetic, 266
    and haloperidol, 279
    and phenothiazine, 277
    side effects of, 278, 285
cholesterol, 276
cholinergic, 376
chorea, 383, 384
chromosome 4, 385, 413
chromosome 6, 41
chromosome 13, 136, 414
chronic fatigue syndrome, 103, 112
cimetidine, 267, 282
cingulotomy, 110
circle of Willis, 367, 396
circular insanity ("folie circulaire"), 22,
        408
citalopram, 81, 242, 272
class inclusion, 319
classic conditioning, 305, 316, 317
clear consciousness, 79
client-centered therapy, 313
clomipramine, 78, 271
clonazepam, 77
clonidine, 135
Cloninger's type 1 alcoholism, 173, 187
clonus, 396

clozapine, 36, 40, 255–256, 280, 284
    and agranulocytosis, 280
    and dibenzodiazipine, 277
    plasma levels of, 50
    side effects of, 280
cluster headache, 337, 377, 378
coarse tremor, 274
cocaine, 49, 180, 182, 205
    crack, 159
cocaine toxicity, 181
cocaine use, 191, 417
cognitive deficits, 382, 414
cognitive development, Piaget's stages of,
        318
cognitive disorders, 50
cognitive distortions, 291–292, 301
cognitive therapy, 145, 155
cognitive-behavioral therapy, 83, 203,
        205, 291–292, 301
comorbid psychiatric disorder, 172
comorbid substance abuse, 276
competency, 148, 158, 161, 165
    determining, 167
    and wills, 168
complete spinal-cord transection, 366,
        396
complex partial seizures, 33
compulsions, 12
compulsive eating behavior, 214
computed tomography scan, 369
concrete operational stage, 318
concrete thinking, 2
conditioned response, 316
conditioning, bell and pad method of, 134
conduct disorder, 139
confidentiality, exceptions to, 148, 157
confusion, 184
    in elderly, 184, 194
    and epilepsy, 380
    versus identity, 323
    and topiramate, 277
confusional state, 268
consciousness, impaired, 335
consultation liaison psychiatry, 141–160
contemplation, 187
continuous performance tasks, 42
Continuous Performance Test, 323
contralateral Horner syndrome, 395
conversion disorder, 94, 107, 108
corpus striatum, 385
corrective emotional experience, 318
cortical atrophy, 385, 390
corticosteroid use, 158
cortisol, 83
cortisol secretion abnormality, 64, 81
Cotard syndrome, 17
cough medicines, 271
countertransference, 295, 300, 303
CPT (Continuous Performance Test), 323
crack cocaine, 159
cranial arteritis, 397
creatinine testing, 79
Creutzfeldt-Jakob disease, 354, 388
crime rate, 348
criminal behavior, 164, 168
criminal offenders, 163, 168
critical comments, 46
CSF (cerebrospinal fluid), 5-HIAA in, 333
CT (computed tomography) scan, 369
Cullen, William, 414
culture-bound disorders, 99, 110
Cushing syndrome, 142, 152
cyclothymia, 84
CYP 3A4 isoenzyme, 259, 282, 283
CYP 2D6 enzyme, 259
cyproheptadine, 203
cyproterone acetate, 60, 79
cytochrome P-450 isoenzyme, 273
cytochrome P-450 system, 230

D2 receptors, 265, 283, 384
DBT (dialectical behavior therapy),
        292–293, 301

de Clerambault syndrome, 38
death, concept of, 127, 136
declarative memory, 320
defense mechanisms, 98, 110, 294, 296
degeneration, subacute combined, 364
deinstitutionalization, 22, 41
déjà entendu, 414
Delay, Jean, 285, 412
delirium, 5, 14, 146
    alcohol withdrawal, 184, 193
    in elderly, 184, 194
    hypoactive, 146, 156
    management of, 157
    in patients with AIDS, 159
delirium tremens, 175, 188
delta 9 tetrahydrocannabinol, 263
delusion of doubles, 12
delusional disorder, 37–39, 50, 412
delusional perception, 11
delusions, 5, 14, 37
    in Alzheimer disease, 119
    bizarre, 49
    in late-onset psychosis, 121
    mood incongruent, 45
    nihilistic, 10
    paranoid, 13
    of parasitosis, 411
    and Parkinson's disease, 384
    of persecution, 50
    primary, 1, 11
    secondary, 11
    in vascular dementia, 119
dementia, 115–116, 121, 149, 357, 397
    in AIDS, 150, 159
    diagnosis of, 120
    distinguished from Alzheimer disease,
        391
    frontotemporal, 358, 391
    of Lewy bodies, 357, 359, 391, 392
    of normal pressure hydrocephalus,
        358, 391
    and Parkinson's disease, 384
    in patients with Down syndrome, 215
    subcortical, 159
    vascular, 113, 119, 356, 359, 390,
        392
dementia praecox, 29
demyelination, 382
    chronic inflammatory demyelinating
        polyneuropathy, 350, 386
denial, 145, 155, 304
Deniker, Pierre, 285, 412
depersonalization, 4, 13
depersonalization disorder, 97, 109
depression, 397
    agitated, 65, 81
    anaclitic, 134
    atypical, 66, 81
    brain imaging studies in, 65, 81
    causes of, 59
    in children, 124, 130
    and cognitive distortions, 301
    defense mechanisms associated with,
        294, 303
    before detoxification, 187
    double, 66, 81
    in elderly, 81, 113–114, 116, 119–121
    endogenous, 53, 76
    epidemiology of, 68, 82
    features of, 216
    immunologic abnormalities in, 65,
        81
    and loss of parent, 86
    major, 85, 203
    and medical illness, 149
    for medical inpatients, 145
    melancholic, 270
    negative cognitive triad as explaining,
        77
    and neurosyphilis, 388
    norepinephrine deficiency hypothesis
        of, 64
    poststroke, 343, 381

psychotic, 2, 12
    role of therapy in, 70
    serotonin deficiency hypothesis of, 63
    and sleep, 74, 218, 221
    and spinal cord compression, 387
    treatment of, 59
    and weight loss, 81
    in women, 56, 77
depressive disorder, 71, 82, 120, 274
depressive illness, 56, 77
derailment (loose association), 50
derealization, 11
desensitization, systematic, 89, 290
desipramine, 135, 269, 270
desmethylimipramine, 135
desmopressin, 134
detoxification, 172, 173, 187, 194
dexamethasone suppression test, 69, 83,
        114, 119, 411, 417
Dhat, 110
diabetes mellitus, 142, 146, 153, 381
diagnosis, psychiatric, reliability of, 4, 13
dialectical behavior therapy, 292–293, 301
dialysis, renal, 145, 155
diazepam, 87, 232, 265, 267
dibenzodiazipine, 277
diffuse brain damage, 79
diphenhydramine hydrochloride, 79
diplopia, 78, 275, 277, 365
discoloration of skin, 285
discontinuation reaction, 244
discontinuation syndrome, 62, 243
discontinuous amnesia, 110
discriminative learning, 413
disinhibition, 392
disorientation to place, 1, 11
dissociative amnesia, 96, 99, 108, 109
dissociative fugue, 100, 109
dissociative identity disorder, 97, 109
dissociative symptoms, 107
distal symmetric polyneuropathy, 389
distortion, 304
disulfiram, 184–185, 193, 194
divorce, and panic disorder, 109
DLB (dementia of Lewy bodies), 357,
        359, 391, 392
doctors, alcohol dependence in, 189
dominant temporal lobe lesions, 360
dopamine, 192
dopamine hypothesis of schizophrenia,
        35, 49
dopaminergic cells, 366, 396
double bookkeeping, 43
double-bind communications, 43
doubles, 12
Down syndrome, 208, 210, 212, 214,
        215, 216
dreaming, vivid, 363, 394
dressing up, and girls, 321
drop attacks, 395
drowsiness, 268, 273
Drummond, Edward, 412
DST (dexamethasone suppression test),
        69, 83, 114, 119, 411, 417
durable power of attorney, 169
Durkheim, Emile, 416
duty to protect, 161, 167
dysarthria, 276, 381
dyspepsia, 276
dysphasia, 157
dysphoric mania, 276
dysthymic disorder, 70, 74, 83, 85
dystonia, 40, 60, 140, 278, 283, 386
    acute, 261, 277–278, 283, 327, 332
    acute form, 261, 277–278, 283, 327,
        332

early-onset Alzheimer disease, 370
eating disorders, 195–205, 203, 301
Ebstein's anomaly, 268
ECA (Epidemiological Catchment Area)
    survey, 404
echopraxia, 16

ECT (electroconvulsive therapy), 28, 70,
        79, 80, 85, 150, 402, 413
EEG (electroencephalogram), 335, 387
egocentric, 308, 319
ego-dystonic, 13
ego(s)
    auxiliary, 288
    function of, 294–295, 302, 303
Ekbom syndrome, 409
elderly
    delirium and confusion in, 184, 194
    depression in, 81, 113–114, 116,
        119–121
    psychodynamic therapy for, 121
    sleep patterns in, 118, 122
    suicide in, 115, 120
    and tardive dyskinesia, 50
    and zopiclone, 79
electroconvulsive therapy, 28, 70, 80, 85,
        150, 402, 413
electroencephalogram, 335, 387
Ellis, Havelock, 304
emergency psychiatry, 325–334
emotion, 321
emotional arousal, 49
emotional intelligence, 404, 413
emotional lability, 7, 15
empathy, 300
Encephalitis
    in AIDS, 147, 157
encephalopathy
    hepatic, 331
    HIV, 359
    Wernicke's, 11, 147, 183
encopresis, 124, 132, 134, 139
enuresis, 124, 134
Epidemiological Catchment Area survey,
        404
epilepsy, 141, 152, 159, 340, 379, 380
    temporal lobe, 51
epinephrine, 332
erectile dysfunction, 275
Erickson, Erik, 304
Erikson's stages of psychosocial and per-
        sonal development, 323
erotomania, 50
essential hypertension, 417
essential tremor, 350, 368, 386, 397
euphoria, 384
executive function, deficits in, 40
existentialism, 298
Exner, John, 413
expert witness, 168
explicit memory, 320
expressed emotion, 29
expressive psychoanalytic therapy, 406,
        414
extinction burst, 317
extrahepatic metabolism, 77
extrapyramidal effects, 50, 260, 283, 397
    acute, 50
extrapyramidal system, 368
extroversion, 321
Eysenck, Hans, 322

face, chorea in, 384
facial movements, 322
factitious disorder (Munchausen syn-
        drome), 95, 102, 104, 108–112,
        224, 226
Falret, Jean-Pierre, 41, 415
family members, of patients with schizo-
        phrenia, 44, 302
family therapy, structural, 293
fatigue, 277
fertility rates, among patients with schiz-
        ophrenia, 47
Festinger, Leon, 322
fetal alcohol syndrome, 185, 194
fetishism, 304
Feuchtersleben, Ernst, 414
first-pass effect, 265
fitness to plead, 164, 168

5HIAA levels, 80
5HT1 mediated prolactin release, 80
5HT platelet uptake, 80
flaccidity, 383
flooding, 291, 300
flumazenil, 327, 332
fluoxetine, 78, 80, 138, 203, 205, 273
flupenthixol, 50, 78
flurazepam, 267
fluvoxamine, 272, 282
"folie circulaire" (circular insanity), 22, 408
formal operational stage, 318
fragile X syndrome, 128, 208
free association, 289
free-floating anxiety, 105
Freud, Anna, 322
Freud, Sigmund, 304, 322
Freudian analysis, 298, 299
Friedman, Meyer, 417
Friedreich ataxia, 376
Fromm-Reichmann, 41
frontal hypermetabolism, 391
frontal lobe
    damage in, 363, 394, 397
    injury to, 359, 388, 392
    lesions in, 158, 361, 381, 393, 399
    tumor in, 152
frontal lobe seizures, 339, 379
frontotemporal dementia, 358, 391
Frotteurism, 204
FTD (frontotemporal dementia), 358, 391

GABA, 383
GABA receptor, 192, 276, 383
GABA-A receptor, 266
gabapentin, 77
gait ataxia, 381
Gajdusek, Carleton, 414
galactorrhea, 278
gambling, pathologic, 410, 417
Ganser syndrome, 102, 111
gender identity, 128, 137
gender identity disorder, 199, 204
generalized anxiety disorder, 88, 91, 106
    with panic attacks, 87, 105
generalized seizures, 339, 379
genetic loading, and bipolar disorder, 76
geriatric psychiatry, 113–122. see also elderly
Gerstmann syndrome, 362, 375, 394, 400
Gestalt psychology, 298
Gestalt therapy, 288
Gilles de la Tourette syndrome. see Tourette syndrome
girls, and dressing up, 321
Gjessing, R., 43
glaucoma
    acute, 396
    acute-angle, 254
gliosis, 48
global confusion, 193
global memory deficits, 394
glutamate, 42, 188
glycine, 192
Goldstein, Kurt, 44
Goleman, Daniel, 413
granular deposits, in anterior lens, 285
Grave's disease, 152, 417
Grisi Siknis, 110
group therapy, 291, 406
guanfacine, 136
guardianship, 167
Guillain-Barre syndrome, 345, 383
guilt feelings, 80

hair loss, 283
Hallervorden-Spatz syndrome, 133, 140
hallucinations
    alcoholic, 6
    auditory, 14, 16, 47, 49

and Parkinson's disease, 384
    reflex, 44
    as running commentaries, 49
    tactile, 10, 17
    visual, 8, 15
haloperidol, 79, 160, 253–254, 257, 265, 269, 277–279, 281
Harris, Tirril, 77
head injury, severe closed, 361
headaches, 273, 277
    chronic, 338
    cluster type, 337, 377, 378
    occipital, 381
hearing difficulty, 213
hearing loss, 215
Heller syndrome, 135
hemianopia, bitemporal, 374, 387
hemiballismus, 349, 385
hemodialysis, 274
hemolytic anemia, 278
hemorrhage
    intracranial, 191
    retinal, 138
    subarachnoid, 378
    vitreous, 396
hepatic disease, 146
hepatic encephalopathy, 331
hepatic extraction, 229
hepatic toxicity, 277
hepatitis, chronic persistent, 273
heroin addiction, 182, 193
heroin dependence, 181
heroin withdrawal, 179, 191
hidden objects, when infants start to search for, 317
Hinckley, John, 412
hippocampus, 48, 398
history taking, 7, 15
histrionic personality disorder, 226
HIV encephalopathy, 359, 392
HIV infection, 147, 149, 150, 157
HIV-associated dementia, 354, 388
HLA DR2, 220
"holding environment," 129
homeless people, 409, 416
homeless shelter, 77
homicide, 164
homosexuality, 200–201, 205
hopelessness, 333
Horner syndrome, 369, 395
hostility, 46
HPA (hypothalamic-pituitary-adrenal) dysfunction, 81
human immunodeficiency virus. see HIV entries
humor, 304
Huntington disease, 346, 348–349, 371, 374, 384, 399
hypercapnia, 397
hyperorality, 391
hyperparathyroidism, 142, 153, 275
hyperphagia, 135
hypersomnia, 135
hypertension, 274, 278, 300, 412
    orthostatic, 248
hyperthermia, 279
hyperthyroidism, 141, 143, 153, 331
hyperuricemia, 386
hypnosis, 295
hypoactive delirium, 146, 156
hypocalcemia, 331
hypochondriasis, 95, 108
hypokalemic alkalosis, 202
hypomania, 71
    antidepressant-induced, 76
hyponatremia, 383
hypoparathyroidism, 397
hypopituitarism, 153
hypotension, 110, 190, 278
hypothalamic-pituitary-adrenal dysfunction, 81
hypothyroidism, 215, 275
hypoventilation, 11

hypoxyphilia, 334

the id, 289, 299
ideas of reference, 6, 15
identity, versus confusion, 323
illicit drugs, 171, 186
illness
    chronic, 49
    depressive, 56, 77
    medical, depression associated with, 149
    psychiatric, 153
imipramine, 134, 281
immigrants, schizophrenia in, 34
immunologic abnormalities, 65
impaired consciousness, 335
implicit-semantic memory, 110
impotence, 269, 278
imprinting, 85, 306, 317
incontinence, 382, 387
India, schizophrenia in, 49
infanticide, 39, 51
inflammatory hair loss, 138
information processing, deficits in, 40
innervation, adrenergic, 90
insanity defense, 162, 167
insidious onset, 44
insight, 10, 17, 43, 157
insomnia, 218, 219, 221
institutional defense mechanisms, 294, 303
intelligence test, 307
intent, 162
interictal behavioral syndrome, 407, 415
International Pilot Study of Schizophrenia, 28
internuclear ophthalmoplegia, 371
interpersonal psychotherapy, 287
intoxication
    alcohol, 167
    barbiturate, 256, 280
    phencyclidine, 330, 333, 401
    water, 276
intracranial hemorrhage, 191
intracranial injuries, 138
intracranial neoplasm, 351
intramuscular injections, 40
introversion, 321
involuntary movement disorders, 382
ipecac, 202
ipsilateral paralysis, 341
IQ test, 414
irrational impulses, 299
isolation, 299

Jacksonian march, 379
jaundice, 277, 278
    cholestatic, 231
jealousy, pathological, 168
Jung, Carl, 304, 321

Kahn, Eugene, 414
Kanner, Leo, 137
Kasanin, Jacob, 50
ketamine, 42
Klein, Melanie, 137, 304, 322
Kleine-Levin syndrome, 124, 135
Kleinian analysis, 298
kleptomania, 410, 416
klismaphilia, 200, 204
Klüver-Bucy syndrome, 350
knife-blade atrophy, 392
Kohlberg, Lawrence, 318, 319
Kohlberg's theory of moral development, 309–310, 319, 320
Koro, 41
Korsakoff syndrome, 147, 157, 177, 185, 189, 194, 376
Kraepelin, Emil, 46, 76
Kuru, 414

LAAM, 185, 194, 245
lamotrigine, 54–55, 76, 79, 251, 277

Landau-Kleffner syndrome, 136
Langfeldt, Gabriel, 415
language ability, 40
language development, 319
lanugo, 202
laryngeal dystonia, 331
Latah, 110
latent meanings, 299
late-onset depressive disorder, 120
late-onset psychosis, 116–117, 121, 122
lateral hypothalamus, 349
lead, toxic levels of, 136
"learned helplessness," 56
Leff, Julian, 285, 412
left frontal lobe lesion, 158, 381, 399
left internal capsule, 382
left temporal lobe lesion, 388
Lennon, John, 412
Leonhard, Karl, 76
Lesch-Nyhan syndrome, 129, 137, 209, 350, 386
lesions
    frontal lobe, 361
    lateral hypothalamus, 349
    left frontal, 158
    lower motor neuron, 368
    midbrain, 377
    multiple ring enhancing, 335
    occipital lobe, 360
    parietal lobe, 360, 363, 368
    of pons, 342
    temporal lobe, 360
    total lesion load, 383
lethargy, 381
leukocytosis, 79
leukopenia, 202
leuprolide, 205
levodopa, 49, 135, 271
Lewinsohn, 85
Lewy bodies, 392
    dementia of, 357, 359, 391, 392
LFTs, elevated, 276
liaison settings, 155
libido, 281
life cycle, stages of, 297, 304
light therapy, 63, 80
Lima, Almeida, 285
limbic system, 395, 396
Linehan, Marsha, 301
lipid homeostasis theory, 69
lipophilic drugs, 229–230, 265
lithium, 55, 235, 245–247, 251
    and aspirin, 275
    as augmenting agent, 80
    and bipolar disorder, 274
    excretion of, 274, 277
    and mania, 79
    and mixed episode, 77
    in presence of liver disease, 156
    and rapid-cycling bipolar disorder, 76
    side effects of, 57, 78, 274, 275
    and suicide rates, 77
    tests before starting, 79
    and tremors, 269
    and weight gain, 277
lithium overdose, 248, 275
lithium toxicity, 246–247, 275, 328, 332
litigiousness, 226
liver disease, 156, 266. see also hepatic
    entries
LKS (Landau-Kleffner syndrome), 136
locked-in syndrome, 343, 382
locus ceruleus, 106
logic-related problems, and children, 318
lorazepam, 45, 79, 257, 281, 333
"low rate of reinforcement," 73
lower limb areflexia, 335
lower motor neuron lesion, 368
LSD (lysergic acid diethylamide), 42, 179
L-tryptophan, 282
lumbar puncture, 354
lysergic acid diethylamide, 42, 179

made experiences, 13
magnetic resonance imagining, 23, 336, 369, 377, 394
magnification, 301
Mahler, Margaret, 137
major depressive disorder, 65–66, 68, 81–82
malingering, 102, 111
Mallenby effect, 415
malpractice, 161, 167
mania, 60, 71–72, 79, 149, 152, 271
manic episode, 68, 84
mannerism, 16
MAOIs (monoamine oxidase inhibitors), 69, 78, 230, 239–241, 265, 270, 271, 278
mature defense mechanisms, 296
MCV, 415
measles, 383
medial temporal lobes, 391
medical emergencies, presenting as psychiatric emergencies, 325, 331
medical illness, depression associated with, 149
medical inpatient unit, 156
medroxyprogesterone, 205
melancholia, 53
memories, recall of, 303
memory, 310–311, 312, 314, 320, 321
    retrieval in, 321
memory deficits, global, 394
men
    alcoholism in, 187
    prion diseases in, 155
    schizophrenia in, 22, 49
    suicide in, 329, 333
meningiomas, 351
meningitis, viral, 388
mens rea, 167
mental retardation, 79, 111, 168, 207–217
    and aggression, 216
    causes of, 208
    children with, 210, 215
    and depressive features, 211, 216
    diagnosis of, 207, 213
    interviewing patients with, 211, 216
    mental age of adults with, 213
    mild, 207, 213
    moderate, 207
    pharmacotherapy in persons with, 216
    and seizure disorder, 210
    severe, 208, 209
mental status examination, 7
Mesmer, Anton, 304
metabolic nitrogen balance, 43
metabolic syndrome, 258, 282
metabolism, 77, 144, 154
methadone, 181, 244–245, 273, 282, 334
methadone withdrawal, 180, 191
methanol ingestion, 396
methyl alcohol poisoning, 176, 189
methyldopa, 78
methylphenidate, 49, 282
metoclopramide, 283
Meyer, Adolph, 412
midbrain lesion, 377, 385
migraine, 337, 377, 378, 381
migraine without aura, 377
mircographia, 383
mirtazapine, 80, 241
mitral valve prolapse, 89, 105, 109
mixed anxiety-depressive disorder, 102
mixed episode, 77, 84
mixed manic episode, 68, 82
M'Naughten, Daniel, 412
moclobemide, 83
Model Penal Code, 169
Moniz, Egaz, 285, 412
monoamine oxidase inhibitors, 69, 78, 230, 239–241, 265, 270, 271, 278
monoamines, 230, 265
monocular amaurosis fugax, 382

monoparesis, 383
monoplegia, 395
mood congruent, 80
mood disorders, 53–86, 81, 82
    affective, 79, 145, 155, 279
mood incongruent delusions, 45
moral development, Kohlberg's theory of, 309–310, 319, 320
moral judgments, children's, 321
mother
    opiate-addicted, 190
    schizophrenic, 21
motivational variables, 227
motor coordination problems, 216
motor neuron disease, 367
motor neuron lesion, 368
motor vehicle accidents, 388
movement disorder, 350
MRI (magnetic resonance imagining), 23, 336, 369, 377, 394
mu receptor, 188, 192
multiple ring enhancing lesions, 335
multiple sclerosis, 344–345, 363, 382, 383, 394, 398
Multiple Sleep Latency Test, 220
Munchausen syndrome (factitious disorder), 108
Murray, Henry, 413
muscarinic receptor blockade, 70
muscle tone, loss of, 220
mutism, akinetic, 349
MVP (mitral valve prolapse), 89, 98, 105, 109
myasthenia gravis, 361
myocardial infarction, 192
myoclonus, 278
myoglobinuria, 40

naltrexone, 333
narcissistic defense mechanisms, 296
narcissistic personality disorder, 224, 227
narcolepsy, 217–218
nausea, 273
nefazodone, 241, 271, 282
negative cognitive triad, 56, 77
negative reinforcement, 317
neurasthenia, 74, 408
neurodevelopmental theory, 106
neurofibromatosis type I, 386
neuroimaging, 121, 389
neuroleptic agent, 151
neuroleptic malignant syndrome, 190, 253–254, 261, 283, 325
    features of, 79
    and mortality, 278
    treatment of, 331
neuroleptics, side effects of, 49
neurology, 335–400
neuropsychiatric complication, 150
neurosis, 405
neurosyphilis, 51, 354, 388
neurotransmitter abnormalities, 88, 105
New Word Learning test, 17
nicotine, 191, 192, 283
night terrors, 217, 220
nightmare disorder, 410, 416
nightmares, 133, 140, 217, 220
nihilistic delusions, 10, 12
NMDA receptor, 413
NMS. see neuroleptic malignant syndrome
Nobel Prize, 263, 285, 402
nocturnal migraine, 337
nondominant parietal lobe lesions, 360
non-rapid eye-movement sleep, 374, 399
noradrenaline, 79
norepinephrine, 43, 231, 266, 269
norepinephrine deficiency hypothesis of depression, 64, 80
norepinephrine reuptake inhibition, 140
normal emotional response, 106
normal pressure hydrocephalus, 398

nortriptyline, 83, 239, 265, 269, 270
Norway, immigrants from, 48
NPH (normal pressure hydrocephalus), 398
NREM (non-rapid eye-movement) sleep, 374, 399
nystagmus, 365, 395, 412

object permanence, 308
obsessional thought, 3, 13
obsessions, 2, 9, 12, 15, 16, 294
obsessive-compulsive disorder, 7, 100, 130, 203, 289
   and behavior therapy, 300
   in children, 138
   and cognitive distortions, 301
obstructive sleep apnea, 399
occipital headache, 381
occipital lobe lesions, 360, 393
OCD. see obsessive-compulsive disorder
ocular muscle, 393
oculogyric crisis, 278
oculomotor nerve neuropathy, 395
Oesterlin, Fräulein, 304
olanzapine, 79, 255, 279, 281
on-off phenomenon, 384
operant conditioning, 305–306
ophthalmoplegia, 193
   internuclear, 371
opiate-addicted mother, 190
opiates, 271
   dependence on, 174
   use of, 182, 192
opioids, 205
   withdrawal from, 328
oppositional defiant disorder, 129, 137
orbitofrontal syndrome, 415
organic anxiety syndrome, 90, 106
organic brain damage, 10, 336
organization, 320
orthostatic hypertension, 83, 248, 273, 327
OTC (over-the-counter) medication, 73
overgeneralization, 301
overinvolvement, 46
over-the-counter medication, 73

P300 wave, 45
pain
   abdominal, 395
   chronic, 159, 238
   spontaneous, 397
pain disorder, 95, 108
pancreatitis, acute, 277
panic attacks, 105, 276
panic disorder, 97, 104, 262
   and behavior therapy, 300
   and mitral valve prolapse, 109
   pathological involvement in, 112
   social factors contributing to, 109
   and suicide, 334
Pappenheim, Bertha, 304
paradoxical suicide, 416
paranoia, 294
paranoid delusion, 13
paranoid ideas, 384
paranoid personality disorder, 224
paranoid schizophrenia, 43
paranoid symptoms, 31
paranoid-schizoid position, 304
paraplegia, 387
parasitosis, delusions of, 417
parenteral vitamin B12, 395
parietal cortex, right, 399
parietal lobe, right, 399
parietal lobe lesions, 360, 363, 368, 393, 394, 397
Parkinson's disease, 346–347, 383, 384, 397
paroxetine, 250, 272, 273, 282
partial complex seizures, 339–340, 379
passive diffusion, of drugs, 265
passivity experiences, 3, 13

passivity phenomena, 12
paternalism, 168
pathologic gambling, 410, 417
pathological anxiety, 90, 106
pathological jealousy, 168
PCP. see phencyclidine entries
PDD (pervasive developmental disorder), 131, 138
pediatric autoimmune neuropsychiatry disorder, 131
pedophilia, 199, 204
Peel, Robert, 412
pemoline, 135, 136
peptic ulcer disease, 417
periodic catatonia, 25
periodic limb movement disorder, 409, 416
peripheral neuropathy, 58, 78, 271, 275
peripheral vasodilatation, 396
Perls, Fritz, 298
perphenazine, 283
Perris, Carlo, 76
persecutory delusions, 50
perseveration, 8, 16
persistent vegetative state, 343
personality change, following head injury, 353
personality disorders, 223–227, 224, 226
   type A, 417
pervasive developmental disorder, 131, 138
petit mal seizures (absence seizures), 340–341, 380, 387
pharmacotherapy, 216
phencyclidine, 181
phencyclidine intoxication, 330, 333, 401
phenelzine, 241, 269, 270, 272, 417
phenobarbitone, 279
phenothiazine, 277
phentolamine, 332
phenytoin, 276, 283
pheochromocytoma, 271
phobias, 89, 98, 106, 303
   behavioral theory of, 110
   blood/injection/injury, 99
   school, 128
   social, 89, 91, 225
   specific, 88
   in women, 105, 106
photosensitivity reactions, 285
physical abuse, 130, 138
physostigmine, 332
Piaget's stages of cognitive development, 307, 318
Piblokto, 110
pica, 132, 139
Pick disease, 359, 375, 400
pindolol, 78, 80
pituitary adenomas, 352
pituitary disease, 143, 153
pituitary tumor, 399
place, disorientation to, 1, 11
plasma tryptophan levels, 80
PMDD (premenstrual dysphoric disorder), 143–144, 153, 154, 256, 281
polycystic ovaries, 283
polyneuropathy, chronic inflammatory demyelinating, 350, 386
pons, lesions of, 342, 385
porphyria, 51, 144, 154, 364
   acute, 364
   acute intermittent, 51
postconcussional syndrome, 353, 388
posterior cerebral artery occlusion, 368
posterior column damage, 367, 396
posterior communicating artery, 396
postinfectious encephalomyelitis, 346
postpartum psychosis, 39, 51
posttraumatic seizures, 339, 379
posttraumatic stress disorder, 92–93, 107, 110–111
postural reflexes, 383
power of attorney, durable, 169

Prader-Willi syndrome, 209, 215
Pratt, Joseph, 415
precipitating factors, absence of, 50
prefrontal cortex, 42
pregnancy complications, 190
pregnancy test, 79
Premack principle, 323
premenstrual dysphoric disorder, 143–144, 153, 154, 256, 281
premorbid asocial characteristics, 49
preoperational stage, 318
priapism, 273
primary delusion, 1, 11
prion diseases, 145, 155
prochlorperazine, 283
progressive agnosia, 394
projection, 302, 304
prolonged QT interval, 273, 278
propranolol, 84, 265
prosocial behavior, 311, 321
prosopagnosia, 371, 392, 393, 398
Protestants, and suicide, 415
Prusiner, Stanley, 414
pseudobulbar palsy, 364, 395
pseudodementia, 2, 12, 115, 120
pseudohallucination, 2, 5, 12, 14
pseudoseizure, 341, 361, 380, 394
pseudotumor cerebri, 387
psychiatric diagnosis, reliability of, 4, 13
psychiatric illness, 153
psychiatrist, in court, 165
psychiatry liaison consultant, 141, 152
psychoanalysis, 289–290, 298, 300
psychoanalytic psychotherapy, 107
psychobiology, 401
psychodrama, 298, 299
psychodynamic therapy, 110, 117, 121, 287
psychology, 305–323
psychometric testing, 121
psychomotor agitation, 412
psychomotor retardation, 32, 76
psychomotor slowing, 277
psychopharmacology, 229–285
psychophysiologic insomnia, 219, 221
psychosis, 39, 51, 116–117, 384. see also individual disorders or syndromes
psychosomatic disease, 417
psychotherapy, 287–304, 300
ptosis of the eyelid, 397
PTSD (posttraumatic stress disorder), 92–93, 107, 110–111
puberty, 321
puerperal psychosis, 39, 51
pyramidal system, 396

QTc interval, 80
quetiapine, 255, 280, 384

raclopride, 41
rapid eye-movement sleep. see REM sleep
rapid-cycling bipolar disorder, 54, 76
rapid-cycling mania, 275, 276
reaction formation, 299, 303
reactive attachment disorder, 132, 139
Reagan, Ronald, 412
reconstructive psychotherapy, 287–288
reflex hallucination, 44
reflexes, absent, 396
reflexive babbling, 319
regression, 300
rehabilitation medicine, 142, 152
REM sleep, 218, 323
   dreaming in, 394
   effect of alcohol on, 189
   and major depressive disorder, 81
   and migraine, 377
   and nightmares, 220
   rebound, 268
remission, early partial, 414
renal dialysis, 145, 155
respiratory depression, 273

restless leg syndrome, 416
restlessness, acute, 278
restraints, 148, 158, 257, 281
reticular activating system, 268
retinal detachment, 396
retinal hemorrhage, 138
retinal pigmentation, 278
retinitis pigmentosa, 263
retrieval, in memory process, 319
Rett syndrome, 123, 134, 209, 214
reversible MAOI, 69
rhinorrhea, 105
"right-wrong test," 165
rigidity, 79, 383
risperidone, 255, 279
Ritalin, 417
Rogers, Carl, 322
Rorschach, Herman, 413
Rorschach test, 404
Rosenman, Ray, 417
rumination disorder, 132, 139
Rush, Benjamin, 415
Russell's sign, 202

Schachter, Stanley, 322
schizoaffective disorder, 38, 47, 274
schizophrenia, 3, 8, 19–51
    acute, 25, 31
    and body type, 29
    brain changes in, 47
    chronic, 31, 37, 48, 50
    cognitive function in, 20, 258, 281
    concordance rate for, 20
    cost of, 20
    and depression, 47, 48
    diagnosis of, 29, 36, 39, 46, 49
    dopamine hypothesis of, 35, 49
    etiology of, 33
    and family members, 32, 44, 47
    family members and, 27
    family therapy for, 293, 302
    and fertility, 47
    forms of, 26
    genetic studies of, 23
    neurotransmitters in, 24
    and nicotine use, 192
    onset of, 22, 46, 123, 134
    prevalence of, 30, 34, 35, 46
    prognostic indicator for, 27, 29, 46
    risk of developing, 31, 32, 47
    and season of birth, 21
    and serotonin, 24, 42
    in socioeconomic classes, 49
    and substance abuse, 182
    and suicide, 34, 49, 328, 333
    symptoms of, 20, 22, 30, 31, 44, 47
    treatment of, 28
    type I, 26
    and violence, 162–163, 167
    in women, 49
schizophrenic mother, 21
schizophrenic patients, chronic institu-
    tionalized, 33
schizophrenic probands, 23
schizophreniform psychosis, 30, 215
schizotypal personality disorder, 226
Schneider, Kurt, 43
Schneider first-rank symptoms, 3, 6, 15
school phobia, 128, 136
seasonal affective disorder, 63, 80
seclusion, use of, 148, 158
secondary amine, 238
secondary delusion, 11
secondary gain, 111
sedation, 275
sedative abstinence, 185, 194
seeing one's body, in external space, 4, 9
seizure disorder, 208, 210, 214, 338, 378
seizure focus, left-sided, 48
seizures, 256, 340, 379
    complex partial, 33
    frontal lobe, 379
    generalized, 379

and Lesch-Nyhan syndrome, 386
and magnesium deficiency, 331
partial complex, 379
as side effect of MAOIs, 271
with temporal lobe focus, 336, 376
withdrawal, 179
selective abstraction, 301
selective serotonin reuptake inhibitors,
    240, 242–243, 252, 256, 272
    adverse reactions with, 273
    and cytochrome P-450 system, 265
    for generalized anxiety disorder, 105
    and increased tricyclic drug concen-
        tration, 282
    and PMDD, 153, 281
    and serotonin syndrome, 282
    side effects of, 272, 277
    switching from, 271
self-mutilation, 214, 386
self-rating scale, 10
Seligman, Martin, 77, 85
sensation, loss of, 387
sensorimotor stage, 317, 318, 319, 321
sensory gating, 42
sensory system, 317
separation, and panic disorder, 109
serotonin, 24, 42, 79, 231, 266
serotonin deficiency hypothesis of de-
    pression, 63, 80
serotonin neurotransmission, 82
serotonin syndrome, 230, 260, 265, 271
sertraline, 107, 111, 203, 282
severe alcohol withdrawal, 172
severe Alzheimer disease, 371
severe closed head injury, 361, 393
severe debilitating OCD, 100
sexual abuse, 130, 138, 210, 215, 226
sexual behavior, 266, 330
sexual disinhibition, 79
sexual disorders, 195–205
sexual dysfunction, 200, 282
sexual impulses, 12
sexual interest, decreased, 203
sexual masochism, 200, 204
sexual offenders, 200
sexual offenses, 168
sexually disinhibited behavior, 79
shoplifting, 168
short-term memory, 314, 321, 323
simple schizophrenia, 43
Singer, Jerome, 322
situational phobia, 106
Skinner, BF, 316
sleep
    abnormalities of, 85
    and depression, 74, 218, 221
    disorders of, 217–221
    NREM, 374, 399
    patterns in elderly, 118, 122
    REM (see REM sleep)
    and serotonin, 266
    stages of, 220, 221
sleep terror, 123, 134, 410, 416
slow language development, 319
smell, loss of, 387
smoking, 303, 377, 381
smooth-pursuit eye movements, 42, 45
social and occupational dysfunction, 84
social contract orientation, 320
social drift theory, 49
social phobia, 89, 91, 106, 203, 224
social referencing, 322
social withdrawal, 47
socioeconomic classes, 49
sodium, 64, 81
sodium valproate, 156
somatic delusional disorder, 50
somatization disorder, 94, 107
somatoform disorder, 94
    undifferentiated, 412
somnambulism, 217, 220
span of apprehension test, 314, 323
specific phobias, 88, 106, 300, 301

speech impairment, 213
SPEM (smooth-pursuit eye movements),
    42, 45
spinal cord compression, 352, 387
spinal epidural abscesses, 363
spontaneous pain, 397
spouse, death of, 321
SSRIs (selective serotonin reuptake in-
    hibitors), 240, 242–243, 252, 256,
    272
    adverse reactions with, 273
    and cytochrome P-450 system, 265
    for generalized anxiety disorder, 105
    and increased tricyclic drug concen-
        tration, 282
    and PMDD, 153, 281
    and serotonin syndrome, 282
    side effects of, 272, 277
    switching from, 271
St. John's wort, 85, 282, 284
stalkers, 167
steroids, 142, 143, 152, 153, 378
Stevens-Johnson syndrome, 77, 277
stimulants, 192, 263, 284
stress disorder, acute, 92
stroke, 149, 342, 343, 372, 381, 391
structural family therapy, 293, 302
subacute combined degeneration, 364
subarachnoid hemorrhage, 378
subcortical dementia, 159
sublimation, 304
substance abuse, 174, 414
substance dependence, 171
substance use, 171–194
subthalamic nucleus, lesion in the, 349
suicidal ideation, 331
suicide
    and alcoholism, 173, 187
    altruistic, 416
    among cancer patients, 158
    and anger, 157
    anomic, 416
    attempted, 148, 157, 329, 333
    and bipolar disorder, 74, 85
    in children, 131, 138, 139
    in different religions, 408
    egoistic, 416
    in elderly, 115, 120
    and epilepsy, 152
    homicide followed by, 164
    and Huntington disease, 384
    in men, 329, 333
    in mentally ill patients, 147
    paradoxical, 416
    predictors of, 329, 333
    and Protestants, 415
    risk factors for, 330, 334
    and schizophrenia, 34, 49, 328, 333
    types of, 416
suppression, 304
sustained attention, 314
symmetric paresis, 383
systematic desensitization, 89, 290, 300
systemic lupus erythematosus, 51
systemic therapy, 293, 302

tachycardia, 269
tacrine, 262
tactile hallucinations, 10, 17
tangentiality, 2, 12
Tarasoff II, 167
tardive dyskinesia, 36–37, 49–50, 59, 79,
    254–255, 278–279
tardive myoclonus, 50
tardive syndromes, 37
TAT (Thematic Apperception Test), 225
TC (therapeutic community), 301
TD (tardive dyskinesia), 36–37, 49–50,
    59, 79, 254–255, 278–279
temperament, 128, 137
temporal lobe, 380, 398
    bilateral lesions, 360, 393
temporal lobe epilepsy, 51

tenth cranial nerve, 380
tertogenicity, 278
thalamus, atrophy of, 385
THC (delta 9 tetrahydrocannabinol), 263
Thematic Apperception Test, 225, 227
therapeutic alliance, 298
therapeutic community, 301
therapeutic index, 258, 282
therapeutic milieu, 303
thiamine, 193
thioridazine, 279, 285
Thomas, Alexander, 137
thoracic region, 394
thought block, 13, 49
thought disorders, 4, 39
Three Essays on the Theory of Sexuality
    (Freud), 304
thrombocytopenia, 276, 283
thyroid-stimulating hormone, 78
thyrotropin-releasing hormone stimula-
    tion, 71, 84
thyroxine, 80
toilet training, 317
token economy, 41
topiramate, 251, 277
torsades de pointes, 278
torture victims, 107
total lesion load, 383
touch, as sensory system, 317
Tourette syndrome, 5, 14, 125–126, 135,
    361–362, 393–394
toxoplasmosis, 386
transactional analysis, 288, 299
transference, 295, 298, 300, 303
transient global amnesia, 342, 362
transient ischemic attacks, basilar artery,
    381
transvestic fetishism, 204
tranylcypromine, 242
traumatic brain injury, 279, 353
trazodone, 220, 244, 273
tremors, 269, 383
    alcohol withdrawal, 178, 190
    coarse, 274
    essential, 350, 368, 386, 397
TRH (thyrotropin-releasing hormone)
    stimulation, 71, 84

trichotillomania, 410–411, 417
tricuspid valve, anomaly of, 284
tricyclic antidepressants, 58, 126, 230,
    236–238
    contraindications for use of, 269
    for depression in elderly, 116
    effects of use of, 270
    overdose of, 237, 269
    plasma drug concentration of, 265
    and weight gain, 277
trifluoperazine, 253, 277, 278
trigeminal neuralgia, 378
trismus, 79
tryptophan, 80
TSH (thyroid-stimulating hormone) lev-
    els, 78
tuberous sclerosis, 129, 137
tyramine, 270

ulcerative colitis, 417
unconscious conflicts, 300
undoing, 299
unilateral electrode placement, 83
unilateral flinging motion, 385
unipolar depressive disorder, 66, 82
upper motor neuron disease, 367
urea testing, 79
urinary retention, 281
UTI (urinary tract infection), 331

valproate, 249–250, 261, 276, 277, 283
valproic acid, 76, 79
variable-ratio schedule, 413
vascular dementia, 113, 119, 356, 359,
    390, 392
Vaughn, Christine E., 285, 412
venlafaxine, 60, 79, 251, 277
ventilation, 300
ventricles, lateral, 32, 385
Veraguth's fold, 86
verbigeration, 6, 14, 44, 49
vertebrobasilar, 380
victim
    duty to protect, 161, 167
    of torture, 107
violence, 162–163, 165, 167, 168
viral meningitis, 388

visual hallucinations, 8, 15, 384
visual impairment, 213
vitamin B12, 395
vitamin B12 deficiency, 143, 153
vitreous hemorrhage, 396
vocabulary
    in adolescence, 321
    of preschool children, 319
von N., Frau Emmy, 304

water intoxication, 276
Wechsler Preschool and Primary Scale of
    Intelligence-Revised, 135
weight control, 303
weight gain, 78, 251, 266, 275–278
weight loss, 65, 76, 81, 277
wellbutrin, 135
Wernicke-Korsakoff syndrome, 193
Wernicke's encephalopathy, 11, 147, 183
Willis, circle of, 367, 396
wills, and mental competency, 168
Wilson's disease, 144, 154
Winnicott, Donald, 137, 304, 322
Wisconsin Card Sorting Test, 23, 45, 377
withdrawal seizures, 179, 191
withdrawal symptoms, 186
women
    alcohol abuse in, 186
    and borderline personality disorder, 226
    Cloninger's type I alcoholism in, 187
    depression in, 56, 77
    drug abuse in, 172
    dystonia in, 79
    late-onset psychosis in, 122
    most common offense committed by,
        164
    phobias in, 105, 106
    physical changes in aging, 120
    and rapid-cycling bipolar disorder, 76
    schizophrenia in, 49
    social phobia in, 106
wrist cutting, frequent, 4, 13

xerostomia, 269

zoloft, 417
zopiclone, 59, 79